W9-CAX-885

Foundations of Professional Personal Training

SECOND EDITION

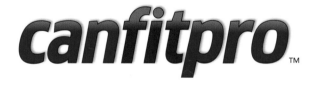

Robert Robinson

Manuscript Coordinator

Rod Macdonald

Daniela Goode

Adam Jongsma

Editors

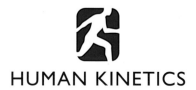

HUMAN KINETICS

Library of Congress Cataloging-in-Publication Data

Names: Can-Fit-Pro (Organization), author. | Macdonald, Rod (Personal trainer), editor.

Title: Foundations of professional personal training / edited by Rod Macdonald, Daniela Goode, Adam Jongsma; Robert Robinson, Manuscript Coordinator.

Description: Second edition. | Champaign, IL : Human Kinetics, [2016] | Includes bibliographical references and index.

Identifiers: LCCN 2015007859 | ISBN 9781450468527 (print)

Subjects: | MESH: Exercise. | Physical Fitness. | Physical Education and Training.

Classification: LCC GV428.7 | NLM QT 256 | DDC 613.7/1--dc23 LC record available at https://lccn.loc.gov/2015007859

ISBN: 978-1-4504-6852-7 (print)

Copyright © 2016, 2008 by Canadian Fitness Professionals, Inc.

All rights reserved. Except for use in a review, the reproduction or utilization of this work in any form or by any electronic, mechanical, or other means, now known or hereafter invented, including xerography, photocopying, and recording, and in any information storage and retrieval system, is forbidden without the written permission of the publisher.

The web addresses cited in this text were current as of October 2015, unless otherwise noted.

Figures 6.9, 6.11, 6.13, 6.15, 6.17, 6.19, and 6.21 reprinted, by permission, from NSCA, 2008, Biomechanics of resistance exercise, E. Harman. In *Essentials of strength training and conditioning,* 3rd ed., edited by T.R. Baechle and R.W. Earle (Champaign, IL: Human Kinetics), 88-89.

Acquisitions Editor: Diana Vincer; **Developmental Editor:** Katherine Maurer; **Managing Editors:** B. Rego, Carly O'Connor and Karla Walsh; **Associate Managing Editor:** Shevone Myrick; **Copyeditor:** Bob Replinger; **Indexer:** Bobbi Swanson; **Permissions Manager:** Dalene Reeder; **Senior Graphic Designer:** Nancy Rasmus; **Cover Designer:** Keith Blomberg; **Photographs (cover):** © iStock.com/Geber86; **Visual Production Assistant:** Joyce Brumfield; **Photo Production Manager:** Jason Allen; **Senior Art Manager:** Kelly Hendren; **Associate Art Manager:** Alan L. Wilborn; **Illustrations:** © Human Kinetics, unless otherwise noted; **Printer:** Walsworth

We thank Microlinks Community Centre in Richmond Hill, Ontario, for assistance in providing the location for the photo shoot for this book.

The video contents of this product are licensed for private home use and traditional, face-to-face classroom instruction only. For public performance licensing, please contact a sales representative at **www.HumanKinetics.com/SalesRepresentatives**.

Printed in the United States of America   10   9   8   7   6   5

The paper in this book was manufactured using responsible forestry methods.

Human Kinetics
P.O. Box 5076
Champaign, IL 61825-5076
Website: www.HumanKinetics.com

In the United States, email info@hkusa.com or call 800-747-4457.
In Canada, email info@hkcanada.com.
In the United Kingdom/Europe, email hk@hkeurope.com.

For information about Human Kinetics' coverage in other areas of the world, please visit our website: **www.HumanKinetics.com**

E6139

Tell us what you think!
Human Kinetics would love to hear what we can do to improve the customer experience. Use this QR code to take our brief survey.

Contents

PART III   Screening and Assessment

PART IV   Program Design and Delivery

All animals seek connection and safety and try to avoid pain. As human beings, we are unique because our intelligence has allowed us to change the world in which we live to make it safer, easier, and more comfortable. But as a result we have inadvertently created a great threat to our own health. Because we have reduced our physical activity and increased our consumption of over-processed, calorie-dense foods, we face a global obesity epidemic. If it is not countered, this epidemic and its related diseases will result in the decline of human life expectancy after centuries of increasing life expectancy. Higher rates of mental health challenges and an increase in environmental toxins should motivate us further to pay more attention to our health. But in this age of access to abundant information, we still desire human interaction to learn and be inspired to achieve change. When it comes to optimizing health, personal training is a key component of that human interaction.

Personal training itself has evolved from its intertwined roots in bodybuilding and sport coaching to become one of the fastest growing, most rewarding careers available. Personal training, as the name implies, is the act of one person guiding another, in this case toward optimal health. No longer confined to the gyms of the rich and famous, personal training has become widely available through a number of channels to assist virtually anyone interested in achieving health and fitness goals.

The fitness industry is composed of many delivery models, from large commercial fitness clubs, to parks and recreation facilities, to small studios, and everything in between. Personal training is available in as many ways as consumers wish to use it. From traditional club models to mobile fitness to virtual or remote personal training, never before have there been as many ways of being a Personal Training Specialist.

About canfitpro

As the industry has evolved and become more diverse, so has canfitpro. In the context of this evolution, we recognize that at our core, our promise is to *inspire healthy living through fitness education*™. To understand where we are going and what we can achieve together, we invite you to understand how canfitpro came to exist.

Founded in 1993, canfitpro was established to support all fitness professionals in their quest for foundational and ongoing education and continued professionalism. As an organization, we meet the needs of Canadian fitness professionals and consumers through our professional fitness certification offerings, conference and tradeshow events, and diverse membership offerings.

Launched in 1998, canfitpro's certification program was created to provide a high-quality nationally recognized fitness certification to produce qualified professionals. Starting with the two programs fundamental to fitness, group fitness instruction and personal training, canfitpro's certification program portfolio has grown to include specialized certifications to meet the increasingly discriminating needs of fitness consumers. Led by our network of qualified course instructors and examiners called PRO TRAINERS, canfitpro's certification programs are designed to meet the certification needs of fitness professionals across Canada by being accessible, attainable, and affordable to all who wish to take them. Through these programs, canfitpro aims to achieve these goals for our certified fitness professionals:

- canfitpro certified fitness professionals demonstrate *commitment to the fitness industry* and show a *high standard of competency and ability.*
- As leaders in the future of Canadian fitness, canfitpro-certified fitness professionals provide a reliable source of *fitness knowledge* and *safe, effective exercise.*
- Achieving this *standard of excellence* makes canfitpro-certified fitness professionals *competitive* and *in high demand for employment* across the country.
- Continuous training shows a dedication to *self-improvement* and a commitment to *providing motivation and information* for all participants.

- Known for *quality* and *enthusiasm*, canfit-pro-certified fitness professionals establish a ***benchmark for excellence and education*** in the fitness industry.

Complementing our certification offerings, canfitpro hosts the world's largest annual fitness professional education conference and tradeshow. canfitpro also hosts a series of regional conference events, webinars, and online learning modules, which allow our certified members to keep their practical skills and knowledge up to date. canfitpro will continue to expand our offerings to provide for the always-growing need for continuing education opportunities for professionals in the fitness industry.

As a canfitpro professional member, you will benefit by becoming part of the largest member-driven fitness organization in Canada, receive discounts on canfitpro certification and conference event registration fees, receive our industry-leading magazine, and have access to discounts with many fitness and non-industry-related vendors.

Personal Training Specialist Certification

The tremendous growth of the fitness industry has increased the number of opportunities for certified Personal Training Specialists. This growth has resulted in a greater need for knowledgeable and qualified people. The fitness profession is continually challenged to maintain consistent, quality leadership and educational programs. The availability of an adequate supply of qualified Personal Training Specialists helps to standardize the services that clubs are able to offer and helps maintain the credibility of the industry as a whole. From working in a fitness facility to starting your own business, the opportunities for Personal Training Specialists have never been greater.

The Personal Training Specialist certification has been developed to provide the participant with the opportunity to become better educated about personal training in a fun, adult-learning atmosphere. This program will enhance your confidence and motivation to lead and motivate your clients to be active, feel great, and get results! The sections that follow summarize what you need to know to become a certified Personal Training Specialist.

Eligibility

canfitpro recommends that participants in the Personal Training Specialist certification course be 16 years of age or older and be professional members of canfitpro. To take part in the exams and thereby complete the certification and be eligible for personal liability insurance, they must be 18 years or older and hold a current (within one year of issue) cardiopulmonary resuscitation (CPR) certificate. Proof of current CPR is required to receive your official certification from canfitpro.

Theoretical Concepts and Practical Competencies

A certified canfitpro Personal Training Specialist must have a solid foundational knowledge of theoretical fitness concepts as well as sound practical competencies to be able to provide safe, effective workouts for clients and have a stable, viable income-earning opportunity. You must know and be comfortable with the following.

Theoretical concepts:
- The benefits of physical activity
- Wellness and holism
- Active living
- Exercise physiology (energy systems, oxygen transport, exercise response)
- Human anatomy (musculoskeletal and cardiorespiratory)
- Biomechanics (joints, levers, modifications, types of contractions)
- Relevance and interpretation of results of fitness assessments
- Principles of conditioning (FITT)
- Training program design
- Injury prevention and safety
- Basic nutrition
- Healthy weight management

Practical competencies:
- Act ethically and in the best interests of the client at all times
- Be able to recommend a variety of exercises and training programs for healthy adults
- Provide safe, effective, efficient, and enjoyable workout delivery

- Demonstrate strong leadership and communication skills
- Demonstrate competent administration of fitness assessments
- Demonstrate proper technique of exercises
- Create a client-centred environment
- Educate clients about how the body responds to exercise
- Monitor client progress and ability
- Self-evaluate training effectiveness
- Be able to put theoretical knowledge into practice
- Present a professional appearance

Tips for Success

At canfitpro, we believe that the best fitness professionals have a lifelong passion for learning. To create the foundation on which to build your career, canfitpro certifications use a hybridized method of instruction including self-study, online learning, one-on-one contact, group learning, and practical experience. On your journey as a fitness professional, to embrace the Myohybrid learning philosophy is to embrace diversity and see value in all methods of learning.

To improve your chance for successful certification, we highly recommend that you prepare for the Personal Training Specialist course with your PRO TRAINER by completing the full online preparatory course available through www.HumanKinetics.com/courses and reading this manual. This approach will ensure that you make the most of canfitpro's Myohybrid learning philosophy, thereby being well prepared for your theory and practical certification exams, as well as a successful career as a Personal Training Specialist. We recommend that you attempt the written theory exam approximately three to four weeks after taking the Personal Training Specialist course. This time frame is designed to help you synthesize the course information while it is still top of the mind.

To ensure that you are ready to demonstrate all the practical competencies required of a canfitpro Personal Training Specialist, we recommend that you invest at least 20 hours honing your professional skills. When ready, you may attempt the practical exam, based on the availability of your PRO TRAINER for the examination.

As you pursue your canfitpro Personal Training Specialist certification, canfitpro and our PRO TRAINERS promise to do the following:

1. **Educate** you to learn the skills you need to provide safe, effective client sessions
2. **Motivate** you by providing a learning environment that is educational and fun
3. **Communicate** with you so that you are directly involved in your own learning process— mentally, verbally, and physically

At the same time, you need to take responsibility for your own learning—to be accountable for your own success and enjoyment. To do that, you should do the following:

1. Commit to attending and actively participating in the entire Myohybrid learning philosophy certification process (take the online course, attend a live course with your PRO TRAINER, adequately prepare for your theory and practical exam).
2. Complete assignments, quizzes, and projects to solidify the theoretical concepts and practical applications.
3. Set goals for yourself so that you meet the timelines for certification completion.
4. Give your best effort by doing the best you can, both physically and mentally.

Using This Book

This text is designed to give you a strong foundation in the theoretical and practical knowledge you need to be a successful Personal Training Specialist. The updated second edition includes new chapters on flexibility and mobility, foundational movement sequences and dynamic assessments, and an expanded section on program design, as well as revisions throughout to provide the most complete and up-to-date information. The exercise and assessment appendices have been updated, and we've added a web resource that includes video clips, printable forms, and other supplemental materials. In addition, the online preparatory course is available through www.HumanKinetics.com to help you build your knowledge through interactive activities that test your knowledge of the important concepts in this text as you prepare for the PTS course and examinations.

This book is divided into four parts. Part I begins by helping you understand yourself and your client as you come to the personal training relationship. It then reviews canfitpro's principles for optimal health, using the concept that health is a continuum that covers overall wellness, not just the absence of disease. In part II you learn to understand the physiology of basic body systems—the bioenergetic, cardiorespiratory, skeletal, and muscular systems—and their relevance for Personal Training Specialists. You'll also learn about the myofascial connections within the body and the foundational movement sequences that are necessary as a starting point for exercise programs and optimal health. In part III we address screening and assessment. The process of building an appropriate exercise program for your client begins with close attention to the client's individual needs through preexercise screening and passive and dynamic assessments. Finally, in part IV you will learn how to apply all the knowledge you have acquired to design and deliver a safe, effective exercise program.

As you work through this text, you will encounter a wealth of information about this fast-paced and constantly evolving industry. In each chapter, you will find learning aids to help you with important concepts, including chapter objectives and summaries, lists of key concepts to review, and review questions. In addition, case studies at the end of each part apply the concepts from that chapter to sample clients to make the connection from theory to practice. A glossary is included to help you learn unfamiliar terms; glossary terms are bolded in the text for reference.

Special traffic light elements are another element that will help you navigate this text. These markers highlight important practical applications for your work with clients. Much like the standard traffic light that it is modeled after, this icon and its colours indicate what you need to do:

Exercise caution when red.

Spend time in critical thinking when yellow.

Put into practice when green.

The traffic light elements both enhance your learning and add some fun to the process.

What Makes a Great Personal Training Specialist

Personal training is a growing profession. The barrier to entry is low, so it is an accessible field to enter. The advantage of this for clients is that they can easily find a personal trainer to work with. The disadvantage is that some of those personal trainers may have little or no foundation in safely and effectively helping their clients. To be an outstanding Personal Training Specialist, you must have a passion for learning and a desire to improve yourself continuously. You need to recognize that although being a Personal Training Specialist may be your source of income, you have taken on a responsibility of care for your clients.

The canfitpro Personal Training Specialist (PTS) certification has been mapped against the set of standards developed by repscanada, the Canadian Register of Exercise and Fitness Professionals, powered by canfitpro. The PTS certification has been identified as meeting standards, meaning that the competencies and evaluations completed within the PTS certification process meet or exceed the professional standards as developed by repscanada. The standards and mapping allow employers and consumers alike to review and understand fitness credentials and the skill set on which you have been assessed. To review the professional standards, please visit repscanada.com

To maintain a consistent standard of quality and excellence from all of our certified professionals, each must observe the *canfitpro Professional Member Code of Ethics* and the *Standards of Practice* related to the designations they hold.

Professional Member Code of Ethics

As a canfitpro professional member, I am committed to abide by the following:

1. I will provide appropriate assistance to any person with an interest in pursuing a fitness program and healthy lifestyle.
2. I will communicate in a genuine, honest, and professional manner.

3. I will not discriminate against any client or participant on such grounds as age, gender, weight, disability, marital status, national or ethnic origin, political affiliation, race, religion, sexual orientation, or socioeconomic status.

4. I will be open to giving and receiving constructive feedback from participants, clients, peers, and allied health professionals.

5. I will collaborate with other fitness and health professionals in the best interests of clients, participants, and the community.

6. I will protect and respect the confidentiality of all professional fitness relationships at all times.

7. I will engage in lifelong learning to maintain and improve my professional knowledge, skills, and abilities.

8. I will respect business, employment, and copyright laws.

9. I will meet or exceed my education provider's professional standards and refer individuals to the appropriate allied health professionals when necessary, if applicable.

10. I will recognize that the self-regulation of the fitness profession is a privilege and that each professional member has a responsibility to uphold this privilege and support the industry.

11. I will comply with canfitpro's noncompliance, complaint, and appeal process:

    1. In the event that a complaint is lodged against a professional member for noncompliance of the canfitpro Code of Ethics, such a complaint will be reviewed by canfitpro for consideration of sanctions against the professional member.

    2. If the complaint represented is of a potentially criminal or illegal nature, the appropriate authorities will be contacted to take over the investigation to pursue the legitimacy of the complaint.

    3. If review of the complaint exceeds 60 days, canfitpro reserves the right to suspend or revoke the enrollment of any professional member, reprimand or issue a formal warning, or take such other action

    as canfitpro may consider appropriate and fair to the issues raised.

    4. If action is taken against the professional member, canfitpro will, within 14 days, issue written notice of the action taken and the professional member's right to appeal, to all parties.

    5. If any party of a complaint is dissatisfied with the ruling by canfitpro, an appeal may be filed with canfitpro in writing within 14 days of the ruling.

    6. Acknowledgement of receipt of the appeal will be sent within 30 days after the date it is received.

    7. canfitpro will review all appeals and a final, binding decision will be reached no later than 90 days after the appeal has been filed.

12. I will act in a professional manner at all times, understanding that I represent the fitness and health industry.

Personal Training Specialist *Standards of Practice*

A canfitpro Personal Training Specialist (hereinafter "PTS") must meet the following *Standards of Practice* based on the canfitpro Personal Training Specialist program.

1. Consider first the well-being of the clients throughout the training session.

2. Work with individuals or small groups of people with varying fitness experience after confirming that clients have completed the Physical Activity Readiness Questionnaire (PAR-Q+) and a health history questionnaire.

3. Provide fitness testing when appropriate to assess clients' current fitness level and, using blood pressure and resting and exercise heart rate, plan a progressive physical activity program.

4. Be competent in planning, preparing, and instructing training sessions using program design concepts, available equipment, and facilities, being mindful of health and safety hazards and risks.

5. Use the principles of fitness, health, and wellness to provide motivation and support

for clients during a progressive physical activity program.

6. Educate clients on the benefits of cardiorespiratory, strength, and flexibility training.

7. Evaluate and manage the effectiveness of a training program using considerations for interval conditioning and educate clients on intensity and the energy systems.

8. Practice as a fitness professional in a manner that treats clients with dignity.

9. In determining professional fees to clients, consider both the nature of the service provided and the ability of the clients to pay.

10. Provide services and assist clients with fitness goals until services are no longer required or wanted, until another suitable fitness or health professional has assumed responsibility for the clients, or until the clients have been given reasonable notice that the PTS intends to terminate the relationship.

11. Recognize your limitations and, when indicated, recommend or seek additional opinions and services from the appropriate professionals.

12. Respect and safeguard the relationship of trust and confidence with clients and not exploit these relationships for personal or financial gain.

13. Give clients clear instructions, explanations, and demonstrations of skills and techniques, giving them the opportunity to practice and correcting what they do with comprehensive feedback.

14. Provide sound nutritional guidance, according only to your qualifications

15. Document client-related data, communications, and progress, and if requested by the clients or an authorized third party, provide a copy unless there is compelling reason to believe that information contained in the records will result in substantial harm to the clients or others.

16. Be truthful about qualifications and the limitations of your expertise and provide services consistent with your competencies.

17. Be competent to deal with emergencies and the immediate management of an acute injury so that the welfare of clients and colleagues is maintained.

The Journey Ahead

The canfitpro Personal Training Specialist certification is designed to be your first step into the fitness industry. We require and encourage you both to maintain your education and to improve on it. We want you to look at your canfitpro certification with pride in knowing that it was your gateway to one of the most rewarding careers available. Because you are dedicated to being a Personal Training Specialist, you will not only help people become more fit but also help them live better, more satisfying lives. At canfitpro we understand that the large array of continuing education available can seem overwhelming to the new Personal Training Specialist; we will support you not only by bringing you closer to world-class education but also by helping you select the best fit to meet your needs and achieve your goals.

Another great advantage of being a Personal Training Specialist with canfitpro is that we have made it simple and incredibly achievable to stay certified. Our national team of CPR PRO TRAINERS make it easy for you to maintain your certification each year. We also provide you with a variety of ways to obtain continuing education credits, or CECs, to remain certified using cutting-edge education and technology. Please visit canfitpro's website or contact our customer relations team for information related to certification programs, conferences and tradeshows, online education opportunities, and much more.

Thank you for being a part of the leading edge of fitness training in Canada. Together as fitness professionals, we will educate, communicate, and motivate fitness consumers everywhere toward a healthier and more active lifestyle.

Accessing and Using the Web Resource

New to this edition is a free web resource, which includes online streaming video of key exercises and assessments, blank forms that can be printed for use with clients, and answers to the review questions that follow each chapter and the case studies. These resources will help you to prepare for your certification exam, master exercise and assessment techniques, and work effectively with clients as a Personal Training Specialist. You can access the web resource by visiting www.HumanKinetics.com/FoundationsOfProfessionalPersonalTraining.

If you purchased a new print book, follow the directions included on the orange-framed page at the front of your book. That page includes access steps and the unique key code that you'll need the first time you access the web resource. If you purchased an e-book from HumanKinetics.com, follow the access instructions that were e-mailed to you after your purchase.

Throughout this text, you will see this icon

when video content, forms, or answers to questions are available in the web resource. Following are the materials that are provided in the web resource:

Forms

Activity preferences form

PAR-Q+

Client health history

Fitness and postural assessment

Client program card

Form to document injury

Form to identify circle of influence

Sample personal training agreement

Video content

Seated spinal rotation test

Straight-leg raise test

Overhead squat test

Push-up test

Sit-and-reach test

Barbell chest press

Incline dumbbell chest press

Push-up (hands and toes)

Push-up (on knees)

Cable lat pull-down

Body bar lat row

Dumbbell biceps curl (standing)

Dumbbell biceps curl (seated)

Cable triceps extension

Dumbbell triceps kickback

Barbell squat

Body bar squat

Body bar stationary lunge

Barbell deadlift

Tubing leg extension

Stability ball hamstring curl

Barbell stiff-legged deadlift

Dumbbell heel raise

Back extension

Modified back extension

Partial abdominal curl-up

Shoulder to knee curl-up

Plank (from elbows, on toes)

Plank (from elbows, on knees)

Bird dog

Dead bug

Other content

Answers to end-of-chapter questions and case study review questions

Comprehensive table of canfitpro's recommendations for optimal health

Photo Credits

Case study photos

Catherine, © iStock.com/Juanmonino

Lisa, © Ginal Santa Maria/Fotolia

Thomas, © clue2305/Fotolia

Photos courtesy of canfitpro

Figure 9.5

Overhead squat test, start positions and bottom positions, chapter 10

Push-up test, chapter 10

Appendix A: Dumbbell chest press, Barbell lat row, Dumbbell lat row, Dumbbell trap shrug, Shoulder press, Dumbbell shoulder raise, Dumbbell rotator cuff external rotation, Barbell or EZ-Bar Biceps Curl, Dumbbell triceps kickback (standing), Dumbbell triceps kickback (kneeling on bench), Barbell triceps extension, Barbell squat, Dumbbell stationary lunge, Dumbbell deadlift, Stability ball hamstring curl, Barbell stiff-legged deadlift, Standing hip adduction, Hip adduction (semiprone), Cable hip abduction, Reverse abdominal curl, Dumbbell oblique lateral flexion, Plank (from elbows, on toes), Plank (from elbows, on knees)

Photos by DIVINEMETHOD Photography, © Human Kinetics

Figure 7.2

Range of motion problem examples, chapter 7

Figure 8.1

Figure 8.2

Seated spinal rotation test, chapter 10

Straight leg raise test, chapter 10

Overhead squat test imbalance examples, chapter 10

Appendix A: Barbell chest press, Dumbbell chest fly, Incline cable fly, Push-up, Push-up (standing, against wall), Double cable lat pull-down, Cable row (underhand, standing), Cable lat row (standing, with rope), Tubing lat row, Tubing shoulder press, Tubing shoulder raise, Tubing rotator cuff external rotation, Tubing rotator cuff internal rotation, Cable biceps curl, Dumbbell biceps concentration curl, Cable biceps single-arm curl, Dumbbell biceps curl, Cable triceps extension, Tubing triceps extension, Bench triceps dips, Barbell deadlift, Dumbbell stiff-legged deadlift, Hip abduction (semiprone), Dumbbell heel raise, Back extension, Partial abdominal curl-up, Stability ball abdominal curl, Shoulder to knee curl-up, Side plank (knees), Side plank (toes), Plank (from elbows, contralateral), Bird dog, Dead bug

Photos by Neil Bernstein, © Human Kinetics

Figure 7.1

Core four on the floor stretches, chapter 7

Appendix A: Machine chest press, Machine chest fly, Cable lat pull-down, Cable lat row, Machine leg press (seated, horizontal), Machine leg press (incline), Machine leg extension, Machine leg curl (prone), Machine leg curl (seated), Machine heel raise (standing), Machine heel raise (seated), Machine back extension

Appendix B: All photos

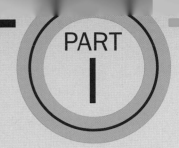

The Journey Begins

Chapter 1 Understanding Yourself and Your Client

Chapter 2 Principles for Optimal Health

As Lao-Tzu said, the journey of a thousand miles begins with one step. So it is with becoming a canfitpro Personal Training Specialist. Whether you are embarking on this certification as your entry point into the fitness industry or you are a seasoned veteran, this section of the manual will assist you in achieving clarity for what lies ahead. From this point forth, you will make choices that will cultivate your reputation as a Personal Training Specialist and influence the way in which you work with your clients. Although you may not have all the answers about where you are headed or when you'll get there, you need to have a destination in mind. This part of the manual will assist you in developing your skills and laying the foundation for strong and fulfilling personal trainer–client relationships.

Understanding Yourself and Your Client

Kim Lavender, FAHP

LEARNING OUTCOMES

After studying this chapter, you will be able to

1. understand your role as a Personal Training Specialist and its effect on your client's mindset;

2. understand your client's role and its effect as it relates to your mindset;

3. understand the skills of listening, being curious, and using your intuition to create fulfilling and rich fitness experiences for your client;

4. adapt and understand key qualities top Personal Training Specialists demonstrate throughout the personal trainer–client relationship;

5. understand the stages of change and ways to work with clients based on the stage they are in and the stage they are striving to achieve;

6. discover what makes clients commit to their workouts and how you can influence exercise adherence;

7. identify how to establish effective goals, such as SMART goals and beyond; and

8. understand how to empower clients and work effectively with various personalities and obstacles that clients commonly encounter in the fitness journey.

Whether it is sport, athletics, joy in movement, or a desire to be fit, many Personal Training Specialists start their journey as avid fitness consumers. People consume fitness in many ways, which include but are not limited to fitness clubs, group fitness, home gym equipment, fitness videos, media influence, and books and magazines. We are inundated with the next best way to lose weight, gain muscle, and reduce stress. Fitness consumers engage in a range of activity from casual walking programs to high-intensity, high-frequency programs. As fitness consumers become more educated and empowered by the knowledge to make optimal health choices, many of them begin to share their knowledge in a more formal and accredited way. They begin to make the transition from consumer to Personal Training Specialist.

In this chapter we reflect on moving from being the recipient of guidance and fitness information to being the one delivering it. The transition from being led to leading others is a pivotal point in a fitness professional's career. The decision to become a Personal Training Specialist is often influenced by a fitness consumer's mentor, personal trainer, or fitness instructor. Someone inevitably asks, "Have you ever thought of being a personal trainer?," thus creating the spark and the first steps to becoming a Personal Training Specialist. In other cases, a keen interest in physical activity and passion for helping others takes a person to a tipping point where he or she is inspired to become a fitness professional. As the person transitions from consumer to specialist, he or she adapts and models the behaviours of other Personal Training Specialists whom the person respects and desires to emulate.

Remembering what it was like to be a first-time exerciser will serve you well as a fitness professional. The challenges, fears, or feelings of being overwhelmed at the beginning of a fitness journey are important for a Personal Training Specialist to reflect on. Understanding this perspective and state with empathy will help you build strong rapport with your clients. We can align the journey of a fitness consumer's transition to becoming a Personal Training Specialist with the stages of change model. This model helps us understand the ways in which a person's mindset affects her or his willingness to adapt a new behaviour. The stages of change are **precontemplation**, **contemplation**, **preparation**, **action**, and **maintenance**. Timelines associated with each stage of change will vary from person to person. This model of behaviour change is discussed in detail later in the chapter, but here is an example of what these stages might look like for someone who is becoming a Personal Training Specialist:

- **Precontemplation**—In this stage, you might develop increased awareness of an opportunity but not be thinking seriously about it yet. You might begin to discuss fears and hopes about becoming a Personal Training Specialist and seek out general education.

- **Contemplation**—You develop increased belief and confidence in the possibility of change. You might evaluate advantages and disadvantages of becoming a Personal Training Specialist, identify your support system, and discuss advantages and benefits.

- **Preparation**—You become informed about the requirements for success and make plans. You might evaluate barriers and opportunities and complete your goal setting and action planning.

- **Action**—You take action. At this stage you would take a course and complete the Personal Training Specialist certification, do business planning, and execute your plan.

- **Maintenance**—This stage happens after change has occurred, continuing with the behaviours required for success. To do this as a Personal Training Specialist, you must maintain certification through ongoing continuing education.

As fitness consumers, people are naturally curious about information and are willing to adapt and try new things; these attributes are also helpful to a Personal Training Specialist. Even after you become a Personal Training Specialist, you need to retain a consumer's mindset and stay current and educated on the evolution of fitness and exercise. This approach will help you better serve your clients.

As the role of the Personal Training Specialist has developed, understanding the mindset of the client has become an integral part of a Personal Training Specialist's approach to servicing clients. Program design appropriate for a client's physical and performance goals encompasses many facets of how you can approach each session, motivate your clients, and keep them on track toward success. Personal training has evolved to facilitate the emotional state and positive mindset that enhances the training experience for clients. To help clients achieve overall success, you need to learn how to coach people to find the focus, determination, or extra effort they need to accomplish their goals and to overcome potential or perceived obstacles.

This chapter reviews the journey of a Personal Training Specialist and his or her client by exploring the multiple stages of the process from before the first session to assisting the client in making sustainable and positive lifelong decisions for optimal health.

Beginning the Personal Trainer–Client Journey

Your success as a Personal Training Specialist will depend on, and be directly aligned with, the success and satisfaction of your clients. The ability to ask powerful questions and understand your client's journey is paramount to achieving long-term suc-cess. To be effective as a Personal Training Specialist, you need a keen understanding of the clients you are working with and the transitions that they will experience. Knowing that the mind and body work as one, you will also understand that the mindset of clients will influence how you, as a Personal Training Specialist, feel, respond, and perform. Your clients' mindset includes such aspects as what motivates them, why they are striving toward their fitness goals, what may hold them back, and what factors influence their success. This understanding will transcend any exercise program and propel canfitpro Personal Training Specialists to be much more to their clients than just instructors of exercise.

Personal Training Specialist's Mindset

Personal Training Specialists should reflect on themselves and their own state of readiness to work with clients. Consider that clients will present themselves

Demonstrating the Mind–Body Connection for Personal Training Specialists

This activity explores how mindset can affect physiology. Note that what we think, we will also feel.

1. Imagine that your future client has shown up late with a negative attitude, is not willing to work, and is challenging to communicate with during each session. When you see the client's name in the appointment book, you dread the session time as it approaches.

Pause here and pay attention to your posture, breathing, and physiology of your body. What do you notice?

2. Take a moment to reset, break state, and literally shake it off. Ensure that you shift your body and take four deep, cleansing breaths. Now imagine that your client shows up early, smiling and excited, fully prepared to accept your guidance, and has fun in sessions while working to reach her or his potential every session. You quickly see changes in the results and look forward to each time you work with the client. You are extremely confident in your program design and the client's ability to adopt positive change and adhere to exercise. When you see the person's name in the appointment book, you smile and immediately imagine hearing the excitement in her or his voice.

Pause again and pay attention to your posture, breathing, and physiology of your body. What do you notice?

3. Reflect on what you observed about your response to the two preceding scenarios. Which assumptions generated a state that would prepare you to service your client well and function at your best?

This exercise can initiate an understanding of the effect that the mindset has on the performance and physiological response of both the Personal Training Specialist and the client. For some Personal Training Specialists, this skill may come naturally, although it can also be developed and improved over time. Consider this as you read through the content of this chapter.

to you as an assimilation of their past exercise, health, and lifestyle experiences. These experiences manifest themselves as memories, attitudes, and preconceived notions that may or may not benefit them. The most important thing to remember is that whatever their history, clients have overcome whatever may have been holding them back to bring them to you as their Personal Training Specialist. Although this insight should not be overwhelming, it should inspire your respect and admiration for their courage and newfound commitment.

After you have learned about the client's past experiences through conversation and the screening process, you will naturally conjure visions of what a pending session will be like, positive or negative. As this plays out in your mind, you explore the sights, sounds, and responses that you expect to fill an experience. These thoughts may generate a physiological response. You can control these images and leverage your ability to create the best possible mindset that will serve you, the Personal Training Specialist, and your client well. This mindset will affect your emotional state and belief in your ability to service your client. Try the activity in the sidebar to explore how your mindset can create a physical and emotional response when approaching a session.

As you anticipate the first session and subsequent sessions with a client, it is useful to establish some key presuppositions or assumptions in advance to establish a positive environment and foundation. A Personal Training Specialist can make the following suppositions to generate a positive state of physiology to operate from. After accepting these assumptions, you can create and find them in your own experiences with clients. When approaching a session with a client, presume the following to be true (O'Connor, 2001):

1. Your clients are doing the best they can with the resources available to them at that moment.
2. Positive intention is behind your clients' behaviour.
3. How your clients behave is not who they are, so you accept them as they are and help to change their behaviour.
4. You respect your clients in their own model of the world.
5. There is no failure—only feedback. You are willing to adapt and change as you go.
6. The mind and body work together, and you work with both as one.
7. Choice is better than no choice, so you will strive and aim to increase opportunities for better choices more often.
8. Change and exercise adherence can be easy and enjoyable.
9. Your client has all the resources needed or can create them.
10. You get what you focus on, so you will maintain an image of a successful personal trainer–client relationship.

Client's Mindset

The role of a Personal Training Specialist is to provide safe and effective exercise programming. Within the instruction of this programming, you can function within your *Standards of Practice* and provide suggestions and questions to help inspire lasting change and exercise adherence. Something new on the outside (e.g., exercising, losing weight, changing body composition) often requires something new on the inside, so your client's mindset will directly affect the results of the program.

If all the suppositions listed previously are true, the questions included in the sidebar can assist clients in developing a focused and positive mindset as they start their personal training journey. This process will enable them to create a positive vision of success, even before they take action. When you adopt this line of questioning, be sure to exercise the skill of active listening, write down the answers that your clients provide, and notice what excites or concerns them.

The questions in the sidebar can assist clients in their journey to reach their fitness goals. By collecting this information, the Personal Training Specialist can leverage this material to inspire change and exercise adherence throughout the personal trainer–client relationship. Asking questions such as these can initiate positive thoughts and a focus on fitness goals, thus serving as reminders of why clients have committed to working out. In turn, this dialogue inspires your clients to show up, work hard, and put purpose into their workouts with you.

Client Fears and Perceptions

You need to understand your clients' perceptions and fears before starting the exercise program. Doing

First Session Questions

"How can I best help you today? What do you want to get out of your workout with me?"

These questions assist in building rapport and empowering clients to take responsibility of their outcomes. A Personal Training Specialist is there to guide and provide safe and effective exercise programming.

"What will it be like when you are following a regular exercise program? Can you describe that for me?"

These questions help your clients look forward to following an exercise program and enjoying exercise adherence.

"When you reach your fitness goals, what will you be able to do?"

This question elicits the clients' feelings of reaching their fitness goals; it is a when question, not an if question. The question also corresponds to the purpose of their goals.

"What fitness accomplishments have you experienced before?" (no matter how far back).

This question helps clients confirm that they do indeed have the resources they need to reach their fitness goals.

this is sometimes difficult because your background and experiences are likely different from those of your clients. In most instances, Personal Training Specialists have a variety of experiences with exercise and are confident in an exercise setting. In contrast, your clients may not have had a lot of experience or may have had experiences that were not entirely positive. These situations may have caused clients to become fearful of many things related to exercise, including fitness facilities, the people who work and work out in them, and even the exercise program itself. If you expect everyone to view exercise the same way you do, then you may be in for a major shock. You need to understand and address your clients' previous experiences and current perceptions of exercise. Only after you do this can you focus on designing appropriate programs for your clients.

Your clients' experiences and feelings in an exercise setting may be significantly different from yours. You need to understand your clients' fears, uncertainties, and any negative perceptions of exercise.

Your clients may have several other beliefs or perceptions:

- Unrealistic expectations for themselves
- Fear of failure
- Fear of not knowing what to do or how to do it
- Perception that everyone will be looking at them
- Belief that they are the only ones who feel the way they do

Personal Training Specialists need to be aware of these possible fears and perceptions. Some are common, especially with clients who are in the early stages of change. The following are actions you can take to help your clients manage these perceptions:

- Get them talking about their previous achievements, no matter how far back.
- Track their success and remind them of their accomplishments along the way.
- Celebrate their success; have fun.
- Ensure them that they are not alone in their journey toward optimal health and that others have felt the same way.
- Ask them whom they want to share their success with.
- Establish a focus that they can use when the way forward becomes difficult. What will motivate them to carry on and move forward?
- Empower them with knowledge and guidance on how to exercise; commend them on remembering key cues and techniques.

- Remind them that their choice to get active and exercise is rewarding.
- Share stories of other clients (with permission) or introduce them to others who have felt the same way so that they believe that success is possible for them too.

When dealing with your clients' negative behaviours or perceptions, using continuing questions can be helpful. For example, when a client states, "I can't," simply ask, "What would it be like if you could? What would that be like?" or "What will it take to accomplish this?" Other empowering questions include the following: "When have you experienced strength before?" (this confirms that they have the resources, although not in the same context). "How can you show that strength again now?" "What will achieving this do for you?" (this question links to their goals or purpose).

Client Empowerment

The experience that clients have with a Personal Training Specialist may influence other aspects of their lives. When clients have a positive experience, make effective choices, and reach their personal fitness goals while working with you, they often experience positive changes in other areas. These changes are often reflected in their view of themselves, their level of self-confidence, and their experience of overall happiness, thus leading to a greater sense of overall fulfillment.

Client fulfillment is the ultimate goal for a Personal Training Specialist, and assisting clients along this important journey is a privilege. Whether clients are just getting started, thinking about making a change, looking for a challenge, or maintaining their exercise adherence, you have the opportunity to be a helpful part of that equation.

Some Personal Training Specialists inappropriately establish relationships in which they insist the client needs the Personal Training Specialist's guidance in order to succeed. This approach does a disservice to the client and can hinder long-term success and fulfillment. Although a Personal Training Specialist can educate and motivate during workout sessions to expedite the client's results, adopting techniques and strategies to endorse positive decision making outside the fitness facility can be long lasting and life changing.

During your training sessions be sure to explain the purpose of each workout component, demonstrate each exercise, cue as necessary, coach to motivate effort, and empower your clients to believe in themselves, their fitness goals, and their ability to achieve success. Table 1.1 gives an example of these types of interactions. Following this process in sequence will ease the adaptation of the clients' learning and fulfillment while affirming their skills and abilities. Leaving out any of these steps could result in clients' becoming disengaged and unsuccessful. See figure 1.1.

A canfitpro Personal Training Specialist's goal is to empower clients to make confident and positive choices in and outside the fitness facility. This goal can be achieved by offering compliments or feedback to clients that confirms and provides evidence

TABLE 1.1   Positive Interactions for Client Fulfillment

Goal	Example comment to client
When explaining exercises, be clear and concise and emphasize key cues for setup, technique, and safety.	"In a squat or lunge, keep your knees tracking over the foot."
When demonstrating and teaching the purpose of the exercise, identify how doing the exercise will benefit the client.	"This exercise targets your leg strength and core stability."
When cueing, ask the client what she or he should remember when executing the exercise. (This questioning enables the client to learn, recall, and remember the key cues for future reference.)	"What should you remember when lowering down into the movement?"
When coaching to motivate the best possible effort from the client, link the purpose of the exercise to the greater purpose of the fitness goals.	"We are including lunges to strengthen your legs and help you accomplish your goal of running a 10K race. Strong now, strong on the course."
Encourage personal empowerment and long-term adherence by offering specific feedback that acknowledges the skill and ability that the client is exhibiting.	"You really dug deep in that set. How do you feel now that you've got through it?"

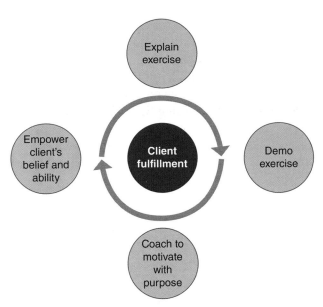

FIGURE 1.1 Cycle of client fulfillment.

of their ability. Doing this increases the likelihood that they will continue with exercise, view themselves as capable, and believe that success is indeed possible. Asking questions also allows clients to take ownership of their success, thereby confirming that they have the resources they need to succeed.

Some examples of empowering feedback are the following:

- "You really focused on the proper alignment throughout that set. That was great!"

- "You found it in you to push through that last 15 seconds of the interval; that took a lot of determination!"

- "You have made fitness a habit. Good for you! I have noticed that you've been really committed to reaching your fitness goals by being active three times per week."

 The Personal Training Specialist should not only educate and motivate clients during sessions but also empower them to take charge of their own fitness goals.

Key Qualities of Effective Personal Training Specialists

To be effective and enjoy great success with their clients, Personal Training Specialists need to have a vast array of skills. Strong subject knowledge pro-vides the programming material necessary. In addition, Personal Training Specialists need the ability to communicate and deliver the training experience so that clients feel successful and enjoy the workout. These qualities and skills should be demonstrated throughout the entire personal trainer–client journey. By exercising these qualities and skills, you, as a Personal Training Specialist, will build strong rapport with your clients and have a positive effect on their overall experience.

Note that should you feel uncomfortable explaining exercises or programming to your client, it is an indication that you need to practice more or refer the client to someone who has the ability and expertise to serve the client's specific needs better.

Throughout your interactions with clients, you need to provide feedback and advice to guide and motivate them in a variety of ways. You should offer feedback during assessments, exercise programming, exercise execution, and ongoing monitoring throughout the program. Communication skills are at the heart of an effective personal trainer–client relationship. You must be able to listen effectively and respond empathetically. If you lack these skills, it will be difficult for you to build the kind of relationship you need with your clients.

Several qualities of effective Personal Training Specialists can enhance the personal trainer–client journey (adapted in part from Howley and Franks, 2003, p. 360):

- **Listening**—Personal Training Specialists need to gather information about clients constantly throughout the training journey. Asking good questions and listening intently will enhance the personal trainer–client relationship and enable you to gather key information that you can leverage in programming and motivating your clients.

- **Curious**—When gathering information about your clients, being curious will lead you to ask good questions and solicit useful feedback about what motivates them, what they are experiencing, and what may be holding them back from further progress.

- **Intuitive**—Throughout the personal trainer–client journey you can trust your intuition to inspire questions that will help your client conjure positive experiences. You may want to put yourself in the position of the client. For example, if you were the client, what would you need to hear, see, or do next?

• **Knowledgeable**—As a Personal Training Specialist, you must know the subject matter you will be discussing with clients. You also need to be knowledgeable enough to stop before giving any advice that is outside your *Standards of Practice*. Personal Training Specialists need to learn constantly and evolve through continuing education.

• **Supportive**—Personal Training Specialists should support clients in their goals and be empathetic to the journey they are taking. Clients will have good and bad days, and you need to be supportive and positive during both.

• **Respectful**—Personal Training Specialists should be respectful of their clients' ideas and approaches to exercise and respectful of their time. You need to focus on the client throughout the entire session and provide the quality experience that the client deserves every time you meet.

• **Model of healthy behaviour**—When you demonstrate healthy behaviours, your clients are more willing to follow your advice and guidance. If you do not model the behaviour you are teaching, you will have difficulty convincing your clients that the program is worth the investment of time, money, and effort.

• **Trustworthy**—Your clients should feel comfortable sharing information related to their health and well-being so that you can make the most informed decisions about their personal training program.

• **Enthusiastic**—As a Personal Training Specialist, you should be motivating and show keen and genuine interest in what clients are doing both inside and outside the fitness centre, supporting their goals of optimal health. Your expression of enthusiasm should be geared to the ways in which your clients like to be motivated and congruent with their personality type.

• **Innovative**—The Personal Training Specialist should constantly be looking for ways to add variety and improve each client's program and ultimate results. Providing safe, fun, effective, and time-efficient choices to clients will empower them and contribute to their long-term exercise adherence.

• **Patient**—Personal Training Specialists work with many types of clients; some will be similar to you, and others may be very different. Regardless of their personality type, level of motivation, and pace of progress, all clients needs your patience as

they progress toward their goals. Some will move quickly, and others will move slowly; all need a certain degree of patience to be successful.

• **Sensitive**—Being sensitive to clients' needs and characteristics is an important quality of a Personal Training Specialist. Whether you can relate to them or not, you need to demonstrate compassion and understanding toward all your clients.

• **Flexible**—Each client is unique and will require you to be flexible in your approach. One style will definitely not fit all your clients. Personal Training Specialists should be flexible throughout workouts and be willing to adjust the plan in the moment if necessary.

• **Self-aware**—As a Personal Training Specialist, you need to be aware of your own strengths and weaknesses and how others may perceive you. You will not be able to grow personally and professionally without a strong sense of who you are and how others view you. Keep this in mind, especially when working out on your own in the fitness facility, because potential clients may be watching and assessing whether they would hire you as a Personal Training Specialist.

• **Resourceful**—You will likely not have answers to all of your clients' possible questions and concerns, so you must be able to refer your clients to other resources or professionals when appropriate. Joining a network of health professionals can become reciprocal; as you refer when necessary, others may begin to refer to you as well.

• **Committed to providing timely, specific feedback**—Your clients need to know how they are doing as they progress toward their goals. Immediate feedback is essential to keeping your clients focused and motivated. The more specific the feedback is, the more valuable it will be to your clients. Be sure to state feedback positively and focus more on what you *want* to see.

• **Capable of providing clear, reasonable instructions and programming**—Personal Training Specialists have a vast knowledge base, most of which your client does not need to hear about in detail. Your responsibility is to communicate your message in a way that clients will easily understand, retain, and find motivating.

• **Able to generate expectations of success**—Personal Training Specialists assist their clients in being accountable for their workouts and healthy lifestyle choices. You also need to demonstrate affirming abilities that lead to success, empower clients, and guide them toward understanding that they are capable of many things they initially thought they could not achieve. The ability to formulate powerful questions helps in generating (and maintaining) clients' expectation of success.

As you can see, Personal Training Specialists need to demonstrate many skills and qualities to work effectively with clients and provide the best possible personal trainer–client experience. You will continue to refine these skills and qualities as you gain experience as a Personal Training Specialist. Over time, you will learn to adapt your skill set to the client you are working with and demonstrate versatility in your style of training, rapport, and communication with each client.

Understanding Behaviour Change

As a Personal Training Specialist you will play a role in supporting and assisting your clients as they progress toward a healthier lifestyle. For this reason, you can benefit from gaining an understanding of the various stages of behavioural change. Knowing where you are personally and where your clients are in their journey will help you implement effective coaching and training techniques.

Transtheoretical Model of Behaviour Change

The most popular way to look at behaviour change is the transtheoretical model, also known as the stages of change model (figure 1.2). This model describes behaviour change as a constantly changing process that follows specific steps. The approach to dealing with transition should therefore vary based on the stage that the client is in. For example, your fitness programming for someone who has been exercising regularly for the past six months would be different from the approach you would use with someone who has not been exercising regularly or has failed at many previous attempts. This model provides specific strategies for progressing through each transitional stage. The sections that follow describe the traditional stages of change as they apply in an exercise setting.

Precontemplation (Not Ready)

A person in this stage is not seriously thinking about changing or starting an exercise program. Potential clients in the precontemplation stage do not intend to start a new healthy behaviour in the near future and may be unaware of the need to change. People in this stage can benefit from learning more about the potential health effects of their current lifestyle, and they should be encouraged to think about the advantages of adopting healthier behaviours.

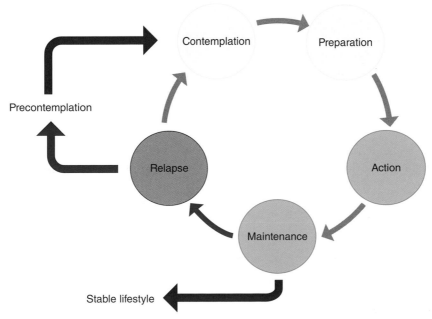

FIGURE 1.2 The stages of change model describes how a person moves through a behavioural change.

Precontemplators typically underestimate the advantages of changing, overestimate the disadvantages, and often are not aware of the consequences of their behaviour.

One of the most effective ways that you can help people at this stage is to encourage them to become more mindful of their decision making and more conscious of the multiple benefits of changing an unhealthy behaviour and adapting a healthier, more active lifestyle. Clients often experience doubt in their ability to make the change, thus leaning more toward the disadvantages. An effective question for these clients would be, "If you could make this change and be active, what would that be like?" This question leads them to generate an image or vision of success and to feel the emotions associated with implementing their new healthy behaviours. This powerful image can expedite their progress toward the next stage of change.

Contemplation (Getting Ready)

In this stage, people have started to think about exercising or changing behaviour and have most likely identified a course of action. At this stage, clients align their intentions to adapt and start the healthy behaviour. Although now they are usually more aware of the benefits of changing, the perceived disadvantages are still about equal to the advantages. They are close to reaching a neutral mindset, and this ambivalence about changing can cause them to continue putting off significant action. Clients at this stage benefit from learning about the kind of person they could be if they changed their behaviour. They will learn more from people who behave in healthy ways. A Personal Training Specialist can help at this stage by encouraging clients to work at reducing the perceived disadvantages of changing their behaviour.

When working with a client at the contemplation stage, the Personal Training Specialist may want to write down the client's expressed advantages and disadvantages, provide strategies to manage obstacles, and emphasize the benefits. Acknowledging the client's progress toward his or her goals will encourage adherence to progressing toward healthy behaviours. Posting the list of advantages in a place where the client can see what he or she is working toward can be helpful for change adaptation.

Preparation (Ready)

Clients at this stage are ready to start taking action. They take small steps that they believe can help them make the healthy behaviour a part of their lives. For example, they tell their friends and family that they want to change their behaviour, and they make statements to demonstrate their growing commitment to change (e.g., status updates on social media declaring and exhibiting their excitement about their change progress). As a Personal Training Specialist, you should understand that clients in this stage may have some lingering doubt about their success. Focusing on the advantages of their changes will serve as confirmation and evidence for them that they are indeed able to make and sustain these changes.

Clients in this stage should be encouraged to seek support from people they trust, to talk about their plan to change the way they act, and to think about how they would feel if they behaved in a healthier way. Their number one concern is often the thought of whether they will fail after they begin to take action. They can benefit from learning that the better prepared they are, the more likely they are to keep progressing. You may find it helpful to ask clients to describe their success and the way they feel about it, and then write it down. A strategy to counteract relapses is important. Clients can refer back to their plans and past success as inspiration to keep exercising. The longer that clients adhere to their plans for healthy behaviours, the more confidence they will gain, as their concerns of failure diminish.

Action (Actively Making Changes)

At this stage, people have begun to take the necessary action, but not much time has passed since they started making the changes. Clients at this stage have changed their behaviour and need to work hard to keep moving ahead. These clients need to learn how to strengthen their commitments to change and to fight urges to slip back or relapse. As their Personal Training Specialist, you can ask them how they think you can best help them stay on track. This assistance may be through reminders of their goals, check-ins on days when they are not in the fitness facility, or off-day exercise planning to keep their momentum and adherence intact.

Clients in this stage can also progress by being taught techniques for keeping up their commitments such as substituting activities related to the unhealthy behaviour with positive ones, rewarding themselves for taking steps toward changing, and avoiding people and situations that tempt them to behave in unhealthy ways. All these strategies keep clients working toward maintenance of their new behaviours.

Maintenance (Adherence to Changes)

This stage begins after the person has successfully adhered to an exercise program for a sustained period, approximately six months or more. People at this stage have changed their behaviour, but they need to be aware of situations that may tempt them to slip back into the old, unhealthy behaviour (relapse)—particularly stressful situations.

People in this stage should seek support from people whom they trust, spend time with people who behave in healthy ways, and remember to engage in healthy activities to cope with stress instead of relying on unhealthy behaviour. Your role as a Personal Training Specialist is not only to highlight the achievements that clients have made so far but also to keep them inspired to stay on track. You can encourage them to set new fitness goals, take on new challenges, or continue to maintain their current level of fitness.

Strategies for Working With the Stages of Change

The personal trainer–client journey can include a couple of sessions for consultation or programming guidance to establish a long-term commitment and build an alliance throughout the stages of change. The Personal Training Specialist can positively affect the likelihood of clients' success by guiding, supporting, and commending them throughout each of the stages of change. A good Personal Training Specialist will be able to identify which stage a client is in at any given time and be able to program and guide the client accordingly. When your client reaches the maintenance stage, she or he has

Intervention Strategies for Stages of Change

Precontemplation
- Increase awareness of the importance of exercise and emphasize the benefits
- Provide general education one on one or through print or electronic publications
- Discuss health risks
- Discuss myths and fears related to exercise

Contemplation
- Make a list of advantages related to regular exercise
- Continue with education and discussion of benefits
- Provide clear and specific recommendations for an exercise program
- Identify social support system (family, friends, coworkers, or other exercisers)
- Build the client's self-confidence

Preparation
- Evaluate support system and barriers
- Provide personalized exercise design
- Work on goal setting and action plan

Action
- Talk to the client about self-monitoring
- Talk to the client about self-reinforcement
- Enhance the client's self-efficacy
- Provide encouragement
- Prepare for relapses
- Help the client prevent relapses

Maintenance
- Review and revise goals and exercise program
- Address concerns that may lead to relapses and strategize how to avoid them
- Set new fitness goals: "What is next?"
- Provide social support; introduce client to others who are in the same phase

demonstrated the ability to sustain the change. You may continue to assist your client by asking, "What is next?" or "How can you see yourself maintaining these changes for the long run?" The overall aim here is to help the client stay in the maintenance stage or set a new goal.

Regardless of which stage your client is in, the potential for relapse always exists. You need to recognize that relapses do occur and be prepared with a strategy for dealing with them. Each client has a different exercise history and needs to be treated individually. Only after you have assessed which stage your client is in can you determine which intervention strategies to use. The sidebar lists intervention strategies that you can use at each stage.

Keep in mind that clients will show up in any of the outlined stages, so you need to be able to work with them according to the stage they are currently in. Clients often get to the action phase and then relapse. For this reason, when you consult with clients you should attempt to provide planning that

reaches a phase of maintenance, provide strategies for preventing relapse, and pursue the client's long-term commitment to a healthy lifestyle and exercise adherence. Recognize that a long-term commitment is not always feasible for clients, but offering the full plan for success serves clients well and informs them of what it will take to reach their goals. Some clients may simply be searching for a limited number of sessions with you to get started, so you need to listen intently and understand what clients are striving for and how you as a Personal Training Specialist can best serve them.

To determine the stage your client is in, you can use the simple questionnaire in figure 1.3.

Influencing Exercise Adherence

Several factors can influence a person's **exercise adherence**, and many clients experience challenges

---

For each of the following questions, please circle yes or no. Be sure to read the questions carefully.

Physical activity or exercise includes walking briskly, jogging, bicycling, swimming, or any other activity that requires similar exertion.

	No	Yes
1. I am currently physically active.	0	1
2. I intend to become more physically active in the next six months.	0	1

For activity to be regular, it must add up to a total of 30 minutes or more per day and be done at least five days per week. For example, you could take one 30-minute walk or take three 10-minute walks for a daily total of 30 minutes.

	No	Yes
3. I currently engage in regular physical activity.	0	1
4. I have been regularly physically active for the past 6 months.	0	1

Note: You may want to cover the following scoring algorithm before reproducing this questionnaire for clients.

Scoring Algorithm
If (question 1 = 0 and question 2 = 0), then you are at stage 1.
If (question 1 = 0 and question 2 = 1), then you are at stage 2.
If (question 1 = 1 and question 3 = 0), then you are at stage 3.
If (question 1 = 1, question 3 = 1, and question 4 = 0), then you are at stage 4.
If (question 1 = 1, question 3 = 1, and question 4 = 1), then you are at stage 5.

FIGURE 1.3 Physical activity stages of change questionnaire.

Reprinted, by permission, from B.H. Marchis, J.S. Rossi, V.C. Selby, R.S. Niaura, and D.B. Abrams, 1992, "The stages and processes of exercise adoption and maintenance in a worksite sample," *Health Psychology* 11: 386-395.

in sticking to their fitness plans. They will inevitably need to overcome and address obstacles to stay on track and achieve their goals. As a Personal Training Specialist you can increase adherence when you use effective strategies to help clients stay motivated, understand each client's preference of motivation techniques, and speak using presuppositions related specifically to their goals.

Motivating Clients

Plan to succeed by helping clients visualize the best possible scenario. When you review clients' fitness goals, it can be helpful to ask more questions about what it will be like when they reach their fitness goals. (Using the word *when* is a presupposition that they will indeed reach their fitness goals and that they have the ability and resources to be successful.) Try asking clients the following: "When you reach your fitness goal of (*insert whatever the client is striving for*), describe what that will look like." "What will you be saying? What will others be saying? How will that feel? What will you do then?" Write down the details, because you can use this information to remind clients of the importance of their goals when they face challenges.

Clients are unique in many ways, including the way in which they prefer to be motivated during a session and outside the fitness facility. To help identify some of the strategies that will aid motivation, you can ask your clients to describe a time in the past when a motivation technique was inspirational. You can also ask what motivation techniques they do not like. Listen carefully, because what they say can tell you what you need to do to motivate them effectively. Asking these questions demonstrates your desire to adapt your methods to match the client's needs and wants, therefore strengthening the personal trainer–client relationship. Be aware of whether they are looking for constant praise, feedback, challenges, high energy, subtle praise, written feedback, or visual metrics.

When clients are struggling with an exercise, they often question why they are doing what they are doing and may search for reasons not to continue. At this time the Personal Training Specialist can remind clients of their expressed goals and the results they are striving for. Clients can then focus on conjuring the mental image of success and exerting the effort necessary to produce and achieve the desired results. Recalling purpose or goals can lead to an increase

in the effort and willingness to adhere to exercise.

The following are some general motivational strategies to increase effort and exercise adherence:

- Recall the purpose or goals they are working toward.
- Make the workouts fun.
- Let clients know what to expect as the workout proceeds and when setting up their next appointment.
- Provide positive behavioural feedback and comment specifically on what clients are doing right (instead of only saying, "Great" or "Way to go"). In addition, comment on what skills and capabilities are leading to their success so that they will repeat the specific behaviours.
- Ask clients how their personal circle is supporting them with the behavioural change.
- Ask whom they are sharing their success with. Encourage group participation and group support to offer the opportunity for social reinforcement, camaraderie, and commitment.
- Include variety and complexity to decrease boredom and increase enjoyment (always keeping safety paramount).
- Provide periodic assessments to give information about progress toward goals and offer positive reinforcement.
- Ask clients what they liked about a workout when they felt successful or strong.
- Use behavioural change strategies, such as personal goal setting, journaling, contracting, and self-management, to foster a greater sense of competency and personal control.
- Always keep workout logs to chart progress. Display progress on record cards or graphs. Note progress daily to give immediate, positive feedback, and provide client with copies that they can keep in sight.
- Recognize goal achievement and progress through appropriate recognition (e.g., newsletters and bulletin boards).
- Ask what healthy rewards they can provide for themselves when they reach milestones or goals along the journey.

- Ask what activities clients enjoy doing and incorporate them in their planned workout programs.

Setting SMART Goals

A key part of a successful Personal Training Specialist's tool kit is the ability to set **SMART goals**. You should use this approach to goal setting whenever you are helping clients set short-term and long-term goals. The acronym SMART stands for the following:

S   specific

M   measurable

A   attainable

R   realistic

T   time sensitive

Specific

Goals should be as specific as possible so that people can picture exactly where they need to be going. Questioning skills are essential to setting specific goals. When clients come to you and say that they want to get in shape and feel better, what exactly do they mean? They could mean that they want to run a marathon, play with their kids, walk up stairs without getting out of breath, or lose weight—the possibilities are endless. The only way to find out what an individual client wants is to ask more questions, such as the following:

- What exactly do you mean by "get in shape" and "feel better"?
- How do you want to feel?
- What do you want to change?

After you have asked these questions, you should have a better idea of what clients want. Their responses will help clarify the nature of their specific goals.

Measurable

Using measurable goals is a great way to give people feedback on their progress. Let's say that your client wants to lose some weight and have more energy. After you know how much adipose tissue (fat) the client needs or wants to lose, you can set a specific goal using a scale and body fat measurement to determine the exact amount of adipose tissue lost. Setting a goal for increased energy is a little differ-ent. When clients have a goal such as this, one that is difficult to measure objectively, you can use a rating scale. For example, ask your clients where they are on a scale of 1 to 10, where 10 is the point at which they have all the energy they desire. If clients say they are at a 5, you could suggest that by their next assessment they will increase their energy level to a 7 or 8. If you can't set a specific numeric goal, then you will need to get your clients to describe how they will feel when they have achieved their goal. For example, clients who want to get in shape might say that they will have achieved this goal after they are able to play with their kids for more than 10 minutes or walk up two flights of stairs without feeling out of breath. If you are not able to set a goal that can be evaluated using either objective measurements or subjective rating methods, then the goal may not be worth setting.

Attainable

When you are setting a goal for your client, you should associate a specific attainable action with it. For example, if your client's goal is to lose 10 kilograms (22 lb) of fat, an action associated with this might be for your client to meet with you three times a week and get in one additional 30-minute session, thereby losing approximately one kilogram (about 2 lb) per week over 10 to 20 weeks.

Realistic

To be motivating, the goal must be believable to clients. If your clients do not think they will be able to reach the goal that has been set, it is not going to be motivating for them. Similarly, if you have set a goal that clients are motivated to achieve but the process involved in achieving it is too aggressive, they will eventually lose motivation because the goal is not realistic for them. You may need to educate your clients on what is realistic for them. For example, if a client has a goal to lose 15 kilograms (33 lb) of fat to get her weight down to 55 kilograms (121 lb) pounds in six weeks, you will need to need to educate her on safe and effective ways to lose body fat as well as the problems with quick-fix programs.

Time Sensitive

The last component to setting an effective goal is the time frame. Every goal you set with your clients should have a date associated with it. The time frame can be long term, short term, or a combination of each. For example, if a person wants to lose 20 kilograms (44 lb) of fat, you might say that doing this is possible in approximately 10 months (long term), but you should also mention the short-term goal of aiming to lose about two to three kilograms (5 to 7 lb) of fat in six to eight weeks. Breaking down long-term goals into short-term goals will keep clients motivated and allow you to give them feedback as they progress toward their long-term goal. A long-term goal by itself may seem too far away, and it may not be motivating because clients know that it will take a long time to get feedback.

From SMART to SMARTERS

The SMART formula is a well-established and widely accepted method of goal setting. Depending on the context of its use, multiple variations can be applied to its standard criteria. As a Personal Training Specialist, after you've established goals using the SMART formula, you can check in with clients to discover the ultimate purpose of reaching these goals and what their attainment will do for them. Through this process, the SMART acronym can be expanded to SMARTERS: **SMART** and

E   Evaluate: At predetermined dates, is the client on track toward the ultimate goal? In what areas has the client succeeded? Where is more attention and effort needed?

R   Realign: After evaluation, if the client is off track, modify the program to ensure timely progress toward the ultimate goal.

S   Success: If progress is on track, be sure to reward the success!

The expansion of the SMART acronym to include ERS ensures that the process of goal setting remains dynamic throughout the personal trainer–client relationship.

Follow-up questions are useful at several times throughout the journey to evaluate clients' success. You can include goal-related questions such as the following:

- "When you lose the 10 kilograms (22 lb) of fat, what will that do for you? Tell me about it."
- "When you run the 5K race in 30 minutes, who are you going to share that with? What else will you be able to do?"

- "When you increase your upper-body strength and core stability, what will that do for you?"

These questions, all based on the presupposition that clients will indeed reach their goals, will help keep them motivated throughout each stage of their program.

You should ensure that when clients are ready to work toward their goals, the projected results are what they truly want. To discover the feasibility of attaining goals and the level of desire that clients have to reach them, you should look at what achieving the goals will cost them. Cost here refers what clients will need to commit to as an investment toward the goal, whether it be time, money, relationships, or other resources. Are clients prepared to do what is necessary, or do they need to adjust their goals?

Clients need to consider two other questions on the journey toward their goals: What do they have now that they want to keep intact? What is currently working that they would like to retain?

Checking in on these aspects will enable clients to look at the big picture of exercise adherence. Doing so can improve the likelihood of reaching their goals with confidence while lessening the chances of relapse. Ensuring that clients recognize when they have reached milestones or had other success along the journey will remind them of the skills and abilities they exhibited to reach each goal. Doing so will help them be able to tap into those skills and abilities when they are needed again. Always remember to celebrate your clients' small victories along the way to achieving their long-term goals!

Other Factors in Exercise Adherence

Many factors affect whether clients will stick to an exercise program. As a Personal Training Specialist, you should understand the challenges that your clients may have to overcome to adhere to their fitness program. Understanding the situations that may help or hinder your clients' success is important, but you should not assume that these factors will prevent clients from achieving their goals. The following paragraphs explain several factors that have been shown to affect clients' adherence. These items can have a positive, negative, or neutral effect on exercise programming.

Individual Factors

Research has shown that a number of individual characteristics affect adherence to exercise. Demographics traditionally have a strong relationship with exercise. In particular, more education, male gender, and higher socioeconomic status have all been positively related to physical activity.

Cognitive and personality variables also play a role. When we look at all the cognitive variables that have been tested over the years, the ones that have been the best predictors of physical activity are self-efficacy and self-motivation. By self-efficacy, we mean the client's belief in being able to do a particular exercise program. A person's level of motivation toward exercise is also a major determinant of success in an exercise program. The more confident and motivated clients are, the more likely they are to be successful in an exercise program. You can facilitate this process by giving them feedback on how they are doing, setting realistic goals, and reassuring them that they can do it.

With respect to behaviour, the best predictor of a person's likelihood to participate in an exercise program is previous experience in an exercise program. Little evidence supports the idea that participation in sport in and of itself will predict future physical activity patterns. Likewise, physical activity patterns in childhood or early adulthood are not good indicators of future activity patterns. The key factor to look at in adults is their recent history of physical activity. Note, however, that when children have a solid social support system that encourages physical activity and have role models to look up to, they are much more likely to be physically active when they are older. This point emphasizes the importance of parental involvement in a child's future patterns of physical activity.

Environmental Factors

Environmental factors play a major role in predicting the likelihood of success. These factors include the social environment (e.g., family and peers) and physical environment (e.g., weather, time, and distance from the facility).

Social Environment   Social support is a critical aspect of the client's environment and plays an important role in the likelihood that he or she will adhere to an exercise program. A spouse in particular has a significant influence. In some cases the spouse's influence can be even stronger than that of the exerciser. As a Personal Training Specialist, you should identify your client's social support system to determine whether it is going to help or hinder the exercise routine. If the social support system is not adequate, consider ways to help the client. One simple approach would be to make sure that the client is introduced to others within the club. Although these introductions will not replace the client's long-established social network, they are a step in the right direction.

Physical Environment   The location of the fitness facility is another important factor in the exercise program of a client. The closer the client's home or workplace is to the exercise setting, the more likely it is that the client will adhere to his or her program.

The most frequently cited reason that people give for not exercising is lack of time. The location of your facility may be tough to get to when you include drive time, getting changed, workout duration, and so on. You may want to provide some time-efficient workout options that clients can do a couple of times per week outside the facility, something that they enjoy and keeps them motivated. You can even request that clients report to you to let you know that they are still on track. This approach provides accountability and increases your service level.

Strive to make appointments as convenient as possible for clients; be sensitive and respect their time by providing time-sensitive and effective workout plans.

Physical Activity Characteristics

The success of an exercise program depends on several structural factors. We will focus on the most important ones, which are exercise intensity, whether the exercise is done in a group or alone, and qualities of the Personal Training Specialist.

Exercise Intensity and Duration   The higher the intensity of the exercise is, the greater the discomfort the exerciser may experience, especially for clients who are starting an exercise program from a relatively sedentary lifestyle. Dropout rates tend to be greater for people in high-intensity exercise (running) compared with low-intensity exercise (walking). Higher intensity exercise also increases the chance for injury, which is another reason to design moderate-intensity exercise programs for many clients. HITT (high-intensity interval training) programs that promise quick results in a short period of work time are also a popular training option. A client's ability and readiness for this type of workout should be considered before introducing HIIT programs. Personal Training Specialists should be aware that as intensity increases, attention to technique often decreases, which may lead to injury and hinder exercise adherence. The challenge is to create a plan with the appropriate intensity and duration so that discomfort is minimized and results are maximized for the client. If the Personal Training Specialist follows the intensity and duration guidelines in this manual, clients are much more likely to be safe and successful.

Group Versus Individual Exercise Programs

Group exercise programs have consistently shown better retention rates when compared with programs in which people exercise on their own. Reasons for this include better social support, more overall enjoyment, increased sense of personal commitment to continue, and opportunity to compare progress and fitness levels with others. Be sure to ask your clients whether group exercise is something they would enjoy. Educate yourself on the options available to complement their training with you, as well as the possibility to implement small-group training programs in which two or more clients train with you simultaneously.

 Small group sessions can increase your client's motivation and decrease financial barriers they may experience, while allowing you the opportunity to maximize your time by training multiple clients in a single session.

Qualities of the Personal Training Specialist

A Personal Training Specialist who exhibits the qualities and skills mentioned earlier in this chapter can support and contribute to clients' exercise adherence in significant ways. Clients often adhere to their workouts when they are constantly looking forward to the time they spend with you. Personal Training Specialists who are lacking in these areas will not have the same level of positive influence on their clients.

Working With Clients

As you work with various clients, you will need to adjust your approach, depending on the unique personality traits, goals, and perceptions of each client. The same approach will not work with all clients. For this reason, Personal Training Specialists need to adopt a supportive and flexible approach with each client and have the ability to empower and work with a variety of personality types.

Personality Traits

As a Personal Training Specialist, you will encounter a multitude of personality types throughout your career, perhaps even during a typical training day. You need to demonstrate flexibility in your training style to mirror and match the characteristics of the client you are training. Note that your client may show more of one personality type than another or express a combination of two or more. Remember that each client is unique and that a personality type is not inherently good or bad. You need to be aware, respect clients as they present themselves, and be prepared to adapt your training style accordingly. Many studios and facilities have assessments available to assist Personal Training Specialists in determining their clients' goals, current state of readiness, and period within which they are looking to achieve their goals. When reviewing the information that follows, consider that clients in each category may be at any of the stages of change. To formulate the most effective response, you may want to refer back to the description of each stage of change and identify the behaviour that your client is currently demonstrating.

The following sections include personality traits that clients might present (generally or on any particular day) and training tips for engaging those clients. These personality traits were first described in the work of Carl Jung, who published the book *Psychological Types* in 1921, and were later expanded into the Myers-Briggs Type Indicator, by Katharine Cook Briggs and her daughter Isabel Briggs Myers.

Energy Expression Preference

Introvert

- A client with this personality trait may have quiet energy, listen intently, and take time to think before acting. He or she prefers to work out at slow times when the facility is not busy. This client likes to know what to expect in each session, demonstrates a keen focus during workouts, and goes with the flow at the pace the trainer sets. To make this client comfortable, use these approaches:

- Use subtle cueing techniques; be mindful of the tone and volume of your voice.
- Schedule sessions for times when the client will feel comfortable in the facility.
- Keep a steady pace during the workout and check in periodically by asking whether instructions are clear or whether the client has any questions.
- Consider calling before scheduled sessions to confirm the schedule and preview what you will be working on so that the client can look forward to it, prepare, and manage expectations.
- Provide home workouts and ask the client to report back to you.

Extrovert

- A client with this personality trait is social and approaches sessions with high energy. She or he is talkative, thinks aloud, enjoys working out in groups, and easily interacts with others, but can sometimes be distracted. This client enjoys intense workouts and an enthusiastic personal trainer who can match her or his energy. To work with this client, use these methods:
  - Use circuit training to keep the client focused during workouts.
  - Stay on track and minimize side conversations.
  - Celebrate success in each session with sincere compliments and recognition of skills. The client may also appreciate written validation of success along the way.
  - Suggest group fitness to complement training days.

Information Perception Preference

Sensors

- A client with this personality trait focuses on the details, appreciates practical solutions, and remembers facts after you have shared them. He or she likes to focus on the moment, leverages established skills and abilities, enjoys a steady, consistent pace, and responds well to step-by-step instructions. To engage this client, use these approaches:
  - Explain each exercise step-by-step, demonstrate focus, and pay attention to ensure the client's comfort during the session. These small details matter to a sensor.
  - Review the client's past workout habits. Align programming to what the client is good at and enjoyed in the past.

Intuitive

- A client with this personality trait enjoys discussing the bigger picture and possibilities. She or he may enjoy workouts that use different tools, will quickly notice anything new or different, and will work at an exercise until she or he perfects it. This client enjoys learning new skills and likes to work in bursts of energy. To work best with this client, try the following methods:
  - Link interim goals to long-term goals.
  - Explore various interval-training styles.
  - Ask how the client is doing and what doing the exercise will help him or her do.
  - Schedule rest periods throughout the workout session.
  - Allow time and provide instruction in sessions to perfect movement patterns.
  - Preview upcoming additions to programming by keeping the client informed of what is to come and what she or he is working toward.

Information Processing Preference

Thinker

- A client with this personality trait appears cool and reserved, appreciates your honest feedback, takes few things personally, is honest and direct, and likes to know the purpose of each exercise. He or she may be motivated by achievement and may enjoy a healthy debate for fun. When working with this client, use these approaches:

○ Be honest and direct with feedback. Be sure to commend the client when he or she makes the recommended correction.

○ Consider providing thought-provoking articles or topics for discussion during sessions to keep the client engaged.

Feeler

• A client with this personality trait makes decisions based on values and feelings. This client is warm and friendly, is in touch with how she or he is feeling, and values harmony and compassion. The client is quick to com-

---

Tips for Working With the Personality Types

Introvert

- Use subtle cueing and low volume
- Make sure the client feels comfortable in the facility
- Ask questions to make sure the client understands your instructions and address any concerns
- Provide home workouts

Extrovert

- Use circuit training to provide variety
- Stay on track and minimize side conversations
- Celebrate success and provide validation
- Recommend group fitness

Sensor

- Explain each exercise step by step
- Focus and pay attention
- Align program with activities the client has enjoyed in the past

Intuitive

- Link interim goals to long-term goals
- Explore variety within interval training
- Allow time for careful technique instruction and to preview upcoming additions to the program

Thinker

- Give honest, direct feedback
- Commend the client for making improvements
- Consider providing articles or additional topics for discussion

Feeler

- Take cues from the client
- Compliment the client as appropriate
- Be easygoing and flexible
- Show gratitude for the client's efforts, and reinforce their goals

Judger

- Schedule training sessions in advance
- Be on time and fully prepared
- Share your plan at the beginning of the session, and follow it as closely as possible

Perceiver

- Help the client stay focused and see things through
- Keep workouts fresh and varied and provide options
- Surprise the client with recognition, fun activities, and challenges

pliment others, is motivated by appreciation, and avoids arguments and conflicts. She or he may schedule personal training appointments on various days and at various times. To work with this type of client, use these approaches:

o Take cues from what the client says and from the people around him or her. The client who compliments others is likely seeking the same for herself or himself.

o Keep the client on track by laying out a training plan and asking whether she or he foresees any problems sticking to the planned appointments. Be flexible when it is necessary to change scheduled appointment times.

o Be easygoing and flexible while keeping the client's goals as a priority. Reinforce the aspects of the fitness goals that the client values.

o Show gratitude for the client's efforts.

Information implementation preference

Judgers

• The client with this personality trait tends to take workouts seriously, is prompt, enjoys having a defined start and finish, and sees the need for rules and structure. He or she likes to make and stick with plans and has a work first, play later attitude. This client will likely have a set training schedule with you each week and will not often change appointment times. Use these approaches to work with this client:

o Schedule training sessions in advance.

o Be on time and fully prepared.

o Take the workout seriously and follow the prompt of the client when she or he eases up; mirror that action with casual conversation.

o Outline your plan and expectations of the session at the beginning and stick with it as much as possible.

Perceivers

• The client with this personality trait is playful and casual, likes to have options, and has a play first, work later attitude. He or she likes to start new things and appreciates the freedom to be spontaneous. To work best with this client, use these methods:

o Help the client see things through; keep records of progress and follow up.

o Keep workouts fresh by regularly introducing new concepts, tools, and exercises.

o When providing options, keep to a this-or-that choice and allow the client to choose.

o Surprise the client with spontaneous events, recognition, and fun activities and challenges.

Building a Programming Alliance

On occasion, a conflict will arise between what clients believe they need to do to achieve their goals and what the Personal Training Specialist has planned. The Personal Training Specialist needs to view the process of program design as an alliance between herself or himself and the client. When clients enjoy and are involved in the experience, they are more likely to want to continue and develop long-term adherence to exercise.

Approaches to Building the Programming Alliance

Seek inclusive and cooperative feedback (supports personal trainer–client rapport).

Example: "Let's work together to find the best solutions for you today."

Provide the rationale for the components of your exercise program design.

Example: "The purpose of implementing cardiorespiratory activity three times a week is to increase your heart and lung capacity while also burning calories."

Ask permission.

Example: "You mentioned that you wanted to shed some weight. Can I explain how building muscle can help you shed the weight and keep it off in the long run?"

The Activity Preferences form, provided in the web resource, will help you establish a productive personal trainer–client relationship by identifying your client's expectations, likes, and dislikes.

As a Personal Training Specialist, you will sometimes notice that what your clients want and what they truly need are two different things. Clients typically come to a Personal Training Specialist with past training experience and some degree of knowledge. Some clients have been influenced by trends or by quick fixes advertised through the media. The Personal Training Specialist has the choice to ignore these desires and preconceptions or work with them to build rapport and a stronger alliance with the client.

When you find yourself in this type of conflict with a client, an educational approach is often helpful. You can often explain why you have chosen a specific exercise or programming concept.

In general, you should deal with potential conflicts ahead of time so that clients know what their boundaries are before they start a program with you. When situations occur afterward, and they inevitably will, you should deal with them immediately. Clients can construe any lack of feedback as an indication that their actions are acceptable, which only makes them more difficult to deal with later. These problems should always be dealt with in a one-on-one meeting when possible so that clients are not made to feel more uncomfortable than they probably already do.

Appropriate Behaviours for Personal Training Specialists

As a Personal Training Specialist, you are responsible for acting in a professional manner. The following are a few behaviours to practice throughout all interactions with clients:

- Maintain a strictly professional relationship with all clients.
- Give exercise-related advice to clients only in areas in which you have received formal training.
- Design programs only for clients who are relatively healthy and free of any special conditions or diseases, unless you have been trained to work with this type of client or are working closely with the client's physician or the appropriate qualified health professionals and following their guidelines.

You need to draw a clear line between what you are trained to do and what you are not. The canfitpro *Standards of Practice and Professional Code of Ethics* elaborates on this, but in some situations you need to use your professional judgment about how you should proceed.

 Self-Reflection

As you begin your journey as a Personal Training Specialist, you should reflect on yourself and what you can bring forth to service your clients. Many Personal Training Specialists have initiated their desire to become a fitness professional with a keen interest in optimal health and a quest to share this passion with others in a helpful manner. You should identify other successful Personal Training Specialists, model their positives behaviours, and implement some of their training techniques and methodologies. By watching and listening to others, you can learn skills and attributes that you would like to emulate. Along with modeling behaviour of successful Personal Training Specialists, you can assess yourself to help guide your journey as a Personal Training Specialist. Knowing where you are and what your *Standards of Practice* are can help define a path of development. Take the time to write down a list of your existing skills and abilities. This inventory will help you understand your unique offerings as a fitness professional. You can also begin to chart your ideas on how you want to develop and evolve your skills and abilities as a Personal Training Specialist. Having a solid grasp on where you currently are and where you want to go can strengthen relationships with your clients and help you stay engaged and motivated throughout your journey as a Personal Training Specialist.

Summary of Main Points

1. Many of the qualities of an effective Personal Training Specialist are intangibles such as trustworthiness, patience, and self-awareness.

2. Personal Training Specialists should be highly aware of their own state of readiness, skills, and capabilities when constructing a plan for their personal training journey.

3. When Personal Training Specialists start with positive presuppositions, they can quickly establish strong rapport with their clients.

4. Successful Personal Training Specialists understand that the mind and body are one, that mindset can affect physiology, and vice versa.

5. Personal Training Specialists can help their clients make consistently healthy choices both within and outside the fitness facility.

6. The stages of change model is a great way for Personal Training Specialists to assess their clients and select exercises based on a person's positioning within the various stages.

7. Many variables determine a client's level of adherence to an exercise program. The variables can be broken down into demographic, cognitive, and environmental factors as well as the characteristics of the actual activity.

8. Setting goals using the SMART (and SMARTERS) formula will help bring structure to the programming plan and provide information that the Personal Training Specialist can use to motivate clients and increase exercise adherence.

9. Successful Personal Training Specialists need to understand how to adapt their style to the individual characteristics of each client's personality.

10. As a Personal Training Specialist, you need to understand the beliefs and perceptions that each client holds.

Key Concepts for Study

Behaviour change
Precontemplation stage
Contemplation stage
Preparation stage

Action stage
Maintenance stage
Exercise adherence
SMART goals/SMARTERS goals

Review Questions

1. What does the acronym SMART represent?

2. Explain the importance of providing the client with the why behind an exercise selected for her or his program. Give an example of a why for a squat.

3. When a fitness consumer is transitioning to becoming a Personal Training Specialist, what stage of change is he or she in when researching certification requirements, completing goal setting, and evaluating barriers and opportunities?

   a. action
   b. maintenance
   c. precontemplation
   d. preparation

4. Which of the following is a useful presupposition for a Personal Training Specialist to have before meeting with a client?

   a. The client will be eager to work hard and then emerge with multiple excuses.

   b. The client will present issues that will be beyond the Personal Training Specialist's *Standards of Practice*.

   c. The client will be on time, enthusiastic, accepting of feedback, and appreciative of the work the Personal Training Specialist has done to prepare for the session.

   d. The client will show up with a negative attitude, and the Personal Training Specialist will do everything possible to change the client's mindset because the Personal Training Specialist has the power to tell the client to change.

5. Which strategy can a Personal Training Specialist use to assist a client in the action stage of change?

   a. Talk to the client about self-monitoring and self-reinforcement.

   b. Provide encouragement.

   c. Be satisfied with results so far.

   d. *a* and *b*

6. What is the most common reason that clients give for not exercising?

   a. It costs too much.

   b. There isn't enough time.

   c. They are nervous to start.

   d. They don't know how.

7. What would be the best way to engage with a client whose personality trait is thinker?

   a. Provide direct and clear feedback.

   b. Give plenty of genuine compliments.

   c. Allow extra time to perfect exercises.

   d. None of the above.

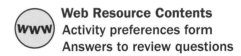

Web Resource Contents
Activity preferences form
Answers to review questions

Principles for Optimal Health

Rod Macdonald, BEd
Kim Lavender, FAHP

LEARNING OUTCOMES

After completing this chapter, you will be able to

1. understand the concept of optimal health and list the nonphysical benefits that a Personal Training Specialist can recognize and influence through the personal trainer–client relationship;

2. understand the difference between the primary and secondary components of fitness;

3. list at least five benefits for each of the primary components of fitness;

4. understand canfitpro's position on achieving optimal health and beyond; and

5. understand each of the nine principles that fall within the canfitpro Personal Training Specialist *Standards of Practice*.

Health is a dynamic process because it is always changing. We all have times of good health, times of sickness, and maybe even times of serious illness. Many of us strive toward optimal health, and as our lifestyle improves, so does our overall health. When people enjoy regular physical activity, they experience a positive effect on their overall health and well-being, thus achieving greater self-confidence, more energy, and a positive attitude.

Performing regular physical activity allows us to experience less disease or illness and enjoy more of the benefits of being active. Those of us who participate in regular physical activity do so partly to improve our current and future health. When asked what it means to be healthy, most people respond by mentioning one or more of the primary components of physical fitness: cardiorespiratory ability, muscular ability, flexibility, and body composition. Although these components are critical aspects to being healthy, they are not the only contributing factors. Physical health is only one aspect of our overall health.

The **optimal health perspective** includes the pursuit of enhanced quality of life, personal growth, and individual potential through positive lifestyle behaviours and attitudes. If we take responsibility for our own health and well-being, we can improve our health on a daily basis. Many factors influence our state of wellness, including nutrition, physical activity, stress-coping methods, sleep habits, relationships, and career success.

Wellness is not an absolute state of being, but rather a continuum that is influenced by our daily behaviours (figure 2.1). Each day we work toward optimal health to live long, full, and healthy lives. When we are in a state of optimal health, we must continue to incorporate behaviours that help us grow toward higher levels of wellness. Thus, to pursue overall health, personal growth, and improved quality of life, your personal training clients will have to maintain a balanced lifestyle. To achieve this balance, canfitpro recommends that we work toward a positive mindset, good nutrition, and intentional physical activity.

Components of Optimal Health

Achieving a state of optimal health requires daily attention to all components of health. As a fitness professional, you have a responsibility to guide and motivate others to improve their choices toward health and well-being. Along with encouraging regular physical activity, Personal Training Specialists should promote this holistic approach to optimal health. As a good role model, you should demonstrate a positive mindset and good nutrition. This practice will improve your personal well-being and provide your clients with a positive model of overall health. If your focus is strictly on the physical benefits of exercise, you are doing a disservice to your clients and not fulfilling your professional obligation as a Personal Training Specialist.

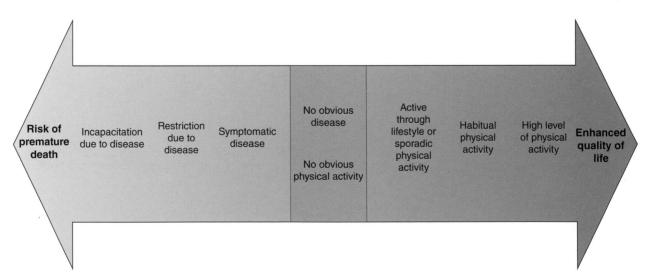

FIGURE 2.1 Physical fitness and overall wellness are best understood as a continuum, rather than an absolute state of being.

When you work with clients on a regular basis, you will begin to learn more about certain aspects of their overall health. Physical fitness can be the catalyst for making other healthy lifestyle choices. By asking questions about all aspects of well-being, you will encourage strong rapport with your clients and address their overall goals for optimal health.

Physical Activity

As Personal Training Specialists, we spend a great deal of time inspiring and assisting others in their pursuit of improved health. Education is an important aspect of this process. We must help people understand why they should be active and promote the benefits of regular physical activity for all clients.

TABLE 2.1   Benefits of Regular Physical Activity

Effect	Benefits
Reduces the risk of premature death	Active people live longer and have better quality of life
Strengthens the heart, cardiovascular system, and respiratory system	Reduces the risk of cardiorespiratory disease
Decreases resting heart rate	Reduces daily wear and tear on the cardiovascular system
Normalizes resting blood pressure	Lessens the stress on the walls of the veins and arteries in the vascular system and reduces the risk of a coronary event or stroke
Improves heart efficiency	Allows a person to perform activities of daily life (ADLs) at higher intensity with greater ease
Decreases body fat	Reduces the risk of major life-threatening diseases such as cardiorespiratory disease and diabetes
Increases HDL ("good") cholesterol and decreases LDL ("bad") cholesterol	Reduces the risk of cardiovascular disease and atherosclerosis (hardening of the arteries)
Keeps body fat in control, increases cellular sensitivity to insulin, and helps to regulate blood sugar levels	Lowers the risk of developing diabetes
Promotes joint stability and increases strength of all connective tissue	Decreases susceptibility to injury
Increases muscular strength	Allows a person to perform activities of daily life (ADLs) with less effort
Strengthens bones	Helps reduce the risk of injuries, broken bones, and osteoporosis
Increases muscle mass and decreases body fat	Creates an improved physique and a more toned appearance, and causes the body to burn more calories during exercise and at rest to sustain the increased muscle
Increases resting metabolism	The body requires more calories at rest, which helps with weight management
Improves core strength by strengthening the abdominal and back muscles	Improves posture and stability and reduces the likelihood of back pain
Improves balance, coordination, and agility	All movements in daily life become easier and safer when the body has better control
Improves body image and self-esteem	Improves mental health and self-image
Reduces depression and anxiety	Improves outlook on life, making all activities more enjoyable
Assists in stress management and gives a person a positive way to deal with stress	Improves the overall quality of everyday life

Physical activity provides many benefits that can have an effect on long-term health. Table 2.1 lists many of the benefits of regular physical activity.

Mindset

Fitness can be defined or expressed in many ways. One definition is that physical fitness is an improved physiological state that leads to improved health and longevity. Note, however, that fitness is a complex concept that also includes the health of the mind (Greenberg, 2004, p. 7), which is just as important as physical health. Understanding these elements is easier when they are further broken down as follows:

- **Social health**—Ability to interact well with people and the environment and to have satisfying personal relationships
- **Mental health**—Ability to learn and grow intellectually through life experiences as well as more formal structures (e.g., school)
- **Emotional health**—Ability to control emotions, feel comfortable expressing them, and express them appropriately

As a Personal Training Specialist, you need to consider each of these aspects as you help clients develop their overall fitness. Although your programs will be focused primarily on the physical components, your clients will also be influenced by the state of their social, mental, and emotional health. Therefore, you need to be aware of how their mindset can positively or negatively affect their ability to achieve and maintain their fitness goals.

As clients make changes to their lifestyle and follow your recommendations, they will certainly encounter difficulties and challenges in the pursuit of optimal health. All clients experience change differently, and numerous variables can affect their ability to adhere to a plan. Many will present themselves with past failures or stories of relapses when they tried to "get fit." They may be feeling defeated and wondering how things could possibly be different and sustainable this time. Other influencers can include but are not limited to social support systems, fitness levels, situations at work, daily challenges, and other unforeseen stressors.

Adapting a positive mindset and a can-do attitude will help increase the clients' confidence in achieving their goals. Even when things go wrong, when they miss a workout or make a bad decision with their nutritional habits, a positive mindset can help clients stay on track and make the small changes necessary to get back in alignment with their goals. Recognizing challenges and addressing them quickly will help clients avoid getting too far off track. You should acknowledge challenges and provide strategies to help your clients cope and move forward. Your role as a Personal Training Specialist is to help your clients adopt a positive mindset toward their health and to offer suggestions for activities or practices that will help them develop further. Embrace the challenges and know that your clients can handle the ups and downs of their journey to optimal health.

Nutritional Health

By combining healthy nutritional choices with well-programmed physical activity, your clients can better attain (and sustain) optimal health. The position of canfitpro on nutrition is based on making healthier choices toward foods that provide the body with the necessary nutrients to maintain an overall healthy lifestyle. As such, Personal Training Specialists are required to understand the basic elements of nutrition (as taught in canfitpro's Fundamentals of Nutrition online modules), so that they are able to provide nutritional guidance to clients based on the recommendations outlined in table 2.3 later in this chapter. You may also use the canfitpro Wheel of Integrated Nutrition (figure 2.2), which illustrates how clients can make healthier choices regarding the sourcing, preparation, and consumption of food.

The Pyramid of Integrated Nutrition (figure 2.3) reflects an eating approach that many of our members have had success with. In general, a healthy approach to eating should focus on fresh, nutrient-dense whole foods and on minimized consumption of highly processed, energy-dense foods and drinks, particularly for clients who need to lose weight. However, specific nutritional needs may vary from client to client.

Some Personal Training Specialists want to provide in-depth nutritional guidance to help clients achieve their weight-loss goals. If you would like to continue your education and be able to address specific questions about nutrition that go beyond the general guidelines previously referenced, canfitpro encourages you to obtain further qualifications that equip you with the required knowledge and skills

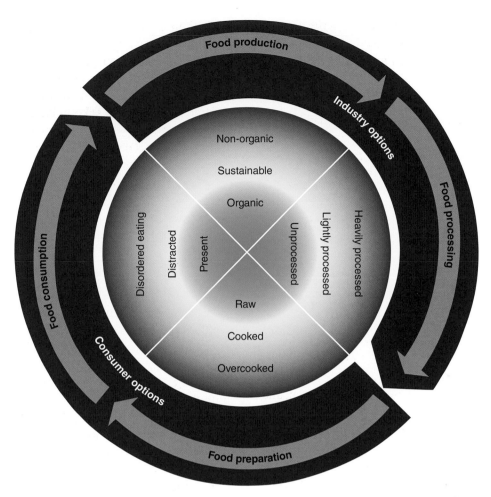

FIGURE 2.2 The Wheel of Integrated Nutrition addresses the nutritional, psychological, and environmental aspects of our food choices.

(such as the Healthy Eating and Weight Loss Coach certification). If you encounter situations that fall outside your Personal Training Specialist certification or additional qualifications you have obtained, then you must refer clients to a suitably qualified nutrition or health professional. The canfitpro Pyramid of Integrated Nutrition and Wheel of Integrated Nutrition are for informational purposes only and do not render medical advice, opinion, diagnosis, or treatment. The information provided through this text and accompanying materials should not be used for diagnosing or treating a health problem or disease. If you have or suspect you or your client(s) may have a health problem or disease, you should consult, or have them consult, the appropriate health care provider. The authors and publishers of this manual assume no responsibility for any circumstances arising out of the use, misuse, interpretation,

or application of any information supplied within this text or accompanying materials. Any application or use of the information, resources, or recommendations presented in this text or accompanying materials is at your own risk.

Physical Activity for Optimal Health

Physical fitness consists of multiple components that must be addressed for your clients to achieve and maintain optimal health. When creating training programs, you need to select activities and exercises that allow your clients to develop in each area. The most important components of physical fitness are divided into two groups—primary and secondary.

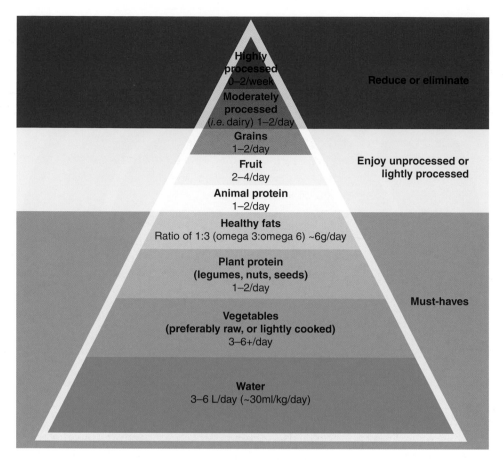

FIGURE 2.3 The Pyramid of Integrated Nutrition provides guidelines on food choices based on the categories each food falls within, as well as the suggested frequency of consumption.

Primary Components of Fitness

The four primary components of fitness that are important to improving overall physical health are cardiorespiratory capacity, muscular capacity, flexibility, and body composition. You need to understand and be able to explain each of these components to your clients and help them understand the positive effect that improvements in these areas will have on their everyday lives.

• **Cardiorespiratory capacity** is the ability of the body to take in oxygen (respiration), deliver it to the cells (circulation), and use it at the cellular level to create energy (bioenergetics) for physical work (activity). Some of the long-term **adaptations** of cardiorespiratory training are decreased resting heart rate, decreased risk of cardiorespiratory disease, improved **endurance**, increased stroke volume, and increased cardiac output.

• **Muscular capacity** is the full spectrum of muscular function, including endurance, strength, and power. This component is trained using various resistance training practices. Some of the long-term adaptations of muscle conditioning are improved functional fitness (the ability to conduct daily activities with greater ease) through increased overall strength, improved muscular endurance, increased basal metabolic rate, improved joint and bone strength, better posture, and decreased risk of injury.

• **Flexibility** is the range of movement or amount of motion that a joint is capable of performing. Each joint has a different amount of flexibility, leading to various levels of mobility. Some of the long-term adaptations of improved flexibility are improved range of motion, improved bodily movements, improved posture, and decreased risk of injury.

• **Body composition** is the proportion of fat-free mass (i.e., muscle, bone, blood, organs, and fluids) to fat mass (adipose tissue deposited under the skin and around organs). Some of the long-term adaptations of improving body composition are decreased risk of cardiorespiratory disease, improved basal metabolic rate, improved bodily function, improved body mass index (BMI), and higher overall self-confidence. As a Personal Training Specialist you will have many clients whose primary fitness goal is to lose weight. You need to educate them on the concept of body composition and draw their attention to the percentage of body fat in addition to their focus on overall weight loss.

Secondary Components of Fitness

The secondary components of fitness are involved in various types of physical activity and are necessary for daily functioning. Athletes in particular experience different levels of success depending on how well they develop these secondary fitness components. Although the primary components are thought to be the most important during a workout, we should not ignore the secondary components because they are important to the completion of daily tasks. As a Personal Training Specialist you can leverage these secondary components of fitness to create engaging workouts for your clients. You may also have clients set goals around them.

The secondary components include the following:

- **Balance**—ability to maintain a specific body position in either a stationary or dynamic (moving) situation, which is critical for all movement patterns
- **Coordination**—ability to use multiple body parts together to produce smooth and fluid motion
- **Agility**—ability to change direction quickly

Explaining the Components of Fitness

You need to explain fitness in terms that clients can understand so that they can make connections to their individual goals. Here are a few examples of how you might communicate the components of fitness and their importance to clients.

Cardiorespiratory Capacity

"When we focus on your cardiorespiratory capacity we will likely notice a decrease in your resting heart rate, which means that your heart is stronger and healthier overall. Training also lowers your risk of cardiorespiratory disease. You will know you are improving when you experience things like not being winded after climbing the stairs or running your first 5K with ease."

Muscular Capacity

"When we focus on muscular strengthening through resistance training, we can target overall strength and endurance as well as ensure that we are balancing our workload among all muscle groups. As we increase your muscle mass you will also burn more calories, even at rest, which will help you with your weight-loss goal. Everyday activities like gardening, cleaning your home, or lifting heavy objects will be easier, and you may notice that your posture improves as well."

Flexibility

"When we focus on your flexibility we will look at improving range of motion in all directions and enhancing your mobility. As your flexibility improves you'll notice that you are able to move your body with ease. Your muscles will feel more relaxed during daily activities. Simple movements like touching your toes, reaching your hand behind your back, or rotating side to side will become smoother and less restricted."

Body Composition

"I understand that your goal is to lose 5 kilograms (11 lb). By focusing on muscle strength and endurance, along with cardiorespiratory training, we can reduce the amount of fat mass you carry, which will improve your overall body composition. Keep in mind that physical activity is only part of the equation. To have long-term success, you will want to ensure you are making healthy nutrition choices as well."

- **Reaction time**—time required to respond to a specific stimulus
- **Speed**—ability to move rapidly
- **Power**—the product of strength and speed
- **Mental capability**—ability to concentrate during exercise to improve training effects

canfitpro's Recommendations for Optimal Health

canfitpro's Myohybrid learning philosophy is an integrative approach for optimizing results in a time-efficient manner. As clients progress toward optimal health, Personal Training Specialists are encouraged to integrate a variety of activities into their programs. For example, approaches such as boot camp, circuit training, and certain group fitness classes will allow simultaneous training of multiple aspects related to optimal health.

 As you read through these sections, you will see several tables summarizing canfitpro's recommendations for optimal health. This information is essential to all canfitpro certifications. Refer back to these tables as you read the other chapters in the book to build your understanding of the recommendations.

Our position on healthy lifestyle choices extends beyond physical activity programming to include guidelines for other positive behavioural changes that your clients should adapt along their journey toward optimal health. The following sections summarize canfitpro's recommendations on physical activity, nutrition, and positive mindset for optimal health in adults aged 18 to 64 years. For additional tools and support, visit www.canfitpro.com.

 The web resource contains a comprehensive table that provides all of canfitpro's recommendations on physical activity, nutrition, and positive mindset for optimal health.

Positive Mindset

Enhancing positive mindset and emotional state can help clients handle daily and unforeseen stressors and increase their personal belief that success is possible. canfitpro recommends adopting daily strategies that help cultivate this positive mindset, such as meditation and positive self-talk (table 2.2). For some clients, working with a mental health professional may be a good strategy to address issues.

The ultimate goal here is to adopt strategies that strengthen positive mindset and reduce or eliminate negative self-talk, replacing it with acceptance and positive self-talk. When starting an effort to improve mindset, clients should seek support from family and friends as they make plans to behave in a healthier way and ask themselves questions that will help define their goals. As they make progress toward optimal health, these questions can be adjusted to strengthen commitment and prevent relapse. Clients should be aware that they may be tempted to slip back into unhealthy behaviour, especially during stressful situations. They should identify unhealthy behaviours, substitute positive ones, and continue to set new goals.

Nutrition

canfitpro's overall recommendation for nutrition is to focus on fresh, nutrient-dense whole foods and to minimize consumption of highly processed, energy-dense foods and drinks (table 2.3). By enhancing nutrition, your clients can improve their overall well-being and optimize their body composition (i.e., balance the proportion of body fat to lean tissue). canfitpro recommends that all adults adopt strategies to improve healthy eating choices.

Clients should start by reducing poor food choices while introducing healthier options. In particular, they should keep themselves well hydrated and aim to increase their daily intake of water, vegetables, and healthy sources of fats. Cruciferous vegetables (broccoli, cabbage, bok choy, and so on) are mentioned specifically, because their consumption can significantly increase the intake of vitamins, minerals, fiber, and phytonutrients that help prevent disease. As clients progress, they should continue to reduce or eliminate unhealthy choices while increasing their choices of healthier foods. After clients establish consistent and healthy patterns, they may not need to make additional changes to their nutritional regimen.

TABLE 2.2   canfitpro's Recommendations for Positive Mindset

Why do it	Enhancing positive mindset and emotional state can assist you in believing that success is possible. You will be able to handle daily and unforeseen stressors more easily.
Recommendations	Adopt strategies that help cultivate positive mindset daily.
Types of activities	Meditation Positive self-talk Cognitive behavioural therapy
Beginners	Seek support from family and friends and plan to behave in a healthier way. Ask yourself questions like these: "When I start being more active, how will I feel?" "What will I look like?"
Intermediate	Make small changes to the questions you ask yourself to strengthen your commitment and to stop you from relapsing. Identify activities related to unhealthy behaviours and replace them with positive ones.
Advanced	Continue to ask yourself questions and be aware that you may be tempted to slip back into unhealthy behaviour, especially during stressful situations. Set new goals and challenges.
Goal	Adopt strategies to strengthen your mindset on a consistent basis. Reduce or eliminate negative self-talk, replacing it with acceptance and positive self-talk.

TABLE 2.3   canfitpro's Recommendations for Nutrition

Why do it	Enhancing nutrition will improve your overall health and body composition (balance of body fat and lean tissue).
Recommendations	Adopt strategies to improve nutritional choices.
Types of activities	Strategically reduce or include specific foods based on the canfitpro pyramid of integrated nutrition.
Beginners	Start by reducing your poor food choices while introducing new, healthier choices. In particular, increase consumption of cruciferous vegetables (broccoli, cabbage, bok choy, and so on) whenever possible.
Intermediate	Continue to reduce or eliminate more poor choices while increasing the frequency of healthier choices.
Advanced	You may not need to alter your regimen. Continue to make few poor choices while increasing the frequency of healthy choices.
Goal	Implement health-promoting nutrition and hydration focusing primarily on fresh, nutrient-dense whole foods. Minimize consumption of highly processed, energy-dense foods and drinks to support your health and healthy body composition.

Cardiorespiratory

Improving cardiorespiratory fitness can reduce your clients' risk of many noncommunicable diseases, such as cardiovascular diseases, cancers, respiratory diseases, and diabetes. canfitpro's position is that all exercise programs for adults should include continuous physical activities involving major muscle groups that increase heart rate and keep it an appropriate intensity for the duration of the workout (table 2.4). Examples of suitable activities to help improve cardiorespiratory health include walking, running, swimming, cycling, and group fitness classes.

People who are just getting started with cardiorespiratory exercise should start with low-intensity activities and gradually increase duration and intensity. The goal should be to perform sessions of 10 minutes or more in duration. As clients progress, they may increase the duration and intensity of exercise sessions as long as they maintain balance across the training program and are careful not to overtrain. The overall goal is to accumulate up to 300 minutes of moderate-intensity aerobic activity per week (about 43 minutes per day) or 150 minutes of vigorous-intensity activity per week (about 22 minutes per day). An equivalent combination of

TABLE 2.4   canfitpro's Recommendations for Cardiorespiratory Fitness

Why do it	Enhancing the health of the cardiorespiratory system (circulatory and respiratory systems primarily) can reduce your risk of several noncommunicable diseases.
Recommendations	Adopt continuous physical activities involving major muscle groups (i.e., the legs) to increase and maintain heart rate at an appropriate intensity.
Types of activities	Walking or running Swimming Cycling Group fitness classes
Beginners	Start with low-intensity activities and increase duration and intensity gradually. The goal should be to perform sessions of 10 minutes or more in duration.
Intermediate	Increase the duration and intensity of your exercise sessions.
Advanced	You may not need to alter your regimen. If you choose to increase volume or intensity, be careful not to overtrain. Strive to achieve balance across all five recommendations.
Goal	Accumulate up to 300 minutes of moderate-intensity aerobic activity per week (about 43 minutes per day) or 150 minutes of vigorous-intensity activity per week (about 22 minutes per day), or an equivalent combination of moderate- and vigorous-intensity activity. Some people (i.e., athletes) may wish to increase time or intensity further.

moderate- and vigorous-intensity activity is also acceptable. In the more advanced stages of training, some people (i.e., athletes) may wish to increase time or intensity further, and others may not need to alter their cardiorespiratory training regimen at all if they continue to make healthy lifestyle choices and minimize the frequency of making poor ones.

Overtraining is doing too much during an exercise program so that daily function is impaired. Both beginner and experienced exercisers should follow the FITT principle for exercise programming (described later in this chapter) in order to prevent overtraining, and beginners should take care to increase their activity levels gradually, working toward the recommended volume of exercise.

Muscle Strengthening

Resistance training activities strengthen muscles, increase muscular capacity, and improve functional fitness (the ability to conduct daily activities with greater ease) while also reducing the risk of several noncommunicable diseases such as cardiovascular diseases, cancers, respiratory diseases, and diabetes. To experience these benefits, canfitpro recommends that all adults participate in physical activities to increase muscular strength and endurance of all

major muscle groups on three or more days per week (table 2.5).

Beginners should start with slow, low-intensity movements and perform three to eight exercises for one set of 12 to 15 repetitions each. They should then add additional sets of each exercise as they master the exercise technique. These exercises can include callisthenic exercise (using clients' body weight, rather than equipment) or resistance training activities. As muscular capacity develops, the volume or intensity of exercise sessions can be gradually increased and more complex movements can be added. The exercises chosen should always be evaluated to make sure that they are appropriate for your clients' goals and abilities. At this stage, momentary muscle fatigue (inability to generate the muscular force required to complete the exercise activity with proper form and technique) should occur before 20 reps have been performed, but no sooner than the 12th rep. Advanced exercisers may not need to alter

Beginners or those trying new activities often feel some soreness one or two days after exercising. If this discomfort prevents comfortable and effective daily function, clients are likely doing too much during their training sessions. Both beginner and experienced exercisers should avoid overtraining.

TABLE 2.5 canfitpro's Recommendations for Muscle Strengthening

Why do it	Muscle strengthening will improve your functional fitness (the ability to conduct daily activities with greater ease) as well as reduce the risk of several noncommunicable diseases.
Recommendations	Adopt physical activities to increase your muscular strength and endurance.
Types of activities	Calisthenic exercise Resistance training
Beginners	Start with slow, low-intensity movements (three to eight exercises) for one set of 12 to 15 repetitions. Build up to workouts of additional sets of each exercise to master the exercise technique.
Intermediate	Gradually increase the volume or intensity of your exercise sessions and add progressively more complex movements appropriate for your goals and abilities.
Advanced	You may not need to alter your regimen. If you choose to increase volume or intensity, be careful not to overtrain. Ensure that you achieve balance across all five recommendations.
Goal	Participate in muscle-strengthening activities involving all major muscle groups on three or more days per week. Momentary muscle fatigue should result before you perform 20 reps. Some people (i.e., athletes) may wish to increase time or intensity further.

their regimen beyond this point, but if they choose to increase volume or intensity further, be careful that they achieve balance across all recommended components and avoid overtraining.

Flexibility

Incorporating activities that enhance flexibility improves mobility and may decrease the risk or severity of injuries. Activities such as stretching and yoga help in achieving optimal range of motion at all joints of the body. canfitpro recommends that adults incorporate stretching into their exercise programs four or more days per week (table 2.6).

Beginners should start with easy-to-accomplish stretches, held statically for at least 20 to 30 seconds each. As flexibility develops, clients can increase the duration of the stretch as well as choose more challenging stretches to increase the intensity of flexibility sessions. Advanced exercisers may not require any further changes to their regimen, but some people, particularly athletes, may wish to increase time or intensity further. In this case they must be sure to avoid overtraining or stretching to the point of hypermobility, which is the rare reduction in stability within a joint because of excessive flexibility.

canfitpro's Training Principles

When designing programs for clients, a Personal Training Specialist must be aware of the following training principles. Although these principles are

TABLE 2.6 canfitpro's Recommendations for Flexibility

Why do it	Enhancing flexibility may decrease the risk of injury and may lessen the severity of injuries.
Recommendations	Adopt physical activities that results in an increase in range of motion at all joints of the body.
Types of activities	Stretching Yoga
Beginners	Start with easy-to-accomplish stretches, held statically for at least 20 to 30 seconds. Increase the duration of the stretches and expand your choice of stretches.
Intermediate	Increase the duration or intensity of your flexibility sessions.
Advanced	You may not need to alter your regimen. If you choose to increase volume or intensity, be careful not to overtrain and ensure that you achieve balance across all five recommendations.
Goal	Enjoy flexibility activities four or more days per week. Some people (i.e., athletes) may wish to increase time or intensity further while avoiding hypermobility.

not new, they have been adapted and assembled to fit within the *Standards of Practice* of a canfitpro Personal Training Specialist. As each component of fitness is examined in this text, these principles will be referred to again where appropriate.

- **FITT**—This principle suggests that when designing a personal training program, the frequency, intensity, time, and type of exercise must be considered. Specifically, frequency is how often clients should be performing a particular component of their program. Intensity is the difficulty level of the program component (as measured by heart rate, load, reps, watts, and so on). Time is how long each component should last and how much rest clients should have (usually measured in minutes or seconds). Type refers to the choice of exercise used for a given component of their program (usually defined as an exercise, piece of equipment, or activity).

- **Individualization**—This principle suggests that program design must accommodate every client's individual needs. For example, two people with the same goal may require very different training programs to achieve the same result. These differences may result from a variety of factors such as available training time, starting fitness level, experience, and other variables.

- **Specificity**—This principle suggests that if clients want to improve a particular aspect of their performance, they have to train that aspect specifically. For example, if a client wants to become a better runner, resistance training will probably deliver measurable improvements, but the client will still have to continue to run to optimize the results.

- **Progressive overload**—This principle suggests that clients must continually challenge their fitness to see significant improvement over time. For example, if the intensity, duration, or complexity of your client's fitness training is not progressively modified throughout the program, the client will eventually plateau, or cease to make improvements. Any overload should be progressive in nature and err on the side of caution. Too much overload can cause the client to become discouraged, or worse, injured.

- **Recovery**—This principle becomes increasingly important as your clients' workouts become more successful. Recovery should not be seen as optional, but as a mandatory principle of training

that must be considered for every program. When working with personal training clients, you must take into account any other activities they are engaged in throughout the week, the type of work they perform, and so on. The recovery period must allow clients to return to the next workout at least as fit as they entered the previous one, if not more. If clients do not recover sufficiently, they are eventually more likely to become ill or injured, and they may discontinue training altogether.

- **Structural tolerance**—This principle suggests that the strengthening of joints (tendons, ligaments, and so on) will result in the ability to sustain subsequently greater stresses in training and to have greater resistance to injury. Although structural tolerance is a positive side effect of most exercise, some clients may require specific activities or exercises that improve the strength of certain joints. For example, a client who has a goal of running a marathon should have some exercises included in her or his program that specifically target the ankles, knees, hips, and back, because marathon training will stress those areas (Zaryski and Smith, 2005).

- **All-around development**—This principle suggests that people who are well developed through all components of fitness are less prone to injury and more likely to perform better in sport and in life. For example, clients who want to train only cardio and dismiss flexibility and resistance training are more likely to become injured should they ever need to call on their strength (e.g., to change a tire, shovel snow, and so on) (Zaryski and Smith, 2005).

- **Reversibility**—This principle suggests that when training ceases, the body will gradually return to its pre-training state. Although the principle of reversibility can be frustrating to clients who face unexpected absences from their exercise programs, it should serve as a cautionary principle in that clients (or Personal Training Specialists) who are not consistent with their adherence to exercise will lose the benefits and return to their pre-training state.

- **Maintenance**—This principle suggests that after a level of fitness has been achieved, it can be maintained with less work than was needed to attain it. As a guideline, to prevent the reversal of adaptation to exercise, clients could train as little as one-third the volume, at the same intensity, for up to 12 weeks (Brooks, 2004).

Summary of Main Points

1. Achievement of optimal health is a dynamic process that involves physical fitness as well as social, mental, and emotional components.

2. A positive mindset is important for both Personal Training Specialists and their clients throughout the personal training journey.

3. To achieve and maintain optimal health, clients need to have a positive mindset, observe good nutritional health, and develop each of the primary components of fitness.

4. The primary components of fitness include cardiorespiratory capacity, muscle strengthening, flexibility, and body composition.

5. The secondary components of fitness are necessary for daily functioning and are important to various types of physical activity.

6. canfitpro's nine training principles are used to design safe and effective personal training programs.

Key Concepts for Study

Cardiorespiratory capacity

Muscular capacity

Flexibility

Body composition

Coordination

Agility

Reaction time

Speed

Power

Mental capability

FITT

Individualization

Specificity

Progressive overload

Recovery

Structural tolerance

All-around development

Reversibility

Maintenance

Review Questions

1. List and explain three of the secondary fitness components.

2. How would you explain body composition to a client who wants to achieve weight loss?

3. Which components of the mind are as important as physical health?

   a. emotional health, heart health, and psychological health

   b. mental health, social health, and emotional health

   c. social health, visceral health, and mental health

   d. emotional health, nutritional health, and mental health

4. What are the primary fitness components?

   a. cardiorespiratory capacity, muscular capacity, flexibility, and body composition

   b. muscular capacity, cardiorespiratory capacity, flexibility, mindset, nutrition, and body composition

   c. cardiorespiratory capacity, muscular capacity, and flexibility

   d. flexibility, cardiorespiratory capacity, muscular capacity, speed, and power

5. Which of canfitpro's nine training principles is best demonstrated by the following example?

   A client who has a goal of running a marathon should have included in the program some exercises that target the ankles, knees, hips, and back because marathon training will stress those areas.

   a. specificity

   b. individualization

   c. structural tolerance

   d. FITT

6. What principle suggests that after training ceases, the body gradually returns to a pre-training state?

   a. reversibility

   b. maintenance

   c. recovery

   d. specificity

7. Which of the following accurately represents canfitpro's recommendations for cardiorespiratory activity?

   a. 300 minutes of moderate-intensity activity per week

   b. 22 minutes of vigorous-intensity activity per day

   c. 150 minutes of vigorous-intensity activity per week

   d. All of the above

 Web Resource Contents

canfitpro's Recommendations on Physical Activity, Nutrition, and Positive Mindset for Optimal Health for Adults Aged 18-64 Years (comprehensive table)

Answers to review questions

CASE STUDIES

Within this manual you will find review questions to help you integrate the information learned in each chapter. The information needed to answer the multiple-choice and most short-answer questions can be found within the corresponding chapter text, and the case study questions are based on the profiles of the three people described in the following sections. These review questions provide a way for you to apply information as you are learning it and to see how you can use it in a practical sense with a variety of clients.

Case Study Profile 1: Catherine Wallace

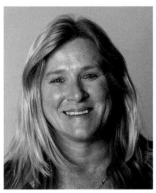
© iStock.com/Juanmonino

Catherine is a 55-year-old woman who is a year away from retirement and currently working part time as a secretary. She is mildly active; she walks her two grandchildren to school every day before going to work. Because she has been working a desk job for the past 30 years, she is concerned about maintaining joint function and mobility. She is overweight and concerned that she may be at a higher risk for cardiovascular disease. Her doctor has suggested that she start an exercise program to decrease her risk of type 2 diabetes. She would like to lose 5 to 7 kilograms (11 to 15 lb) and wouldn't mind gaining some muscle mass. She would like to see changes as soon as possible but trusts that a Personal Training Specialist will help her establish appropriate time frames for her goals.

Catherine has never before been a member of a gym, so she does not have any major preferences in terms of equipment. She would like to work with a Personal Training Specialist twice a week to achieve her goals, and she is committed to working out two more times per week on her own if necessary, after she is comfortable with the new exercises she is learning.

Catherine has no major medical conditions and is looking forward to enjoying the benefits of increased exercise, although she is somewhat nervous about getting started. Having never worked out in a gym before, she is worried about the possibility of hurting herself. Her other major concern is that the gym members may be far younger and more fit than she is. She enjoys interacting with people but does not think that many people in the gym will be like her.

Catherine often skips breakfast, has two or three coffees per day, takes her lunch to work most days, eats a large dinner, and snacks on high-calorie foods throughout the day. She is aware that she needs to make some changes with respect to nutrition and is open to suggestions.

Case Study Profile 2: Lisa Bryant

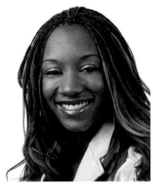
© Ginal Santa Maria/Fotolia

Lisa is a 24-year-old graduate student. She is in her second year of a master's program in kinesiology, which takes up almost all her spare time. She recently decided to join the university gym and take advantage of discounted student rates on personal training. She loves to play sports but hasn't participated in any organized sports since starting university. She is concerned that she is now gaining weight and has noticed changes to her figure over the past few years. In high school, she was on the basketball and volleyball teams and trained three or four times each week. Lisa would like to get back to the way she looked and performed in high school. Her main goals are to improve her skills in sport, lose 7 kilograms (15 lb), and increase her flexibility and endurance. She would love to lose the first 5 kilograms (11 lb) within the next two months because she will be attending a friend's wedding at that time. She also wants to improve her eating habits and metabolism because her previous nutritional lifestyle included eating anything she chose to, leading to undesired weight gain.

Lisa has no outstanding medical conditions, loves exercising, and looks forward to making training a regular part of her lifestyle again. Her perception is that she will need to work out for about an hour and a half on four or five days per week to achieve her goals. She would like to work with a Personal

Training Specialist once a week to achieve her goals and plans to work out on four additional days per week, using the program you create for her. Her preferences are jogging, body-weight training, and taking group fitness classes. Outside her regular fitness routine, she would like to start playing volleyball again once or twice a week.

Case Study Profile 3: Thomas Yang

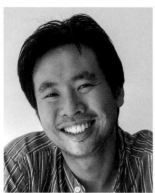

© clue2305/Fotolia

Thomas is a 39-year-old career and family man. He works full time for a bank and takes care of his family, which includes three young children. Because he works long days (and sometimes on weekends), he is extremely busy and finds that he is usually exhausted by the end of the day. He takes great pride in having won the National College Swimming Championship as a student, but he has not been involved in intense physical activity since he graduated. He has no known medical conditions. He would like an easy workout to increase endurance, strength, and muscle tone. In terms of equipment preferences, he thinks that he would like the elliptical machine and rowing ergometer for his cardio workouts.

Thomas' major barrier is time. He has not been able to overcome this hurdle in the past and has been unable to maintain a consistent training schedule. He does not have any other major obstacles that prevent him from exercising on his own or with a Personal Training Specialist. He has recently joined the gym but can work out only once or twice a week for 30 to 45 minutes, although he may be able to add a third weekly workout. He prefers to work out when there aren't a lot of people around. He would also like suggestions on ways to work out on his own outside the gym (i.e., at work or home). He has good nutritional habits and is fairly well read with respect to exercise. Even so, he is a little confused about what he needs to do to achieve his specific goals, so he would like to work with a Personal Training Specialist at least once a week.

PART I   Case Study Questions

1. Using the information provided in the three case study profiles, create an individualized SMART goal for each of these clients: Catherine, Lisa, and Thomas.

2. Catherine has expressed her hesitancy both to exercise and to be in a gym. What strategy would you use to help Catherine overcome this hesitancy and increase her commitment to her goals? (Include in your answer questions or phrases that you would say to her during this conversation.)

3. What is one presumption that you have about Lisa, based on her profile, and how will you work to counter it?

4. Thomas listened intently during your first meeting. When asked about his exercise preferences, he highlighted his lack of time and mentioned that he prefers to work out on his own. How would you adjust your style to Thomas' personality, and what would you do to work optimally with him?

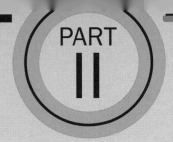

PART

II

Understanding the Body

With the foundation of better understanding yourself and your client in place, you can now add the requisite theoretical knowledge of the body that every successful Personal Training Specialist must have. The material found herein will provide you with knowledge of the major systems of the body and the way that they work, as well as an introduction to foundational movement sequences. This information will give you the confidence to continue on your journey.

Bioenergetics

Brian Justin, M.Kin
Gregory S. Anderson, PhD

LEARNING OUTCOMES

After completing this chapter, you will be able to

1. understand the source of energy for exercise;

2. explain homeostasis and metabolism as they relate to physical activity;

3. understand the structure of ATP;

4. explain the difference between aerobic and anaerobic production of energy;

5. explain how the three energy systems produce ATP; and

6. understand the development of the energy systems through interval conditioning.

Food begins its journey into the body in the mouth. As we chew, we mechanically break down the food and mix it with saliva, which both provides lubrication for swallowing and helps to break down carbohydrate chemically, by the enzyme amylase. After this, the chewed food, called a bolus, is swallowed down the esophagus and then further broken down in the stomach. Protein is the primary foodstuff broken down in the stomach through mechanical churning and the action of digestive enzymes and stomach acid. The protein is broken down into strings of amino acids called peptides. Digestion further continues in the small intestine where enzymes work to break down fat and carbohydrate into smaller particles that your body can absorb, transport, and use for various functions. Dietary fat is broken down by enzymes called lipases into fatty acids and monoglycerides, and carbohydrate breaks down into simple sugars (namely glucose) through amylase enzymes. Protein is further broken down from peptide chains into amino acids and di- and tripeptides amino acids through protease enzymes.

After the food has been effectively digested, it must be absorbed into the body. This occurs primarily in the small intestine (90% of all absorption occurs here). With its increased surface area created by fingerlike projections known as villi, the small intestine absorbs glucose and other simple sugars, amino acids, peptides, and short- and long-chain fatty acids. Water is also absorbed in the small intestine. These absorbed particles are transported to the liver and then on to the areas of the body where they will be either used or stored.

The next stop in the digestive process is the large intestine, also known as the colon. The major events that happen here are water absorption, bacterial breakdown of peptides to amino acids, and the absorption of several vitamins (including B and K). Any remains in the colon after this point are typically excreted with the next normal bowel movement.

How do the food particles we absorb through digestion then get used to fuel our physical activity? This question is answered through the concept of **bioenergetics**—the study of how energy flows in the human body. In this chapter we are concerned primarily with the conversion of food as large molecules of carbohydrate, protein, and fat into a useful form of energy for exercise or activity.

The molecule that the body uses as its energy currency is called **adenosine triphosphate**, or ATP. Figure 3.1 shows an overview of how food is broken down and distributed through the body to fuel activity.

Bioenergetics Terminology

In this chapter you will frequently see the terms *energy* and *metabolism*. In bioenergetics, these terms are defined as follows.

Energy is the ability to do physical work. In daily life we see many forms of energy, such as electrical energy (light), heat (fire), chemical energy (gasoline), and mechanical energy (water to turn a turbine). In examining how the body is capable of performing muscle contraction, we analyze the conversion of chemical energy (food) into mechanical energy (muscle contraction).

Metabolism is the sum of all chemical reactions in the body that either use or create energy. In some cases, large molecules are broken down into smaller ones (through a *catabolic process,* such as the digestion of food), and in other cases the cells build larger molecules from smaller ones (through an *anabolic process,* such as the use of amino acids to build muscle). The combination of these catabolic and anabolic processes in the body is collectively called *metabolism.* The energy either used or created from all the metabolic processes is called adenosine triphosphate (ATP). When the demand for energy is comfortably met by the supply of available ATP, all body functions can occur with relative ease because the body is in a state of balance and stability. This state is called **homeostasis**. Although the concept suggests stability, all body functions are constantly changing to adapt to the environment and maintain an overall balance of metabolic processes.

Although metabolism is the sum of anabolic and catabolic processes, you will see in other parts of this text the terms **aerobic metabolism** and **anaerobic metabolism**. These terms refer to the specific subsets of metabolism that occur in each of those two contexts. Aerobic metabolism is the sum of anabolic (the creation of ATP) and catabolic (the breakdown of food substrates) processes that occur in an aerobic context (i.e., using oxygen.) Anaerobic metabolism does not require oxygen in order to produce ATP. Note that metabolism is happening all the time, not just during exercise.

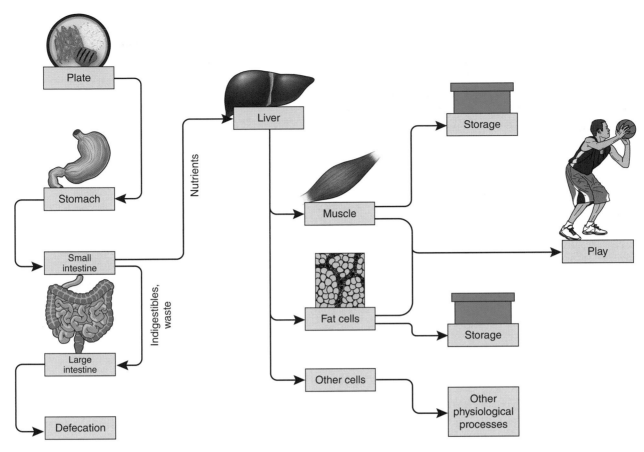

FIGURE 3.1 From plate to play—a summary of the process by which food is digested and converted to energy, as well as being used for other physiological processes such as building and repairing cells.

When speaking about metabolism in this chapter, we focus primarily on the creation of adenosine triphosphate (ATP) for physical activity, either through aerobic pathways, which use oxygen, or through anaerobic pathways, which occur in the absence of oxygen. ATP is a chemical compound made up of adenosine and three phosphate molecules. ATP is the energy currency of the body. Therefore, if you want to perform any activity, you must pay for it with ATP.

The chemical form of ATP looks like this:

$$\text{Adenosine-P}\sim\text{P}\sim\text{P}$$

Note that [-] represents a low-energy bond and [~] represents a high-energy bond. When food is broken down, the released energy is stored in the high-energy bonds of the ATP compound and then used to power all cellular needs.

Every movement we make requires the production and use of energy. The human body has the capacity to create and store its own ATP to use for energy. Whether at rest or when exercising at extreme intensity, the muscles and functions of the body require a specific amount of ATP to accomplish each task. The body does not use only one method to produce ATP. At any time, all the energy systems are being used to produce energy, and the demand of a particular movement dictates which system will dominate in this **energy continuum**. Our bodies are capable of movements of various intensities and durations, so a Personal Training Specialist needs to understand energy production. Depending on the intensity, duration, and availability of oxygen during activity, the cells of the body can produce ATP using both anaerobic and aerobic metabolic methods.

Introduction to the Energy Systems

The human body uses four systems when forming ATP:

1. ATP–CP (phosphagen) system
2. Anaerobic (glycolytic) system
3. Aerobic (glycolytic) system
4. Fatty acid oxidation system

The ATP–CP and glycolytic energy systems are both *anaerobic* systems, meaning that they operate without the use of oxygen. *Aerobic* means "with oxygen," and the aerobic (or oxidative) system uses oxygen to create ATP for muscular contraction. The anaerobic systems are limited and efficient for only short bouts of activity, whereas the aerobic system uses an abundant supply of fat and carbohydrate to create ATP to fuel long bouts of activity. Although all four energy systems function together at any one time to provide the energy that the body requires, at times certain systems become predominant. For example, the anaerobic systems provide much of the energy needed at the start of exercise, when intensity increases, and during high-intensity activity (e.g., sprints, agility drills, heavy lifts; see table 3.1).

Anaerobic Metabolism Systems

As mentioned earlier, in anaerobic metabolism, ATP is made through a chemical reaction that does not require oxygen. It provides energy when the activity is so intense that the body cannot get oxygen to the muscles in time to produce ATP aerobically. ATP must therefore be made without the presence of oxygen. The process of anaerobic respiration can be completed entirely within the cytosol of the cell. Let's look at the two subcategories of anaerobic metabolism that can create ATP.

ATP–CP (Phosphagen) System

This system provides fuel for up to 10 seconds at maximal intensity. ATP and CP are high-energy compounds stored in limited amounts within the muscle. Although the total amount of ATP and CP varies based on the type of muscle fiber, the amount of stored CP is about four to five times greater than the amount of stored ATP. For the startup of intense movement, and especially for brief, intense activity, this system provides the ATP for muscle contraction to occur. The system works in two phases.

ATP–CP phase 1 uses stored ATP and provides enough fuel for one to two seconds of maximal muscle effort. When the nervous system signals a muscle to contract, the ATP is split, forming ADP and P (adenosine diphosphate and phosphate):

$$ATP \text{ (splits)} \rightarrow ADP + P + energy$$

If we remember that ATP is adenosine triphosphate, or adenosine plus three phosphate molecules attached with high-energy bonds, we can rewrite the equation like this:

$$Adenosine\text{-}P{\sim}P{\sim}P \rightarrow Adenosine\text{-}P{\sim}P + P + E$$

with the E representing the energy released when the bonds in ATP are broken. The release of energy

TABLE 3.1   Comparison of Energy Systems

| Parameter | ANAEROBIC SYSTEMS | | AEROBIC SYSTEMS | |
	ATP–CP (phosphagen) system	Anaerobic (glycolytic) system	Aerobic (glycolytic) system	Fatty acid oxidation system
Main energy source	ATP, creatine phosphate	Carbohydrate	Carbohydrate	Fat
Type of energy	Immediate	Short term	Long term	Long term
Intensity level	Highest (maximal)	Very hard to vigorous	Vigorous to light	Light to very light
ATP production rate	Highest	High	Low	Lowest
ATP produced	1 ATP/molecule of CP	2 ATP/glucose molecules 3 ATP/glycogen molecules	38 ATP/glucose molecules	100 or more ATP/fatty acid molecules*
Capacity of ATP production	Lowest	Low	High	Highest
Endurance capacity	Lowest	Low	High	Highest
Time consideration	1–10 sec	10 sec–2 min	>2 min**	
Example activity	50–100 m sprint	200–400 m sprint	800 m marathon**	

*ATP production using fatty acid oxidation can vary depending on the length of the fatty acid chain, so the number produced is 100 or more.

**This is dependent on the available supply of muscle and liver glycogen.

from the splitting of ATP allows the muscle to contract.

ATP–CP phase 2 creates energy by breaking down **creatine phosphate (CP)**, and it is known as the phosphagen system. CP is the backup for ATP. It is a high-energy chemical compound stored in the muscle cell in greater quantities than ATP. With the aid of an enzyme called creatine kinase, CP splits (releasing energy and a phosphate) to provide energy to re-form ATP from ADP. Creatine kinase is stimulated by the increased concentration of ADP in the cell. This provides a feedback mechanism for rapidly forming ATP from the high-energy phosphates, which allows the muscle to keep contracting until the ATP and CP levels decline to the point that the body must slow down and draw on another energy system to continue. This reaction is outlined here:

$$ADP + CP \rightarrow ATP + creatine$$
$$\uparrow$$
$$creatine\ kinase$$

This chemical reaction may be easier understood, if you consider it as

$$Adenosine\text{-}P{\sim}P + C{\sim}P \rightarrow Adenosine\text{-}P{\sim}P {\sim}P + C$$

Remember that the breakdown of stored ATP and the resynthesis using CP are both anaerobic chemical reactions that occur within a muscle cell. In other words, the reaction occurs without oxygen being available to the cell.

The total amount of stored ATP and CP is limited to approximately 10 seconds of intense effort. When the storage is depleted, the cells will no longer be able to provide ATP at the same high rate, and the body will have to slow down so that metabolism can match energy needs through glycolysis (or the glycolytic system), the next fastest method to synthesize ATP.

Anaerobic (Glycolytic) System

This system provides fuel for up to two minutes at maximal intensity. The glycolytic energy pathway is a series of 10 enzyme-driven reactions that cause the breakdown of carbohydrate in the form of glycogen stored in the muscle cell or glucose found in the blood. These reactions take place in the cytoplasm of the cell. This method of metabolism creates energy in the form of two or three ATP molecules,

depending on the source. From glucose, it produces two ATP molecules, and from glycogen stored in the muscle, it produces three ATP molecules. The reason for the difference is that the process of glucose breakdown requires one more ATP molecule to be invested than does the breakdown of glycogen. In both instances, a three-carbon compound called pyruvate is also formed. The breakdown of glycogen or glucose to form two or three ATP molecules is called glycolysis. Because it occurs without oxygen, it is an incomplete chemical reaction. After glycogen stores within the muscle are depleted and the glycolytic energy system uses glucose from the bloodstream to produce ATP, the pathway results in the breakdown of pyruvate to form a cellular by-product called lactic acid (LA). The chemical reaction for the breakdown of glucose is

$$Glucose \rightarrow 2ATP + 2LA + heat$$

The point at which the body begins to form lactic acid, beyond what it can metabolize with the oxygen present, is called the **lactate threshold** (LT). As more glucose is metabolized, more lactic acid is produced. It gathers in the muscle cell, which lowers the cellular pH (becoming more acidic) and begins to slow the speed and strength of muscular contraction. This process is, in part, felt as a burning sensation in the muscle after high-intensity exercise. Eventually, the lactic acid can reach a level high enough to cause temporary muscle failure (meaning that no further contraction can occur). This point is called **lactic acidosis**.

The production of ATP using the glycolytic pathway is limited because lactic acid accumulates, potentially resulting in the need to cease exercise if intensity is not reduced. The muscle cells can be trained to improve this energy pathway so that they produce less lactic acid at the same intensity, thus allowing us to exercise harder for longer. This process occurs because glycolytic enzymes increase by 10% to 25% when training this system through high-intensity exercise. Over time, cells also become more efficient at working with lactic acid in the cellular environment and may last longer at higher intensity.

Glycolysis is the prime producer of ATP from 10 seconds to two minutes of intense exercise. Beyond two minutes of intense exercise, either the muscle will shut down or, if the speed or intensity of contraction is reduced, the blood will be able to deliver adequate oxygen, thereby allowing the aerobic metabolic system to produce additional ATP.

Aerobic Metabolism System

When sufficient oxygen is available to the muscle cells for a given intensity of exercise, an abundance of ATP is produced in the cells. In this case, the supply of oxygen is delivered by the cardiorespiratory system to meet the demand for oxygen in the exercising muscles so that ATP can now be made in the presence of oxygen. Two subcategories of aerobic metabolism can create ATP—aerobic glycolysis and fatty acid oxidation, both of which contribute to this category of metabolism.

Aerobic (Glycolytic) System

This system provides fuel for more than two minutes of exercise at moderate intensity. Aerobic metabolism begins in the same way as the glycolytic pathway in that glycogen or glucose is broken down into pyruvate to produce two or three molecules of ATP. But because oxygen is present, instead of being converted to lactic acid, pyruvate enters a series of reactions known as the *Krebs cycle* and the *electron transport chain*. Oxygen is made available to the muscle cells from nearby capillaries, and the cell is able to take in that oxygen. The muscle cell can now begin to use the available oxygen to produce additional ATP aerobically. Mitochondria, the cellular structures with specialized enzymes to assist in aerobic metabolism, use either glucose or fat for fuel to create ATP.

With this continuous supply of oxygen, the muscle cell begins to break down glucose in the presence of oxygen to produce ATP. This series of aerobic chemical reactions (including the combination of glycolysis, the Krebs cycle, and the electron transport chain) is efficient and produces large amounts of ATP (one unit of glucose equals up to 38 ATP). The waste products of this complete breakdown of glucose are carbon dioxide (CO_2) and water (H_2O) as well as heat. These by-products are simply diffused into the bloodstream and taken away for disposal (carbon dioxide is exhaled, and water is used elsewhere or lost through sweat). The net chemical reaction to break down glucose and glycogen for ATP is

$$\text{Glucose} + O_2 \rightarrow 38\text{ATP} + CO_2 + H_2O + \text{heat}$$

This system of ATP production is limited only by the ability of the cardiorespiratory system to deliver oxygen. If oxygen is available, then glucose and glycogen are metabolized to make ATP. This system is especially useful for producing energy for long, continuous, moderate- to low-intensity exercise (see figure 3.2).

Fatty Acid Oxidation System

The muscle cell is capable of using fatty acids to make ATP, and this aerobic metabolic pathway is called fatty acid oxidation. This system provides fuel during low-intensity exercise lasting longer than two minutes. It also occurs in the mitochondria of the muscle cells when a continuous supply of oxygen is present. This aerobic metabolism of fat produces a large amount of ATP (one unit of fatty acid equals 100 or more ATP depending on the length of the fatty acid chain). Fatty acids are a high-energy fuel, but they are difficult to metabolize because a large amount of oxygen is required for this reaction to occur. The chemical reaction for oxidation of a typical fatty acid is as follows:

$$\text{Fatty acid} + O_2 \rightarrow 100^+\text{ATP} + CO_2 + H_2O + \text{heat}$$

This chemical reaction produces carbon dioxide, water, and heat, and these by-products are easily disposed of elsewhere in the body. The fatty acid oxidation energy system is rarely limited by the supply of fatty acids in the body; its main limitation is the lengthy duration of low-intensity exercise necessary to use it effectively as the primary energy source of a training session. Few people exercise for these extreme durations, but those who do (such as conditioned marathon runners) use a great deal of body fat to fuel activity.

At rest and during low-intensity exercise, muscle cells can use fatty acids as fuel because the demand for energy is low and the supply of oxygen is adequate. But because intensity is low, the amount of fatty acids used is low. In addition, because energy demand is low and each unit of fatty acids produces a large amount of energy, few units of fatty acids are used at rest.

When a person goes from rest to exercise, the body adjusts its supply of energy to meet the required demand by automatically shifting the emphasis between the different energy systems. As exercise intensity increases, the cardiorespiratory system is limited in its ability to supply the required

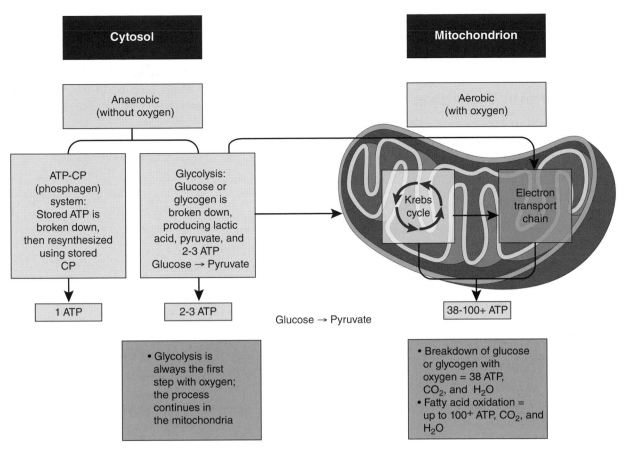

FIGURE 3.2   Pathways for ATP production in a muscle cell.

amount of oxygen quickly enough to allow fatty acid oxidation to occur. The metabolism of glucose and glycogen requires less oxygen, so glucose becomes the preferred fuel for the creation of ATP, in both the aerobic and anaerobic systems. Understanding exercise intensity becomes the key to understanding what method the muscle cell will choose to produce the necessary ATP for muscle contraction.

Interaction of the Energy Systems

The following sequence describes the transition from rest to exercise and back to recovery, illustrating how the three energy systems work together.

• **At rest**—Only small amounts of energy are needed, and they are supplied almost exclusively using aerobic metabolism of fatty acids.

• **At the beginning of exercise**—Depending on the difference between resting state and the level of exercise during the warm-up, the primary energy system used may vary. If the energy demand is only slightly higher than at rest, the aerobic system will continue to be used. If the energy demand is immediate and high, stored energy or ATP will be used (CP may also help to create more energy anaerobically until the aerobic system catches up or until the anaerobic glycolysis system kicks in after 20 to 30 seconds). This underscores the importance of a proper warm-up since commencing exercise that is too intense may result in the accumulation of lactic acid and impairment of the ability to continue exercise.

• **During steady-state exercise**—After the supply of oxygen meets the demand, the muscle cell creates ATP using the breakdown of glycogen and glucose through the aerobic system. This system works as long as needed, provided enough glucose and oxygen are available. Note that for extremely long-duration exercise, the presence of adequate glucose and glycogen may become a limiting factor, pushing the emphasis toward the fatty acid oxidation system (if the athlete is well conditioned) or the glycolytic system if intensity is too high for the use of fatty acids. If the intensity of steady-state exercise is low enough, fat metabolism can occur as long as enough oxygen is available.

• **During strenuous exercise**—When energy demand increases rapidly and intensity is high, the anaerobic system will have to provide ATP. When the ATP–CP phosphagen system is fatigued (after approximately 10 seconds), the glycolytic system takes over the responsibility to produce ATP. The production and accumulation of lactic acid along with exercise intensity dictates the longevity of this system. Fatigue or failure may result if high-intensity exercise continues beyond two minutes or if the intensity is moderate but oxygen demand exceeds supply.

• **During recovery**—Although the need for a higher supply of energy is reduced or eliminated immediately after an exercise session, the body continues to take in a higher level of oxygen than it needs at rest, to be able to pay off the oxygen debt that occurred at the beginning of exercise as well as to facilitate recovery from the exercise session.

None of the energy systems works independently. All systems are working at the same time, but the intensity of the activity determines which system is predominant. The basic idea is that if you need energy quickly (power, or energy per unit of time), the anaerobic systems will be used predominantly. If you need a lot of energy (capacity, or amount of ATP) but you do not need it quickly, such as for a long-distance hike, the aerobic system will be used predominately.

In discussing the interaction of the energy systems, the conditioning of clients for recreational and elite athletics becomes relevant. Table 3.2 shows the estimated contribution of each system for the performance and duration of common sports or activities. These system contributions can change from moment to moment depending on the player position and game intensity. As a Personal Training Specialist, you still want to train all three systems, but your emphasis on a particular system should reflect the estimated contribution of each system for the given sport or activity.

Oxygen Deficit

At the beginning of an exercise session, your body does not have the required amount of oxygen to maintain homeostasis and meet the needs of the increased level of activity. This state is known as the **oxygen deficit**, and it explains why the respiration rate and depth of breath increase during the warm-up phase of your workout. After your oxygen supply has increased enough to meet the demand of steady-state moderate-intensity exercise, homeostasis is maintained through the aerobic energy system. As mentioned earlier, whether for anaerobic or aerobic exercise, after the workout is complete and the need for a higher supply of energy is reduced or eliminated, the body continues to take in extra oxygen (more than would ordinarily be consumed at rest).

Lactate Threshold

An important concept to understand regarding strenuous exercise is the lactate threshold (LT). As mentioned before, the LT is the point at which the aerobic system cannot supply enough ATP for the needs of the body, forcing the anaerobic systems to increase their contribution of ATP. When the LT is surpassed, anaerobic metabolism dominates and a significant accumulation of lactic acid begins to occur as a by-product of high-intensity exercise. If the exercise remains above the LT, this accumulation leads to muscle fatigue, discomfort, and possibly failure. This point occurs at approximately 85% to 90% of maximum heart rate or approximately 80% to 85% of $\dot{V}O_2$max in conditioned clients and 60% to 65% of maximal heart rate or 50% to 55% of $\dot{V}O_2$max in untrained clients. Note, however, that these values may vary 5% to 10% from client to client.

The point or intensity at which clients reach their lactate threshold depends on their fitness level and will change over time as they achieve greater fitness. More fit clients have better oxygen delivery and extraction mechanisms and therefore have greater tolerance for lactic acid compared with deconditioned clients. The more conditioned you are, the harder you can exercise before you surpass the lactate threshold.

TABLE 3.2   Primary Metabolic Demands of Various Sports

Sport	ATP–CP (phosphagen) system	Anaerobic (glycolytic) system	Aerobic (glycolytic) system
Baseball	High	Low	—
Basketball	High	Moderate to high	—
Boxing	High	High	Moderate
Diving	High	Low	—
Fencing	High	Moderate	—
Field events	High	—	—
Field hockey	High	Moderate	Moderate
Football (American)	High	Moderate	Low
Golf	High	—	—
Gymnastics	High	Moderate	—
Ice hockey	High	Moderate	Moderate
Lacrosse	High	Moderate	Moderate
Marathon	Low	Low	High
Mixed martial arts	High	High	Moderate
Power lifting	High	Low	Low
Skiing:			
Cross-country	Low	Low	High
Downhill	High	High	Moderate
Soccer	High	Moderate	High
Strength competitions	High	Moderate to high	Low
Swimming:			
Short distance	High	Moderate	—
Long distance	—	Moderate	High
Tennis	High	—	—
Track (athletics):			
Short distance	High	Moderate	—
Long distance	—	Moderate	High
Ultraendurance events	Low	Low	High
Volleyball	High	Moderate	—
Wrestling	High	High	Moderate
Weightlifting	High	Low	Low

Note: All types of metabolism are involved to some extent in all activities. Fatty acid oxidation is limited as intensity increases.

Reprinted, by permission, from NSCA, 2008, Adaptations to anaerobic training programs, N.A. Ratamess. In *Essentials of strength training and conditioning*, 3rd ed., edited by T.R. Baechle and R.W. Earle (Champaign, IL: Human Kinetics), 95.

This oxygen uptake is known as excess post-exercise oxygen consumption (EPOC), or recovery oxygen uptake, and it helps your body repay the oxygen debt created during the exercise session. With mild aerobic exercise of relatively short duration, about half of the recovery oxygen consumption occurs within 30 seconds, and complete recovery occurs within several minutes. The oxygen debt in this case isn't large, because steady state (homeostasis) is reached quickly in mild aerobic exercise, resulting in faster recovery. With strenuous exercise, anaerobic metabolism increases along with increased levels of lactic acid, body temperature, and hormone levels. During exhaustive exercise, steady state is not reached, so greater oxygen debt is created. Depending on the intensity and duration of the exercise, up to 24 hours may be needed to return to pre-exercise oxygen consumption because of the larger oxygen debt. Notice in figure 3.3 that EPOC is high immediately after exercise, and although it decreases rapidly,

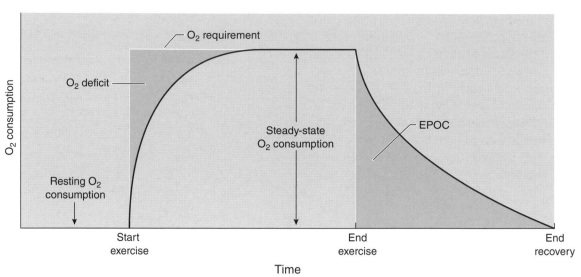

FIGURE 3.3 Oxygen deficit and EPOC.

Calculating Caloric Expenditure From Exercise

Personal Training Specialists are often asked by clients how many calories they burn during a certain activity. For activities such as walking, running, and cycling, caloric expenditure can be estimated with a reasonable amount of accuracy. Note, however, that estimating caloric expenditure becomes more complex as the skill level requirement of an activity increases.

To calculate the caloric expenditure of an activity, you can use the metabolic equivalent of the activity. A metabolic equivalent (or MET) is a term used to represent resting metabolism and is accepted to be 3.5 ml of oxygen per kilogram of body mass per minute (or 3.5 ml/kg/min). So a person weighing 75 kg (165 lb) would be consuming 262.5 ml of oxygen per minute (75 × 3.5) at rest:

3.5 ml × 75 kg = 262.5 ml/min

See the table for various MET levels of common activities.

MET Levels of Common Activities

Activity	MET level
Running (8.0 kph)	8.3
Running (12.1 kph)	11.8
Walking (3.2 kph, level firm surface)	2.8
Walking (5.6 kph, level firm surface)	4.3
Hiking	6.0
Bicycling (16.1–19.2 kph, light effort)	6.8
Bicycling (22.5–25.6 kph, vigorous effort)	10.0
Swimming (freestyle, light or moderate effort)	5.8
Swimming (freestyle, vigorous effort)	9.8

Data from B.E. Ainsworth et al., 2011, *The compendium of physical activities tracking guide*. Healthy Lifestyles Research Center, College of Nursing & Health Innovation, Arizona State University. Available: https://sites.google.com/site/compendiumofphysicalactivities

Our next step is to convert METs into calories (commonly abbreviated as kcal). If you remember the relationship that 1 MET = 1 kcal/kg/hr, then you will have an easy time calculating this conversion. If your 75 kg (165 lb) client was performing an activity at 4.5 METs for 30 minutes, you would calculate as follows:

4.5 METs = 4.5 kcal/kg/hr
Energy expenditure (kcal/min) = (4.5 kcal x 75 kg) ÷ 60
= 337.5 ÷ 60
= 5.625 kcal/min

Considering the total duration of activity in this example is 30 minutes, this client's total caloric expenditure for activity = 5.625 × 30 = 168.75 kcal.

some increase in oxygen consumption occurs for a time. The higher intake immediately after exercise is associated with the restoration of ATP and CP, as well as the oxygen stores within muscles. The prolonged moderate increase in oxygen consumption is related to the removal of lactic acid from muscles or blood and facilitation of the conversion of lactate to glucose in the liver to replenish glycogen stores. The amount of EPOC is greater with heavier, more exhaustive exercise. This occurrence can lead to the burning of additional calories during and after interval-training sessions, commonly known as the after burn.

EPOC is used for ATP and CP replenishment and resynthesis of a small portion of lactic acid to glycogen (although most of the glycogen is restored from dietary carbohydrate). All systems that are activated during exercise increase the need for oxygen during recovery. This creates a disequilibrium of physiologic functions during steady-state aerobic exercise, which EPOC helps resolve. Recovery oxygen uptake also helps to

- reload oxygen to the blood returning to the lungs from active muscles;
- replenish oxygen in the myoglobin in muscles;
- repay energy costs of ventilation above rest;
- meet the energy requirements of a harder working heart;
- repair tissue through the redistribution of calcium, potassium, and sodium ions within muscle and other body compartments; and
- support the elevated metabolism because of the thermogenic hormones released during

exercise (epinephrine, norepinephrine, thyroxine, and glucocorticoids).

In summary, EPOC is used for the recovery of activities that use both anaerobic and aerobic metabolism to produce energy. The more anaerobic or intense the exercise is, the greater the oxygen debt is, and therefore the more EPOC is required to return the body to a pre-exercise state.

Developing the Energy Systems

Although you will likely be training all the energy systems regardless of the type of program you design for your clients, you can design a program that specifically addresses one of the energy systems more than the others, if so desired. You may want to consider this when your clients' goals are sport and performance specific, rather than a more traditional fitness or health goal. For example, the client who is training for a 5K run will need to train the glycolytic system after developing the aerobic system to ensure that she or he has the ability not only to sustain a high level of effort but also to manage the inevitable lactate buildup resulting from comparatively short but intense exertion. One of the best ways of accomplishing this is through interval training.

Your client will need to develop a base of continuous training to become accustomed to exertion before undertaking an interval-training program. Table 3.3 shows the program variables involved in designing safe and effective interval-training programs. The following sections provide more context for understanding the table.

TABLE 3.3   Program Variables in Interval-Training Programs

Energy system trained	Work interval time	Work-to-rest ratio	Work volume	Type of relief	Intensity	Set and rest times
ATP–CP (phosphagen)	10–20 sec	1:3–1:6 (e.g., 10 sec work: 30–60 sec rest)	2–8 min of accumulated work time	Rest relief (walking, stretching)	Maximal	One set of intervals equals 60 sec work (e.g., 6 reps of 10 sec work time, or 3 reps of 20 sec work intervals). Rest 5–10 min between sets. Perform as many sets as necessary to achieve desired total work volume.

> continued

TABLE 3.3   *> continued*

Energy system trained	Work interval time	Work-to-rest ratio	Work volume	Type of relief	Intensity	Set and rest times
Anaerobic (glycolytic)	20 sec–2 min	1:2–1:5 (e.g., 20 sec work: 40–120 sec rest)	2–12 min of accumulated work time	Work relief (light exercise, jogging)	Maximal	One set of intervals equals up to 3 min work time (e.g., 6 reps of 30 sec intervals). Rest 10-12 min between sets. Perform as many sets as necessary to achieve desired total work volume.
Aerobic (glycolytic)	>2 min	2:1–1:1 (e.g., 10 min work: 5–10 min rest)	20–60 min of accumulated work time	Rest relief	Upper edge of comfort zone or sport specific	Set should not exceed 60 min work time. Rest 10–15 min between sets. Perform as many sets as necessary to achieve desired total work volume

Work-to-Rest Ratio

The **work-to-rest ratio** designates how much rest your client should have in relation to the amount of work completed during the work interval. For example, a work-to-rest ratio of 1:3 suggests that after completing an interval of 10 seconds, a client must rest 30 seconds before the next interval of work. The length of rest will also depend on the fitness level of the client (a less-conditioned client needs more time). Therefore, a range is given in the table.

The length of work and rest intervals depends on the training goals and the intensity of the work interval but also on the fitness level of the client. More intense work intervals require relatively longer rest intervals, and less-conditioned clients will need more rest.

Type of Relief

Relief between exercises can consist of either rest (e.g., light active stretching or slow walking) or work (e.g., fast walking or slow jogging). When training the ATP–CP (phosphagen) system, you want to give your client rest relief. If work relief is used instead, some of the ATP that would be replenished for the next work interval will be used to support the activity of the relief. This inhibits the reloading of intramuscular ATP and CP stores. If these stores are not replenished, the body will have to rely more on the anaerobic glycolytic (lactic acid) system for the next work interval and the intensity will have to be lowered. Thus, you will no longer be developing the ATP–CP (phosphagen) system.

For glycolytic intervals, work relief has been assigned because it will inhibit or partially block the complete restoration of the ATP–CP (phosphagen) system, and as a consequence the lactic acid system rather than the ATP–CP (phosphagen) system will dominate the subsequent work interval. Also, work relief aids the clearance of lactic acid, which encourages the improvement of this system and the ability of the body to handle lactic acid.

Activities included in aerobic intervals use rest relief. The rationale for this is that with rest relief, the lactic acid developed during intense aerobic intervals will not be cleared effectively and therefore the anaerobic glycolytic system will not provide aid during the next work interval. This method gives a stronger training stimulus to the aerobic system during the next work phase.

Monitoring the Intensity of an Interval

One simple way to monitor intensity is through heart rate (HR) monitoring. For the ATP–CP and anaerobic glycolytic systems, the intensity given in table 3.3 is maximal; cardiorespiratory training is slightly lower in intensity. Table 3.4 gives age-adjusted HRs that you can use while monitoring interval conditioning. The work interval relates to a maximal exertion (up to 90% HRmax), while the relief interval represents a HRmax up to 70%. The relief between sets represents a moderate level of

exertion (up to 60%). Note that fitness level and activity specificity may alter these numbers.

Important Considerations for Interval Training

When implementing interval-training programs for your clients, keep these guidelines in mind.

1. Fitness interval conditioning can be as simple as adjusting the intensity up and down to challenge the client's anaerobic system in an informal way.

2. If you are training an athlete, the previous parameters may be useful. Alternatively, you can complete a specific assessment of

TABLE 3.4   Age-Adjusted Heart Rates Based on HRmax

Age (years)	Work interval HR (BPM)	Relief interval HR (BPM)	Relief HR between sets (BPM)
Under 20	190	150	125
20–29	180	140	120
30–39	170	130	110
40–49	160	120	105
50–59	150	115	100
60–69	140	105	90

HR = heart rate; BPM = beats per minute.

From E. Fox and D. Mathews, 1974, *Interval training* (Philadelphia, PA: W.B.Saunders), 60. By permission of Donald Mathews.

Arranging Work and Rest Times

During interval training, a set consists of a series of both work and rest intervals (e.g. six intervals of 10-second sprints, each followed by 30 seconds of rest). Repetitions are the number of work intervals within one set.

As an example, let's say you ask your 26-year-old client to complete two minutes of work intervals for the ATP–CP (phosphagen) system, and you would like to use a 10-second interval time. This would amount to 12 intervals to achieve the total two minutes of work. Based on table 3.3, one set of intervals for the ATP–CP (phosphagen) system is 60 seconds of work. Therefore, if using a 1:3 ratio, your client would have to complete two sets, each containing six repetitions. In this example the 10-second work interval plus 30-second rest interval is one repetition. Accounting for both work and rest, each set of six repetitions would take four minutes to complete.

Based on this client's age (26 years old), the work interval should raise the HR to approximately 180 beats per minute (BPM), and the HR should fall to 140 BPM during each rest interval. After completing all six reps for the first set, the client would rest 5 to 10 minutes to get the HR down to 120 BPM. After this extended rest period, you would have the client perform another full set of repetitions (i.e., six 10-second intervals with 30-second rest intervals between repetitions). When you calculate the total time for this interval workout, you will see that 13 to 18 minutes of your training session will be used to produce the goal of two minutes of work for the ATP–CP (phosphagen) system.

the client's sport demands to ensure that you understand the specific requirements.

3. Exhaustion is not the goal of an interval-conditioning program. It should be challenging but also safe and enjoyable.

4. Be sure that the client completes a warm-up of at least 5 to 10 minutes before interval conditioning and performs a cool-down of at least 5 minutes afterward. Ideally, the HR should feel like the pre-exercise level by the end of the cool-down.

5. Beginning exercisers should not participate in anaerobic intervals.

6. Anaerobic interval training should only be completed two or three times per week. Inter-sperse these sessions with lighter intensity cardiorespiratory training sessions.

7. Many activities can be used for interval conditioning.

Developing all three energy systems will help with recreational sport performance as well as daily activities (such as playing with children or running to catch a bus), and it will provide a good foundation for all-around development of cardiorespiratory fitness. As a Personal Training Specialist, use this style of training to your clients' advantage, being sure that the exercises and intervals progress in a safe and logical manner.

Summary of Main Points

1. Energy is defined as the ability to do physical work. The body needs ATP to convert the chemical energy from food into muscle contraction for movement.

2. Metabolism includes all chemical reactions that allow large molecules to break down and other molecules to build up.

3. Energy is produced in the cells of the body in the form of ATP using anaerobic metabolism (without oxygen) and aerobic metabolism (with oxygen).

4. The duration and intensity of exercise dictate which energy system produces the necessary energy for specific activities.

5. Interval conditioning is an effective method of developing the energy systems.

Key Concepts for Study

Bioenergetics

Energy

Metabolism

Homeostasis

Adenosine triphosphate (ATP)

Creatine phosphate (CP)

Lactate threshold (LT)

Anaerobic glycolysis

Aerobic system

Work-to-rest ratio

Energy continuum

Oxygen deficit/debt

Excess post-exercise oxygen consumption (EPOC)

Review Questions

1. Describe the relationship between metabolism and the energy used for muscle contraction.

2. Describe EPOC and its role in exercise recovery.

3. The ATP–CP (phosphagen) system produces _____ ATP per molecule of creatine phosphate.

   a. 1

   b. 2

   c. 20

   d. 3

4. What type of relief makes up the rest interval for developing the anaerobic glycolytic system?

   a. rest relief

   b. work relief

   c. passive relief

   d. hard jogging

5. EPOC is used for all the following processes *except*

   a. ATP replenishment

   b. CP replenishment

   c. digestion of carbohydrates to glucose

   d. conversion of lactate to glucose

6. The aerobic (oxidative) energy system is fueled by _____ and produces up to _____ ATP per unit of fuel.

   a. fat; 39

   b. glucose or glycogen; 2 to 3

   c. glycogen; 100 or more

   d. glucose and fat; 100 or more

7. What terminology best describes the point at which the aerobic system cannot supply enough ATP for the needs of the body, forcing the anaerobic systems to increase their contribution of ATP?

   a. homeostasis

   b. lactate threshold

   c. anaerobic glycolysis

   d. catabolic metabolism

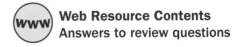

Web Resource Contents
Answers to review questions

Cardiorespiratory Concepts

Gregory S. Anderson, PhD
Brian Justin, M.Kin

LEARNING OUTCOMES

After completing this chapter, you will be able to

1. describe the anatomy of the heart;

2. explain the flow of blood from the heart to the body and back again;

3. discuss the mechanics of the cardiovascular system and its response to exercise;

4. explain the function and anatomy of the respiratory system;

5. discuss the mechanics of the respiratory system and its response to exercise;

6. identify the major benefits of cardiorespiratory training;

7. identify basic differences in developing cardiorespiratory training programs for beginner, intermediate, and advanced clients;

8. explain the major issues that affect the design of cardiorespiratory training based on the FITT formula; and

9. determine appropriate exercises for cardiorespiratory warm-up and recovery.

The cardiovascular and respiratory systems are essential to body motion. They work together as the combined cardiorespiratory system to deliver oxygen and nutrients and remove wastes from body tissues. The respiratory system adds oxygen and removes carbon dioxide from the blood, and the **circulatory system** transports these substances along with nutrients to and from body tissues.

Increased physical activity strengthens the heart, circulatory system, and lungs. As a Personal Training Specialist, you must understand how these systems assist in producing movement and how they adapt to training to make people feel healthier, move more easily, and live longer.

Cardiovascular System

The cardiovascular system is composed of the heart and a network of arteries and veins (blood vessels) that carry blood throughout the body; blood trans-ports nutrients, oxygen, carbon dioxide, metabolic waste products, and key chemical messengers (i.e., hormones). The circulatory system is also involved in maintaining the core temperature of the body by transporting heat from the core to the skin, where it can dissipate.

Cardiovascular Anatomy

The heart is a muscular pump that creates the pressure required to move blood through the circulatory system (figure 4.1). It has four chambers and functions as two pumps, one on the right side and one on the left. The right atrium and right ventricle form the right pump, collecting blood returning from the tissues and moving it through the lungs (referred to as **pulmonary circulation**). The left atrium and left ventricle combine to make the left pump, which receives blood from the lungs and moves it through the tissues of the body and back to the right side of the heart (referred to as **systemic circulation**).

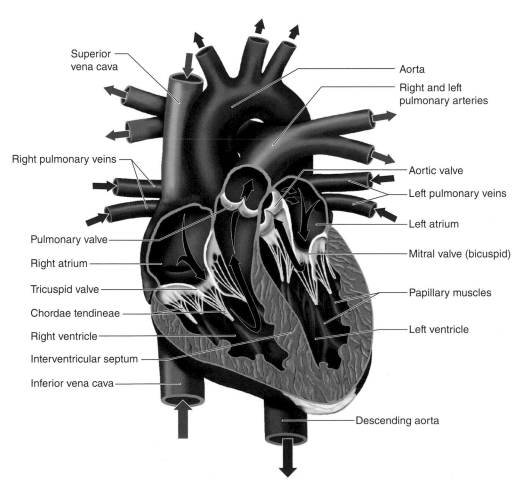

FIGURE 4.1 Structure of the human heart and course of blood flow through its chambers.

In the four-chamber system, each **atrium** receives blood returning to the heart through veins and passes the blood into the **ventricles**, which are the muscular pumps that move the blood away from the heart through the arteries. Blood moves through the pulmonary circuit to the lungs and then through the systemic circuit to body tissues.

Circulation

Blood travels in arteries either to the lungs from the right side of the heart or to body tissues from the left side. It returns to the heart through veins, which bring blood back to the left atrium from the lungs or to the right atrium from body tissues. At the start of this loop, the oxygenated blood leaves the heart from the left ventricle through the aorta and travels from the arteries to microscopic vessels called **arterioles**, which then branch into even smaller vessels called **capillaries**. Capillaries are the smallest and most numerous of blood vessels. At the capillary level, the blood passes by cells, where oxygen and nutrients are dropped off and carbon dioxide and other waste products are picked up for transport. After this gas exchange, the deoxygenated blood carrying the extra carbon dioxide leaves the arterial system and begins making its way back to the heart by way of veins. Major veins from the upper and lower halves of the body empty directly into the right side of the heart. The blood passes from the right atrium to the right ventricle, where it is then pushed out to the lungs. In the lungs, the blood picks up oxygen and drops off carbon dioxide through diffusion. Oxygenated blood then returns to the left atrium through pulmonary veins to start the circuit over again.

In a typical adult, five litres of blood circulate every minute at rest and up to six or seven times a minute during maximal exercise. The function of the left ventricle is to force blood out of the heart through the aorta. Oxygen-rich (red) blood travels out of the aorta and is sent under pressure to all parts of the body (figure 4.2).

Blood Pressure

Blood pressure (BP) is the result of blood being pumped out of the ventricles and exerting force against the arterial walls. In a healthy person at rest, blood in the circulatory system is forced through the arteries at an average pressure of 120/80 millimetres of mercury (mmHg). The top number, or **systolic**

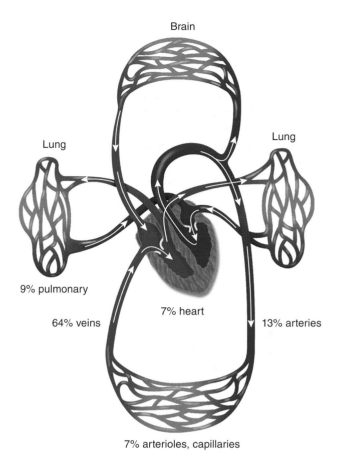

Brain

Lung

Lung

9% pulmonary

7% heart

64% veins

13% arteries

7% arterioles, capillaries

FIGURE 4.2 The arterial (right) and venous components of the circulatory system. The percent values indicate the distribution of blood volume throughout the circulatory system at rest.

pressure, is the pressure exerted on the walls of the arteries as the heart contracts, representing peak pressure in the system. The bottom number, or **diastolic pressure**, is the pressure exerted on the walls of the arteries as the heart relaxes and fills again, representing the lowest pressure in the arteries. Training increases the ability of the heart to pump blood, but as a client becomes more fit, resting BP remains constant or may even decrease because exercise also helps maintain the elasticity of vessels and keeps the circulatory system healthy.

During exercise, the heart must pump harder to deliver the oxygen required by the working muscles, and volume of blood pumped out of the left ventricle increases. As more blood is pumped into the aorta, the aorta is distended a greater amount, and thus BP normally increases during exercise. During moderate exercise, systolic pressure rises quickly to values above 200 mmHg and then levels off, whereas diastolic pressure remains relatively stable because of the opening of more capillary beds. During straining exercises such as weightlifting, BP may spike to much higher levels as the muscular contractions compress the arteries and produce a much greater resistance to blood flow. During such nonrhythmic activities, the low-pressure veins are also compressed and blood flow back to the heart and brain may be reduced, resulting in dizziness or faintness. For people with hypertension, these types of activities may be dangerous.

During activities such as resistance training, arteries are compressed, increasing blood pressure and potentially compromising circulation. If these straining activities are done improperly, they may cause dizziness or faintness and can be dangerous, especially for people with high blood pressure. It is important that Personal Training Specialists coach appropriate breathing during exercise training, and follow the FITT principle, to ensure client safety.

Heart Rate and Output

The heart pumps approximately 72 beats per minute (BPM) at rest. Each time the heart pumps, it forces blood into the arteries to deliver oxygen and nutrients to the metabolically active tissues of the body. The wave of blood moving through the arteries can be felt as a pulse at any of the major arteries that are close to the skin (i.e., radial artery in the arm, temporal artery of the head, and carotid artery in the neck). The radial pulse is taken at the wrist along the outer edge of the lateral tendons and is the preferred location for manual **heart rate (HR)** measurement. The link between metabolic demand and HR allows Personal Training Specialists to use HR as an indicator of exercise intensity. As the demand for oxygen increases with activity, the heart must pump faster to provide more oxygen. Thus, monitoring HR is

When monitoring a client's HR manually, place your fingertips (and not your thumb) over the artery, as the thumb has a very strong pulse of its own and could cause an error in calculation.

a basic requirement for working with clients in a personal training environment.

HR monitors (worn on the wrist or across the chest) are more reliable than the sensors on cardio machines and provide excellent alternatives to taking HRs manually.

In addition to heart rate, the amount of blood that the heart pumps can be used to measure the function of the heart. **Stroke volume (SV)** is the amount of blood that the left ventricle ejects in one beat. Resting stroke volume for a typical male averages around 70 millilitres. As a client becomes more fit, the ventricles become larger, allowing them to hold more blood and contract with more force. This causes stroke volume to increase; thus, a trained person will be able to deliver more blood per heartbeat than an untrained person of the same body size. Therefore, a well-conditioned heart does not have to work as hard to deliver the amount of blood required by the body at rest or during exercise.

Cardiac output (Q) is the amount of blood that the heart ejects in one minute. It is the product of HR and stroke volume (SV); that is, how many times the heart beats and how much blood it ejects per beat. The equation for cardiac output is

$$Q = SV \times HR$$

As demands for oxygen and nutrients increase during exercise, so does cardiac output (by increasing both HR and stroke volume). Stroke volume increases early in exercise and continues to rise through moderate exercise, after which it plateaus. HR increases with exercise intensity to maximal levels, where it plateaus before exhaustion.

While at rest, the cardiac output required by the body is about five litres of blood circulated per minute. The trained heart is a more efficient pump and can create a greater contraction to pump out more blood per beat (i.e., larger stroke volume) than the untrained heart. With improved fitness and increased stroke volume, resting HR decreases. For this reason, during rest the trained heart beats at a slower rate and gets more rest between beats, beating 28,000 fewer times in a day. During exercise, the trained heart is capable of delivering greater amounts of oxygen to meet the demands of the exercise. To offer an example, we can compare the rest and exercise responses of a trained person and an untrained person.

Rest

Untrained: 5,000 millilitres =
70 BPM × 71.4 millilitres

Trained: 5,000 millilitres =
50 BPM × 100 millilitres

Maximal Exercise

Untrained: 20,000 millilitres =
195 BPM × 102.6 millilitres

Trained: 35,000 millilitres =
195 BPM × 179.5 millilitres

Increasing cardiac output during exercise means that the trained person is able to deliver more oxygen and nutrients to the working muscles. Further, during exercise the body redistributes blood from less active tissues, such as digestive organs and kidneys, to the heart and skeletal muscles (table 4.1).

Respiratory System

The pulmonary or respiratory system is made up of the left and right lungs and a network of air passageways. This system exchanges gas between the bloodstream and the environment, and it provides a large interface between the air we breathe and

TABLE 4.1 Distribution of Cardiac Output at Rest and During Strenuous Exercise

Body tissue	Rest	Strenuous exercise
Muscle	20%	84%
Liver	27%	2%
Kidneys	22%	1%
Brain	14%	4%
Skin	6%	2%
Heart	4%	4%
Other	7%	3%

the blood circulating through our lungs. It is at this interface that oxygen is brought into the bloodstream and carbon dioxide is removed from the blood. This exchange of gases occurs because of ventilation and diffusion. **Ventilation** refers to the mechanical process of moving air in and out of the lungs, whereas *diffusion* refers to the way gases are exchanged in the lungs.

Respiratory Anatomy

The respiratory system consists of the mouth, nose, nasal cavity, pharynx, larynx, trachea, bronchial tree, and lungs (figure 4.3). Air (containing 21%

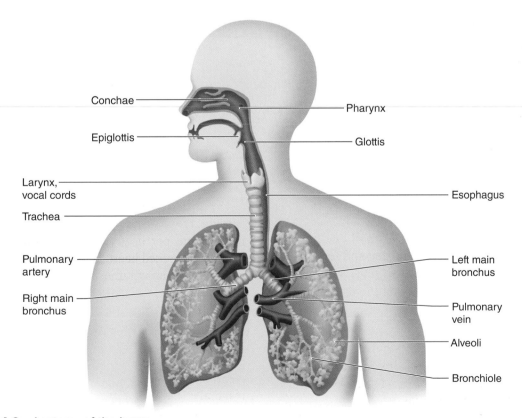

FIGURE 4.3 Anatomy of the lungs.

oxygen) is inhaled from the atmosphere by the mouth and nose, travels through the trachea, and enters the primary bronchi and their subdivisions— the secondary and tertiary bronchi. The ends of the tertiary bronchi branches contain bronchioles, which have tiny air sacs called *alveoli* at their ends. These alveolar sacs are microscopic, thin-walled elastic sacs where gas is exchanged. Air fills the alveoli, which are surrounded by capillaries, where oxygen rapidly moves from the alveoli into the blood by a process called *diffusion*. At the same time, the alveoli receive carbon dioxide from the capillaries, for removal through exhalation. This respiration process is a continuous cycle.

The average adult has a lung volume of four to six litres of mixed air. The term *mixed air* refers to ordinary room air, which contains nitrogen (78%), oxygen (21%), and a small amount of carbon dioxide (0.04%). The lungs contain over 300 million alveoli, providing a very large surface area for diffusion to take place. If the alveolar surface were spread out flat, it would cover 60 to 80 square metres, an area the size of a tennis court.

Ventilation

Air moves in and out of the lungs along pressure gradients created by diaphragm contraction and relaxation. Inspiration, the process of air moving into the lungs, occurs when lung pressure is below atmospheric pressure. This low pressure is created by the diaphragm contracting and pushing down into the abdomen while other inspiratory muscles lift the ribs upward and outward, increasing the volume of the thoracic cavity in which the lungs sit. This creates a partial vacuum and the lungs are sucked open, increasing their volume because of the enlarged chest cavity and falling air pressure within the lungs. Because inspiration uses muscle contractions, it requires energy expenditure. Figure 4.4 summarizes the movement of oxygen through the respiratory system, beginning with inspiration.

Expiration is the passive process of air moving out of the lungs that occurs when lung pressure exceeds atmospheric pressure. When the diaphragm and the other inspiratory muscles relax and the stretched lungs recoil, the chest cavity decreases in volume, lung air pressure increases above atmospheric pressure, and air is forced out of the lungs.

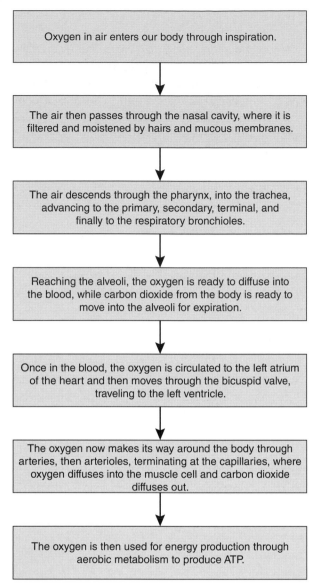

FIGURE 4.4 This diagram summarizes the path of oxygen from its entry into the body to its use in aerobic metabolism.

Cardiorespiratory Response to Exercise

At the onset of exercise, the cardiorespiratory system responds to a change in demand for oxygen. This response begins immediately, but a delay may occur in accommodating this increased requirement, depending on the difference between the oxygen demand before exercise and during exercise (oxygen deficit). This is the rationale in support of a thorough warm-up, which prepares the cardiorespiratory system to generate ATP through the aerobic systems after a few minutes of moderate activity.

When a person begins exercise, the brain recognizes a need for more oxygen in the muscles. It signals the heart to increase HR and stroke volume, which increases cardiac output. The increase in cardiac output increases the amount of blood (and therefore oxygen) that is carried to the exercising muscles. Blood flow redistributes away from the abdominal area by vasoconstriction (narrowing of the arteries) and increases to the working muscles by vasodilation (widening of the arteries). A change also occurs in BP to accommodate the increased demand for oxygen. As the demand for blood flow increases, systolic pressure elevates as blood is forced out of the heart at a faster rate and higher pressure. Diastolic pressure should stay the same or even slightly decrease because of vasodilation of vessels in the exercising muscles, which reduces the resistance and pressure of the blood.

At the onset of exercise, the rate of respiration also increases. This change in breathing rate and depth helps meet the demand for additional oxygen to be used in energy production. During the first few minutes of exercise, pulmonary ventilation increases in a similar manner to exercise HR. At rest, ventilation is approximately 10 litres per minute. In the first minute of exercise, it can increase to approximately 45 litres per minute. After two minutes, when a person reaches steady-state exercise, it can increase to approximately 60 litres per minute. Pulmonary ventilation may increase to 220 litres of air per minute in well-conditioned endurance athletes in response to maximum metabolic demands. Figure 4.5 shows typical HR and ventilation responses for a fit person who is jogging on a treadmill.

Systems Integration

Cardiorespiratory fitness reflects the efficiency of the cardiovascular, respiratory, and muscular systems. It reflects the ability to perform continuous, repetitive movement using the large muscle groups of the body for an extended period without fatigue by generating energy for physical work through the aerobic energy pathways. This capacity is often described using terms such as *cardiorespiratory endurance, cardiorespiratory capacity,* and *maximal oxygen consumption.*

Cardiorespiratory capacity, abbreviated as $\dot{V}O_2max$, is defined as the maximum amount of oxygen the body can extract and use in the process of energy production. $\dot{V}O_2max$ reflects the amount of energy that can be generated through the cardiorespiratory energy pathways, and it depends on the ability to ventilate the lungs, the ease at which oxygen moves from the lungs to the blood, the capacity of the blood to carry the oxygen, the ability of the heart to pump blood (cardiac output) and distribute it to the working musculature, and the ability of the muscles to extract and use the oxygen delivered. For this reason, $\dot{V}O_2max$ reflects the ability to integrate the responses from various systems required to support increased activity. It can be measured in maximum volume of oxygen per minute in litres or relative to body mass (millilitres per kilogram per minute). Normal values for a fit male and an unfit male who both weigh 70 kilograms (154 lb) are presented in table 4.2.

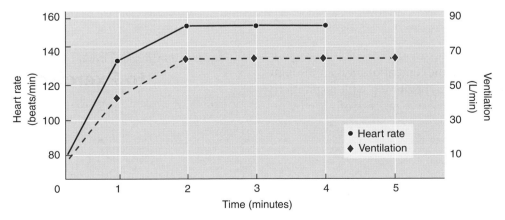

FIGURE 4.5 A concept diagram of HR and ventilation response.

TABLE 4.2   Oxygen Uptake During Rest and Maximal Exercise

	Fit participant (70 kg [154 lb])	Unfit participant (70 kg [154 lb])
Resting $\dot{V}O_2$max		
Relative (ml/kg/min)	3.5 ml/kg/min	3.5 ml/kg/min
Absolute (L/min)	0.25 L/min	0.25 L/min
Maximal $\dot{V}O_2$max		
Relative (ml/kg/min)	60 ml/kg/min	35 ml/kg/min
Absolute (L/min)	4.2 L/min	2.5 L/min

Factors that contribute to cardiorespiratory capacity can generally be divided into two categories: a central component involving the heart and its ability to distribute blood (and therefore oxygen) and a peripheral component involving the muscles and their ability to extract and use oxygen in the production of aerobic energy. This distinction is important because the components respond to different training regimes; what best develops the central component does not necessarily develop the peripheral component.

Oxygen Uptake During Recovery

After exercise stops, oxygen consumption remains elevated above resting levels for a while despite the fact that the oxygen demands placed on the body during exercise are no longer present. Referred to as *EPOC* (see chapter 3), this oxygen is used for recovery processes that bring the body back to homeostasis. The magnitude of the recovery process varies based on the intensity and duration of the exercise. Light activity causes little disturbance in the body and requires a recovery period that is usually short and relatively unnoticeable, whereas intense exercise can result in a recovery period lasting many hours, sometimes even days.

The rate of recovery is rapid for the first few minutes after exercise and then slows for the remainder of the recovery period. The fast portion of recovery helps replenish the ATP–CP stores and remove lactic acid, and the slower portion of recovery supports muscle tissue repair and adaptations that occur because of the exercise. EPOC has been shown to be smaller and occur at a faster rate for the same exercise following many weeks of cardiorespiratory training; thus, training can affect recovery rate. In addition, active recovery, such as light cardiorespiratory exercise, has been shown to be better than passive recovery, supporting the need for a cool-down period after training. Active recovery, when the person keeps moving instead of stopping, assists the heart and circulatory system in redistributing blood to all parts of the body. This prevents blood from pooling in the exercising muscles and helps cells reduce the oxygen debt created during exercise when oxygen supply does not meet demand. Abruptly stopping activity (for example, suddenly ending a high-intensity run) places considerable stress on the cardiorespiratory system. Just as the warm-up gradually increases exercise intensity, active recovery, including a gradual decrease in the intensity of exercise, reduces the stress on the cardiorespiratory system, ensuring a safe and effective recovery.

The primary method of cardiorespiratory recovery is to gradually reduce exercise intensity. As a Personal Training Specialist, you can assist this recovery by
- reducing the intensity and impact of the exercise,
- reducing the range of motion of movements, and
- instructing clients to begin an active recovery.

Benefits of Cardiorespiratory Training

Many studies have shown the benefits of cardiorespiratory training, especially for helping to reduce the risk of heart disease. Cardiorespiratory training also reduces resting HR, normalizes resting BP, and improves the ability to perform daily activities. Physiological improvements and their related benefits are listed in table 4.3. These physiological benefits lead to an overall improvement in both oxygen

TABLE 4.3   Physical Improvements and Benefits as a Result of Cardiorespiratory Training

Improvements	Benefits
Delivery of blood (central training effects)	
Increased stroke volume	Greater delivery of oxygen and nutrients
Stronger heart muscle	Increased blood delivery
Increase in red blood cells	Greater capacity for carrying oxygen throughout the body
Extraction of oxygen (peripheral training effects)	
Increased capillary density	Provides more vessels for efficient nutrient delivery and waste removal
Increased size and number of mitochondria	Improved aerobic production of ATP
Increased aerobic enzymes	Enhanced ability to use oxygen

delivery and oxygen extraction. The result is an increase in cardiorespiratory capacity, or $\dot{V}O_2max$:

$$\dot{V}O_2max = oxygen\ delivery \times oxygen\ extraction.$$

Program Design for Cardiorespiratory Training

For client to have success in an exercise program, the Personal Training Specialist must make correct decisions about program design. If a Personal Training Specialist does not interpret a client's expectations, experience, fitness level, and training goals correctly, the training program will not be effective.

When designing programs for clients, consider the FITT formula: frequency, intensity, time, and type. The canfitpro guidelines for cardiorespiratory training recommend 300 minutes of moderate-intensity activity or 150 minutes of vigorous-intensity activity (or a combination of the two) to be accumulated per week. The activity can be accumulated in 10-minute sessions or in longer bouts of exercise. In designing programs for your clients, you can use the FITT formula to create a program that allows them to reach this goal progressively or even go beyond it, if appropriate. The development of an individualized FITT design is influenced by many factors. Personal Training Specialists must develop a strong knowledge base regarding each component of the FITT formula. The following sections examine the four components of the FITT formula as they pertain to the development of cardiorespiratory fitness.

Frequency

Frequency refers to the number of times that the cardiorespiratory system is intentionally stressed each week. The frequency of activity depends on the intensity and duration of each training period. The number of workouts you program per week will vary depending on the duration of your clients' cardiorespiratory sessions. The goal is to accumulate the guidelines stated earlier. So, if you are doing only 10-minute sessions, more frequent sessions will

Considerations for Cardiorespiratory Exercise Frequency

When deciding on the exercise frequency for a client's cardiorespiratory training program, consider the following factors:

- **Number of sessions that a client is able to commit to**—Various factors affect this choice, including family, work, social, and financial commitments. As a Personal Training Specialist, you should work with the capabilities and availability of the client to establish a reasonable expectation regarding frequency.

- **Client's current fitness level**—If the client is not a regular exerciser, recommend a slow increase in activity level. If the client is already fit, the number of sessions can be more frequent.

- **Client's goals for cardiorespiratory conditioning**—If the client is interested in weight reduction, recommend more frequent training to enhance results. Clients who seek improved health and fitness also need to exercise more frequently.

be required. If you program longer sessions, then frequency can be decreased. Exercise frequency is influenced by the client's lifestyle. Ideally, all clients would have the time and motivation to exercise every day, but the reality is that most people lead busy lives and have a limited amount of free time to dedicate to exercise.

When counseling clients about exercise frequency, encourage them to modify their current activity patterns for improvement. Regular physical activity helps establish exercise as a habit and minimizes the risk of injury. Research shows that people can improve cardiorespiratory health in two exercise sessions per week (Garber et al., 2011). This approach leads to health benefits, fat reduction, and lowered risk of injury. As exercise frequency increases, results improve. Research indicates that dramatic improvements in cardiorespiratory fitness and cardiorespiratory health occur as training sessions increase from three to five sessions per week (Garber et al., 2011). A common recommendation is to exercise one day and rest the next. Note, however, that improvement levels off; few extra cardiorespiratory effects occur by increasing from five to seven sessions per week. Therefore, optimal cardiorespiratory training effects occur in three to five training sessions per week using a combination of moderate and vigorous activity.

 Closely observe clients who wish to exercise every day to ensure that they do not overtrain. Frequent exercisers must pay close attention to exercise intensity to maintain positive adaptation to exercise.

Intensity

Intensity refers to the rate of work being performed. The rate of work can be described as a speed (such as running 10 km in an hour) or relative load placed on the cardiorespiratory system (percentage of maximum HR). Training intensity can have a significant effect on the success of the workout because it has considerable physiological and psychological effects on the client. For example, if the workout is too difficult, the client may be unable to complete the planned activity. From a physiological standpoint, the client's body is unable to supply the required energy, and from a psychological standpoint, the client might not enjoy the exercise session

because it is too difficult. The result is a client who does not have fun and may want to avoid future workouts. When this occurs, you may have lost a client. On an opposite note, if the intensity is too low, the client will not realize the training goals from a physiological perspective. From a psychological standpoint, the client may become bored. Finding a balance between these polar ends is the art of program design.

Because intensity is so closely linked to client success and enjoyment, you need to understand the major ways to determine and evaluate exercise intensity. The three primary methods of planning and detecting exercise intensity are based on the physiological response of the body to exercise: oxygen uptake, HR monitoring, and perceived exertion. Physiological (HR) and psychological (perceived exertion) responses to exercise are intensity specific and act as adequate markers in the design of exercise intensity during cardiorespiratory training sessions. Most Personal Training Specialists cannot monitor oxygen uptake during a client's exercise session; this option is available only to elite athletes who have access to laboratory testing and training.

The most common method of evaluating intensity during cardiorespiratory training is exercise HR. Heart rate increases linearly with oxygen uptake (or exercise intensity) throughout the majority of the exercise range. Most clients understand what their HR is and can be trained to use a heart rate monitor or take their HR manually, so HR is a natural indicator to use for designing exercise intensity. The two primary ways of using HR for designing exercise intensity are a percentage of HR maximum or a percentage of HR reserve. Both rely on knowing the client's maximum HR, or HRmax.

Most clients will not know their HRmax, and determining it can be dangerous for many clients. But a general indicator of HRmax can be found by using the following equation:

$$HRmax = 220 - age$$

Because of changes in the nervous system, the capacity of the heart decreases with age. The previous equation determines a theoretical HRmax and provides a good guess as to what a client's HRmax may be. But these values can be incorrect, and you should observe clients carefully to determine the appropriateness of the exercise intensity. For example, in theory a 20-year-old should have an HRmax of 200 BPM, but maximum HRs as low as 180 and as high as 220 are common. Using this equation will overpredict the intensity for people with a lower HRmax and underpredict the intensity of people with a higher HRmax. Ratings of perceived exertion can also be used to estimate a client's exercise intensity. These scales are described in detail later in this chapter.

Percentage of Maximum Heart Rate

Using HRmax to determine exercise intensity provides an estimate of how hard the client should exercise. In general, research shows that an appropriate range of recommended exercise intensity falls between 55% and 90% of HRmax, a range known as the target heart rate **training zone**. This range encourages clients to exercise hard enough to achieve cardiorespiratory gains, but not so hard that the aerobic energy system is unable to provide enough energy, which would make the exercise anaerobic. Where a client belongs in this intensity range is based on exercise experience, exercise goals, and current fitness level. This method is not the most accurate way to set exercise intensity, but most clients understand it.

You can use this equation to determine a target heart rate training zone using the percentage of HRmax method:

$$\text{Target HR} = (220 - \text{age}) \times \text{percent}$$

For example, for a 40-year-old client:

$$
\begin{aligned}
\text{Lower target HR} &= (220 - 40) \times .55 \\
&= 180 \times .55 \\
&= 99 \text{ BPM}
\end{aligned}
$$

$$
\begin{aligned}
\text{Upper target HR} &= (220 - 40) \times .9 \\
&= 180 \times .9 \\
&= 162 \text{ BPM}
\end{aligned}
$$

Based on the preceding calculations, using the HRmax method and the 55% to 90% range, this client's target training zone is 99 to 162 BPM.

If the client is a beginner or has a low fitness level, we would use exercise values near the lower end of the full target HR zone (55% to 64% of HRmax). For an intermediate-fitness client, we would use values in the middle (65% to 74% of HRmax), and for an advanced-fitness client, we would use values in the upper range (75% to 90% HRmax). Table 4.4 shows recommended HRs for various ages and training zones.

TABLE 4.4 Heart Rate Chart

Age	Percent (%) HRmax	HR (BPM)
20	55	110
	60	120
	70	140
	80	160
	90	180
30	55	105
	60	114
	70	133
	80	152
	90	171
40	55	99
	60	108
	70	126
	80	144
	90	162
50	55	94
	60	102
	70	119
	80	136
	90	153
60	55	88
	60	96
	70	112
	80	128
	90	144

If clients do not have a HR monitor, they can take an exercise pulse at the radial or carotid pulse site. Ask them to count the number of beats in 15 seconds and multiply that number by 4 to determine BPM. Be aware, however, that this method can be inaccurate by as much as 10 to 15 BPM.

To determine how hard clients should exercise, consider their current fitness level. The more fit the client is, the more stress the body is capable of handling. The more stress the body can handle, the more intense the workout should be. Fit clients need to train at higher intensity to continue to develop the cardiorespiratory system.

Heart Rate Reserve

A second method of determining exercise intensity is heart rate reserve (HRR). This calculation takes resting HR into account and calculates the number of beats your client can safely increase HR during exercise (HRmax minus resting HR). It also con-

Considerations for Cardiorespiratory Exercise Intensity

When deciding on the exercise intensity for a client's cardiorespiratory training program, consider the following factors:

- **Client's exercise experience**—Clients with minimal exercise experience should begin training at the lower end of the intensity spectrum (55% to 64%).
- **Client's current fitness level**—More fit clients should work in the moderate (65% to 74%) to high (75% to 90%) range of the target zone.
- **Client's goals for cardiorespiratory conditioning**—Improving cardiorespiratory health requires clients to exercise in their target zone. Fat loss requires increased total caloric expenditure overall.

siders fitness, based on the understanding that as people become more fit, their resting HR decreases. Using the HRR calculation is most appropriate when you know your client's resting and maximum HRs, exercise experience, and current cardiorespiratory fitness level. In addition, the client should have been working out with you for a while.

As compared to HRmax, for which the range is 55% to 90%, when using this method to determine intensity, target HRs during cardiorespiratory training should fall between 50% and 85% of HRR. This is to ensure the target HR is not overestimated. For **target heart rate** calculations using the HRR method, use the following equation, also known as the Karvonen formula:

Target HR = [(HRmax − resting HR) × percentage] + resting HR

For example, the following is the calculation of target training zone for a 40-year-old client with a resting HR of 75 BPM:

Lower target HR = ([(220 − 40) − 75] × .5) + 75
= [(180 − 75) × .5] + 75
= (105 × .5) + 75
= 52.5 + 75
= 128 BPM

Upper target HR = ([(220 − 40) − 75] × .85) + 75
= [(180 − 75) × .85] + 75
= (105 × .85) + 75
= 89.25 + 75
= 164 BPM

Therefore, the client's training zone should be 128 to 164 BPM, based on the HRR equation.

When both maximum and resting HRs are known, HRR may be a good option, but when calculating HRmax, the same error (10 to 15 BPM) is added as when using percentage of HRmax, and the HRR

method will not produce better results than the simpler method. Further, cardiorespiratory fitness must be known and percentage values for lower target HR must be adjusted accordingly; otherwise, as clients gain fitness, their lower target HR would decrease, which is incorrect. Using our previous example, let's explore this concept after the person has considerable training experience and has reduced resting HR to 62 BPM:

Lower target HR = ([(220 − 40) − 62] × .5) + 62
= [(180 − 62) × .5] + 62
= (118 × .5) + 62
= 59 + 62
= 121 BPM

Therefore, if we were to still use 50% HRR as the client's lower HR, we would get only 121 BPM for the lower end of the client's training zone.

In this situation, as the person became more fit, the estimated lower target HR decreased. Thus, to be accurate, we need to increase the percentage of HRR as clients become more fit. In this example, because the client is now well above average fitness, we might choose to use a percentage value of 75% for her lower target HR. Recalculating the HRR equation now using .75 instead of .50, we would get a lower target HR of 151 BPM. Note that this value is significantly higher than the 121 BPM we initially calculated for her lower target. The HRR method must be interpreted with caution unless all the variables are known to be true and the Personal Training Specialist has experience in determining the lower target HR multiplication (percentage) factor based on measured aerobic capacity.

Rating of Perceived Exertion

Many Personal Training Specialists use HR monitors with clients. An HR monitor gives the client immediate, accurate, and continual feedback about exercise intensity. Personal Training Specialists can combine HR monitoring with **rating of perceived exertion (RPE)** to establish an understanding of how their clients' bodies respond to exercise. Research has demonstrated that a person's RPE during exercise, on a 6–20 scale, is closely related to exercise heart rate.

Encourage your clients to communicate with you about intensity throughout the exercise session. They can do this by rating their exertion using a numeric system and descriptive statements. Dr. Gunnar Borg developed a scale for rating perception of physical effort, which can be used to help clients express their level of fatigue during the workout. The original Borg scale has perceived exertion values of 6 through 20 and can be easily compared with the client's heart rate. The average young healthy adult's HR can be approximated by multiplying the person's RPE by a factor of 10. For example, a client's report of being at 11 on the RPE scale corresponds to a heart rate of approximately 110 BPM. Simply adding a zero to the Borg scale figure gives you the corresponding estimated heart rate value. When clients are used to comparing the values, they can become proficient at estimating their heart rate based on their level of exertion.

When your clients are at the target heart rate you have calculated for them and they report a lower or higher value on the RPE scale, then you will know whether their calculated zone is underpredicting or overpredicting their intensity. You may find it easier to accurately assess your clients' rate of perceived exertion using a scale modified to values of 0 through 10 or by simply asking them to describe the way the activity feels in terms of intensity (e.g., light, moderate, hard, and so on). Reevaluating this relationship after training adaptations have occurred is recommended because both heart rate response and perceived exertion will change for a given intensity.

A person's RPE has been shown to be correlated to several physiological markers, but it is not recommended as the primary method of designing exercise intensity (Garber et al., 2011). As a Personal Training Specialist, you can combine the use of HR and RPE to monitor your clients' workout intensity.

Comparing the Methods

The relationships among RPE, percentage of HRmax, percentage of HRR, breathing rate, and energy system involvement are relatively stable across the population. These associations are detailed in table 4.5.

TABLE 4.5 Expressions of Exercise Intensity

RPE (6–20)	Approximate heart rate	%HRR	% HRmax	Predominant energy system	Breathing rate	RPE (0–10)	RPE descriptions	Descriptors
6	60	<20	<45	Aerobic	Normal	0	Nothing at all	All-day pace approaching the intensity of active recovery activities, "Comfortable"
7	70					1	Very easy	
8	80							
9	90					2	Somewhat easy	
10	100	20–39	45–59		Slight increase			
11	110					3	Moderate	
12	120	40–55	60–69		Greater Increase			Tempo or threshold pace, "Comfortably uncomfortable"
13	130					4	Somewhat hard	
14	140	55–80	70–85	Aerobic or anaerobic*	More out of breath			
15	150					5	Hard	
16	160					6		Anaerobic capacity Neuromuscular power "Push," "Go hard"
17	170	>80	>85	Anaerobic	Almost completely out of breath	7	Very hard	
18	180					8		
19	190					9	Very, very hard	
20	200	100	100	Anaerobic (ATP–CP)	Completely out of breath	10	Maximal exertion	

*Fitness-level dependent.

Adapted, by permission, from D. Warburton et al., 2006, Prescribing exercise as preventative therapy, *Canadian Medical Association Journal* 174 (7): 961–974.

Considerations for Cardiorespiratory Exercise Duration

When deciding on the exercise duration for a client's cardiorespiratory training program, consider the following factors:

- **Client's exercise experience**—Beginner clients should start with 10 to 15 minutes of activity and then gradually increase exercise time in small increments (5 minutes) every week until they reach the total goal time.
- **Client's current fitness level**—Beginner clients can start with a manageable amount of activity and add duration toward a goal of 15 to 30 minutes as they adapt to the increased workload.
- **Client's goals for cardiorespiratory conditioning**—More fit clients may exercise between 30 and 60 minutes as desired. Improving cardiorespiratory efficiency requires more than 20 minutes of elevated HR. Weight reduction requires longer exercise time to maximize caloric expenditure.

Time

Exercise time, often also referred to as duration, reflects the length of time that a training stimulus is applied without rest. For example, if you warm up for 10 minutes, jog for 25 minutes, and cool down for 5 minutes, the duration of the cardiorespiratory training is 25 minutes, because that is the amount of time that the body is stressed enough to stimulate an adaptation or improvement in fitness. Although the warm-up and cool-down will have a small effect, it is not enough to be considered actual exercise time.

Exercise time is linked to intensity because the harder the exercise is, the shorter the duration typically is. You must establish a proper combination of intensity and duration to produce fitness gains for clients based on their needs and goals.

canfitpro's *Recommendations on Physical Activity, Nutrition, and Mindset for Optimal Health* suggest a range of exercise duration depending on the effort of the activity. In general, for health benefits to occur, intensity and duration are inversely related—the easier the exercise is, the longer it should last. Research shows that health improves with approximately 20 to 30 minutes of exercise in the target HR zone.

To determine appropriate exercise duration, consider each client's current level of fitness, goals, and needs. To impose overload for positive adaptation, duration can increase as the client becomes more fit. Be aware that as exercise duration increases, the risk of injury also increases. Careful consideration is required when determining proper exercise time.

Type

Exercise type refers to the mode of activity performed. To maximize client success, you must match the activities to the client. An obvious starting point is to choose an activity that the client enjoys or has performed previously with some success. Many people choose not to exercise because they do not find it enjoyable. Your goal is to find fun in all activities for clients; incorporating fun into each workout improves your clients' chances for success.

Different types of equipment and exercises have varying levels of difficulty. Factors that affect exercise difficulty include skill, coordination, and caloric expenditure. Training modes and equipment should be based on the client's current fitness level, fitness experience, goals, and needs. Many clients prefer activities that are continuous in nature, such as walking, swimming, running, stepping, cycling, and skating. Clients can perform many continuous cardiorespiratory activities outdoors or indoors on machines such as treadmills, stair climbers, and cross-trainers. This type of training allows clients to build gradually to steady-state exercise and stay there before cooling down. Activities such as tennis, squash, basketball, in-line skating, skiing, aerobics, step aerobics, and swimming require greater levels of skill and coordination.

The caloric expenditure required to perform an activity is another consideration. The two major factors that affect caloric expenditure are the amount of muscle mass used and the type of movement. As a rule, more muscle mass and more movement (espe-

Considerations for Cardiorespiratory Exercise Type

When deciding on the exercise type for a client's cardiorespiratory training program, consider the following factors:

- **Client's exercise experience**—Beginner clients should start on equipment that requires minimal skill, coordination, and caloric expenditure.

- **Client's current fitness level**—Beginner clients should choose exercises that limit movement in the vertical plane and involve less muscle mass. More conditioned clients can be challenged with equipment and activities that involve complex movements in horizontal and vertical planes.

- **Client's goals for cardiorespiratory conditioning**—Clients working to improve cardiorespiratory conditioning can experiment with many types of exercise equipment. When weight reduction is the goal, clients should perform the type of exercise that maximizes caloric expenditure.

cially in the vertical plane) require more effort. The greater the effort is, the more calories are burned. As a Personal Training Specialist, you should closely examine the exercises you recommend to clients to determine which exercise type is best for maximizing their desired results.

Putting It All Together

Before you design your client's program, he or she should undergo an assessment of cardiorespiratory fitness. One simple test is the Rockport Walking Fitness Test. You simply instruct the client to walk 1,600 metres (1.6 km), which is equal to four laps around a 400-metre track, as quickly as possible and record his or her heart rate and time. You can estimate the client's cardiorespiratory fitness by a simple calculation (found in chapter 9). This test provides a baseline that you can use to track progress and provides some information by which you can set the initial intensity of the program.

When preparing your client's cardiorespiratory training program, you will need to consider all the components of the FITT principle. Research has determined guidelines for the optimal combinations of exercise frequency, intensity, time, and type for general fitness programs (Garber et al., 2011). Table 4.6 provides general guidelines for program development using the FITT acronym for program design (frequency, intensity, time, and type). Each client will respond differently, and keeping communication channels open with clients will allow you to modify programs before problems arise. Figure 4.6 shows the expected fitness improvements as clients

are able to increase their frequency, intensity, and duration of exercise.

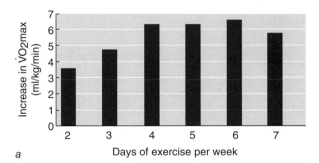

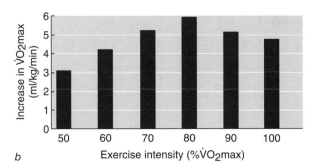

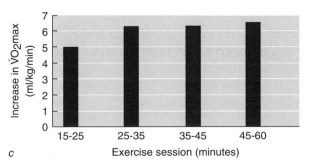

FIGURE 4.6 Fitness improvements with increases in *(a)* frequency, *(b)* intensity, and *(c)* duration.

TABLE 4.6 Cardiorespiratory Training Guidelines

	Client type	Physical activity profile	Possible program focus	Frequency	INTENSITY %HRmax*	HRR*	RPE* (0-10)	Time	Type
Target training zone: beginner	Nonexerciser	No habitual activity and extremely deconditioned	Sedentary	• Improve health profile • Increased energy • ADLs made easier • Weight reduction • Increased endurance	1–4 workouts/week	55–64%	50–85%	2–4	10–30 min	Simple movements that require minimal challenge to balance, stability, and coordination (e.g., walking, stationary cycling, swimming, water aerobics, and basic fitness classes)
	Occasional exerciser	Minimal current exercise and moderately to highly deconditioned	Minimal activity						15–30 min	
Target training zone: intermediate	Recreational exerciser	Suboptimal exercise frequency and mildly to moderately deconditioned	Sporadic physical activity	• Improved health profile • Increased endurance • Improved overall fitness • Weight reduction • Program variety	3–5 workouts/week	65–74%	50–85%	4–6	20–45 min	Any of the previous and movements involving moderate challenge to balance, stability, coordination, and muscular capacity (e.g., stair climbing, treadmill, fitness classes, cycling classes, interval training, cross-training)
Target training zone: advanced	Committed exerciser or athlete	Regular moderate to vigorous activity	Habitual physical activity		3–5 workouts/week	75–90%	50–85%	4–9	20–60 min	Any of the previous and complex movements that challenge multiple components of fitness (e.g., cross- training, interval training, advanced circuits, sport-specific training)
	Dedicated exerciser or elite athlete	Regular vigorous activity	High amounts of physical activity	• Increase $\dot{V}_2$ max • Weight maintenance • Program variety • Sport training						

*The HRmax, HRR, and RPE values listed in this table represent the average intensity for the stated duration of exercise. Note that clients may exceed the recommended range for short periods during a workout, based on their fitness level and the type of cardiorespiratory exercise they are performing. In addition, many less-conditioned clients initially report a higher perceived intensity as they adjust to a new cardiorespiratory program.

When you consider the concepts of bioenergetics (chapter 3) alongside the physiological effects of cardiorespiratory training, you will better understand the process of oxygen delivery and energy production, as outlined in figure 4.7. This information will help you design your clients' cardiorespiratory training sessions. Keeping in mind the various changes that occur during and after exercise, each cardiorespiratory training session should begin with a warm-up (to prepare the body for the increased demands of the training session) and should be followed by a progressive cool-down (to lower the heart rate and redistribute blood flow accordingly). Additional recommendations for warm-up and cool-down are discussed in chapter 11 of this text.

6 The deoxygenated blood is pumped from the right ventricle to the lungs via the pulmonary artery. Carbon dioxide is exhaled and fresh oxygen is supplied to the blood. The cycle begins again. At rest, this cycle of oxygen transfer and energy creation takes about 20 seconds to occur.

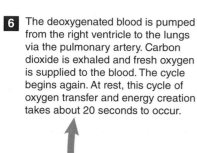

At rest

1 Air is breathed in through the airways to the lung alveoli. A rich supply of oxygen surrounds the alveoli and permits the exchange of oxygen from the lungs to the capillaries. Carbon dioxide is exhaled. Hemoglobin in the red blood cell binds with the oxygen and carries it.

2 The oxygenated blood is carried via the pulmonary vein to the left atrium of the heart. The left ventricle of the heart pumps the oxygenated blood through the aorta to all parts of the body, including the exercising muscles.

5 Carbon dioxide and water are the waste products and are carried away in the blood. Veins carry the deoxygenated blood back to the right atrium of the heart.

3 The oxygenated blood is sent through the arteries, arterioles, and capillaries to the muscle. The oxygen diffuses through the capillaries to the muscle cells. Dissolved nutrients from food are also delivered.

4 The muscle cell breaks down stored glycogen or glucose in the presence of the oxygen to produce ATP (if using aerobic metabolism).

a

---

6 When steady state is reached, oxygen supply meets demand and aerobic metabolism supplies the needed ATP. The faster a person reaches steady-state exercise, the smaller the oxygen deficit. A less fit person takes longer to reach steady state and therefore creates a greater oxygen deficit and must produce more ATP using anaerobic methods. When exercise stops, there is still an elevated oxygen delivery. This extra oxygen is used to help the body recover from anaerobic and aerobic metabolism.

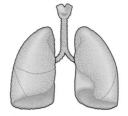

During exercise

1 The respiratory rate and depth of breathing increase. The rate of gas exchange across the alveoli increases. More capillaries open to allow better gas exchange to occur in the lungs. The hemoglobin in the blood is saturated with oxygen.

2 The left atrium of the heart fills to a greater capacity with oxygenated blood. More blood is pumped with each beat (stroke volume) and the heart rate increases, producing a greater output of blood (cardiac output) each minute. Blood pressure rises so that the blood is pumped out of the heart with more force (systolic pressure rises), but the pressure in the heart as it fills stays the same (diastolic pressure stays the same).

5 Exercising muscles force the veins to return the deoxygenated blood to the heart faster.

3 The arterioles and capillaries dilate to carry more blood. Blood is shunted toward areas of need (muscles) and away from areas of low activity.

4 At the muscle cell, the rate of gas exchange increases to deliver more oxygen. But, at the beginning of intense exercise, the cardiovascular and respiratory systems cannot instantaneously increase the delivery of oxygen to the muscles to meet the ATP demands aerobically, so the anaerobic energy systems supply the ATP. The volume of oxygen missing in the first few minutes of exercise is the oxygen deficit.

b

FIGURE 4.7 An overview of oxygen delivery and energy production *(a)* at rest and *(b)* during exercise.

Summary of Main Points

1. The cardiorespiratory system is a transport system for oxygen. It picks up oxygen in the lungs and takes it to cells in the body.

2. Resting HR for the average person is 72 BPM; average resting BP is 120/80 mmHg.

3. At the onset of exercise, the cardiorespiratory system responds to the increased demand for oxygen by increasing HR, stroke volume, and cardiac output.

4. The respiratory system provides oxygen to the body and gets rid of carbon dioxide.

5. At the onset of exercise, the respiratory system provides additional oxygen to the working muscles by rapidly increasing the rate of ventilation (similar to the increase in HR).

6. Aerobic capacity is measured by the amount of oxygen that can be delivered to the muscle cell compared with the amount of oxygen used by the muscle cell to make energy for muscle contraction ($\dot{V}O_2$max).

7. The cellular benefits of cardiorespiratory conditioning include an increase in the number of aerobic enzymes, an increase in the number and size of mitochondria, improved blood delivery, and increased capillary density.

8. The decisions you make in developing thorough cardiorespiratory training programs for clients are crucial.

9. Cardiorespiratory training design should be based on the client's experience, current fitness level, and goals.

10. Follow the FITT formula for cardiorespiratory program design (frequency, intensity, time, and type).

11. Exercise frequency should range from one to five sessions per week.

12. Exercise intensity should range from 55% to 90% of HRmax, or 50% to 85% HRR.

13. Exercise time should range from 10 to 60 minutes per session.

14. Exercise type should match the client's needs.

15. Energy or ATP is produced through anaerobic and aerobic metabolism. When oxygen supply can't meet activity demand, the client reaches the anaerobic threshold and can no longer produce energy aerobically.

16. Recovery is the final phase of cardiorespiratory exercise. Its primary purpose is to assist the body in recovering from exercise and gradually return to pre-exercise state.

Key Concepts for Study

Pulmonary circulation

Systemic circulation

Atrium

Ventricle

Blood pressure (BP)

Cardiac output

Ventilation

Diffusion

$\dot{V}O_2$max

Central training effects

Peripheral training effects

Target heart rate (HR)

Training zone

Review Questions

1. Explain the difference between systolic and diastolic blood pressure.

2. List appropriate program focus areas for a client who is deconditioned and has minimal exercise experience.

3. Stroke volume is the amount of blood _____.

   a. ejected per hour

   b. ejected by the right ventricle per beat

   c. ejected by the left ventricle per beat

   d. ejected per minute

4. Why should the Personal Training Specialist never take the client's pulse with the thumb?

   a. It has a pulse of its own.

   b. It gives too much pressure and will occlude the radial artery.

   c. The thumb should be used only if the client is measuring her or his own pulse.

   d. The other fingers have a stronger pulse than the thumb.

5. Cardiac output is equal to:

   a. SV × HR

   b. SV × BP

   c. BP × HR

   d. HR × BP

6. The value 3.5 ml/kg/min represent the volume of oxygen consumed

   a. at rest

   b. during steady state exercise

   c. during vigorous exercise

   d. during body-weight-supported exercise

7. Which of the following is the most accurate description for the acronym RPE?

   a. rate of physical exertion, the primary method of designing exercise intensity

   b. rate of perceived exertion, the primary method of designing exercise intensity

   c. rate of physical exertion, closely related to the client's heart rate

   d. rate of perceived exertion, closely related to the client's heart rate

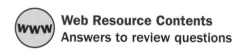

Web Resource Contents
Answers to review questions

5

Skeletal Anatomy

Gregory S. Anderson, PhD

LEARNING OUTCOMES

After completing this chapter, you will be able to

1. list the primary functions of bones;

2. identify the classifications of bones;

3. locate and name major bones in the body;

4. define anatomical position;

5. locate important structures in the body using proper anatomical terms;

6. identify classifications of joints and types of synovial joints;

7. describe joint movement using correct terminology;

8. identify movements that occur in the major joints;

9. understand the role of the core muscles and spinal stabilization system; and

10. describe some of the causes of lower back pain as well as factors involved in maintaining overall health of the back.

The skeletal system consists of a framework of bones and their **articulations** at joints. The study of bones is referred to as **osteology**, and the study of joints is referred to as **arthrology**. Together, the rigid structures of bone and the articulations of these bones at joints work to provide both mechanical and physiological functions.

The skeletal system provides several functions:

- **Support**—supports the weight of the body by providing a framework that allows upright posture
- **Movement**—allows movement by providing a rigid lever system for muscle attachment across joints
- **Protection**—protects vital organs and soft tissue with bony encasements
- **Mineral deposit**—stores required minerals in the body and maintains mineral balance in the blood
- **Blood cell formation**—forms red blood cells within the red bone marrow of the long bones
- **Energy reservoir**—stores energy in the form of fat in the yellow bone marrow and adipose tissue

Bones

Bones play an important role in movement by providing a series of independently movable levers that the muscles can pull to move various parts of the body. But the skeleton is not just a movable frame. The human body needs bones to stand as well as create movement.

The average human adult skeleton has 206 bones (with variability in the fused vertebra that make up the "tailbone"). Babies are born with 270 soft bones, but many of these fuse together by about age 25 into the 206 hard, permanent bones of the adult skeleton (see figure 5.1). Bones are living tissue that grows, changes, and adapts just like any other tissue in the body. Bones are 50% fluid and 50% solid. Minerals make them rigid, and protein makes them strong.

In children, for example, bones grow in length and diameter; then, as we age, mineral density declines and our bones become more brittle.

In infants and very young children, the long bones in the body are primarily cartilage, which allows them to be flexible and pliable. As the child grows, the cartilage cells divide and enlarge, allowing large increases in bone length, seen as increases in height. After the cartilage cells develop, they die, and the space is invaded by bone-building material. Thus, the process of ossification, or laying down of the bone mineral, occurs as the human skeleton matures from childhood to adulthood. Full ossification ends between the ages of 16 and 25 years old.

The hard mineral component of the bone is a combination of mineral and salts, such as calcium and phosphate. This component of bone, referred to as the inorganic component, provides bony strength for compressive forces, such as those produced while standing. But without the softer, more pliable component, the bone would break easily. This softer component, the organic component, is made up of living cells, fibers, and a sticky protein substance within the extracellular matrix. This organic component gives the bone flexibility and tensile strength to resist pulling and shearing forces. The rest of the bone is water.

Bones in the body can be grouped into categories based on appearance (table 5.1). Long bones, which are longer than they are wide, are found in the arms and legs. They act as long levers that the muscles pull on to produce large movements. Short bones are roughly cube-like, such as the bones in the wrist and ankle. These bones offer a great deal of stability, strength, and shock absorption and typically allow movement in many directions. Flat bones are broad, thin layers of bone such as those of the skull or sternum that offer protection to vital organs, but little motion, as well as bones such as the ribs and scapula, which provide protection and a broad site of muscular attachment. Irregular bones, such as the vertebrae, do not fit any other description. The vertebrae make up the spine—the long, weight-bearing pillar that supports the body's mass in an upright position and functions as a site for muscle attachment and shock absorbers.

Parts of the Skeleton

Structurally, the human adult skeleton consists of 206 bones divided into the **axial skeleton** and **appendicular skeleton** (figure 5.2). The axial skeleton includes the skull, spine, ribs, and sternum (breastbone) and consists of 80 bones. It provides the longitudinal axis of the trunk to which the limbs attach, and it protects the vital organs of the body.

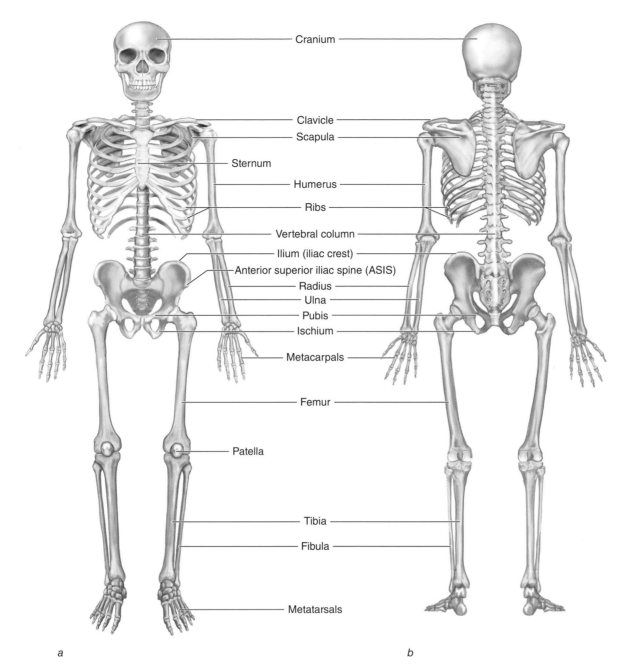

a   b

FIGURE 5.1   The human skeleton with its *(a)* anterior and *(b)* posterior views.

TABLE 5.1   Classifications of Bones

Classification	Examples	Function
Long bones	Femur Humerus	Serve as levers for movement
Short bones	Tarsals (ankle) Carpals (wrist)	Give strength to joints but with limited mobility
Flat bones	Ribs Scapulae	Provide a broad site for muscle attachment, protect internal organs
Irregular bones	Ischium Pubis Vertebrae	Protect internal organs, support the body

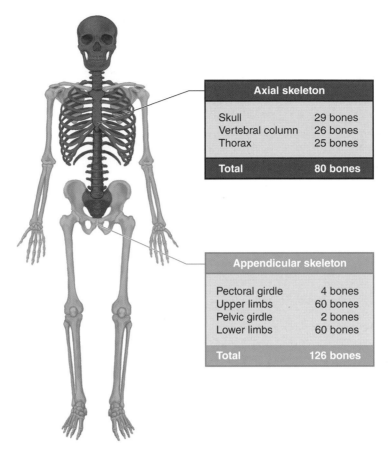

Axial skeleton	
Skull	29 bones
Vertebral column	26 bones
Thorax	25 bones
Total	**80 bones**

Appendicular skeleton	
Pectoral girdle	4 bones
Upper limbs	60 bones
Pelvic girdle	2 bones
Lower limbs	60 bones
Total	**126 bones**

FIGURE 5.2   The axial and appendicular skeletons.

The appendicular skeleton includes the bones of the appendages (i.e., upper and lower limbs) and the bony girdles to which they attach (the shoulders and pelvis). This part of the skeletal system contains 126 bones: 64 in the shoulders and upper limbs and 62 in the pelvis and lower limbs.

Joints

The bones of the skeleton are held together at joints. Different joints allow different types of movement, and they are classified into groups according to their structure. There are three classifications of joints: fibrous, **cartilaginous**, and **synovial**. Joint capsules and ligaments are forms of fibrous connective tissue that support the articulations between bones at joints. The joint capsule of synovial joints holds the bones together and is filled with synovial fluid. **Ligaments** are tough, short bands of fibrous connective tissue composed mainly of long, stringy collagen molecules. Ligaments connect bones to other bones,

holding them together in an articulation, and they are much stronger than the joint capsules. When the ligaments are damaged, the injuries are referred to as sprains.

Fibrous Joints

Fibrous joints connect bones to one another with fibrous connective tissue and allow very little, if any, movement. The bones of the skull and pelvis are held together by fibrous joints. The long bones of the forearm (radius and ulna) are also held in relation to one another through fibrous tissue.

Cartilaginous Joints

Cartilaginous joints are ones in which the bones are separated by cartilage. These joints allow for a little or no movement, and they are found in areas of the body where protection, stability, and strength are required, such as between the ribs and sternum, and between the vertebrae.

Synovial Joints

Synovial joints allow much more movement than cartilaginous joints do. These freely movable joints have cartilage along the surfaces where bones join to reduce friction and absorb shock. They are also enclosed by an articular capsule that holds synovial fluid (a lubricating fluid produced by the synovial membrane) inside the joint cavity. The six types of synovial joints provide various amounts of movement. The three most common types of synovial joints you need to be familiar with as a Personal Training Specialist are the hinge, condyloid, and ball-and-socket joints. The six types of synovial joints are described in table 5.2.

 Most of the movements of the limbs are movements of synovial joints. Knowing the range of motion of each joint will help you to understand your clients' movements and identify restrictions in their mobility.

Describing Movement

The skeleton and joints define the shape and basic movements of the human body. Researchers, Personal Training Specialists, and other professionals who deal with movement should know the standard terms for describing parts of the body and their movements.

The point of reference used to describe body parts or movements is called the anatomical position. The anatomical position is one in which a person stands with arms at the sides and palms facing forward. From this position, parts of the body can be described in relation to one another, and movement can be described using standard terms. The three cardinal **planes of movement** shown in figure 5.3

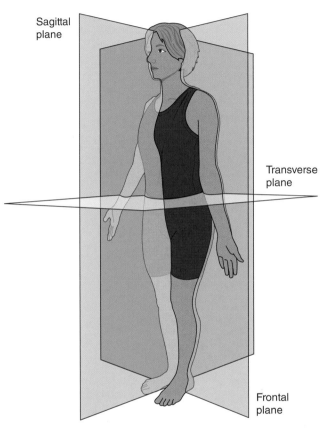

FIGURE 5.3 The sagittal, frontal, and transverse planes are used to provide standardized descriptions of body movements.

TABLE 5.2 Six Types of Synovial Joints

Type	Movement	Examples
Gliding	Allows minimal movement in one plane, with rotation	Bones within the wrist and ankle (carpals and tarsals)
Pivot	Allows rotation along a long axis	The radius and ulna (at the elbow) allowing pronation and supination of the forearm
Hinge	Allows movement in one direction or plane of motion	Elbow and knee joints, allowing flexion and extension
Condyloid	Allows movement in two directions or planes of motion	The "knuckles" in each finger and in the wrist and ankle
Saddle	Allows movement in several directions similar to but greater than condyloid joints	The thumb moving in various directions
Ball and socket	Allows movement in three directions or planes of motion	The shoulder and hip joints allowing free movement in all directions (circumduction) with large ranges of motion

provide a reference point to understand the three dimensions of movement in the body. The **frontal plane** divides the anterior and posterior aspects of the body. It is the dominant plane for movements such as adduction and abduction (as seen in a lateral arm raise exercise). The right and left sides of the body are divided by the **sagittal plane**, which corresponds with movements involving flexion and extension (e.g., squat). The third plane is the **transverse** (horizontal) **plane**. It divides the superior and inferior parts of the body. Movements in this plane typically involve twisting or rotation.

Spatial Terminology

Spatial terms describe the relationship between two structures. True anatomical terms do not change with movement (i.e., distal), although some lay terms may (i.e., medial). For example, when a person stands in the anatomical position and places the hand on the heart, the hand is medial to the elbow, although it remains distal (farther from the torso in the chain). The following terms are used to describe the position of body parts during both static posture and movement.

- **Anterior and posterior**—Anterior describes the front of the body; posterior describes the back of the body.
- **Medial and lateral**—Body parts that are closer to the midline of the body are medial; parts that are away from the midline of the body are lateral.
- **Superior and inferior**—When one body part is above another, it is superior; when one body part is below another, it is inferior.
- **Supine and prone**—When the body lies face up, it is supine; when the body lies facedown, it is prone.
- **Dorsal and plantar**—The top of the foot is referred to as the dorsal surface; the bottom of the foot is called the plantar surface.
- **Proximal and distal**—The end of a bone or muscle that is closer to the midline of the body (torso) is called the proximal end; the end that is farther from the body is called the distal end.

Joint Movement Terminology

To describe movement at a joint, we use specific terminology to identify the direction in which the movement occurs. These terms are used throughout the text, so you need to become familiar with them. Table 5.3 gives an overview of the joint movements allowed by each of the major joints of the body.

- **Flexion, extension, and hyperextension**—Bending a joint is called flexion (i.e., the joint angle decreases). Straightening a joint is called extension (i.e., the joint angle increases). Movement that occurs beyond the normal joint range of motion (ROM) is called hyperextension, or hyperflexion.
- **Abduction (protraction) and adduction (retraction)**—Abduction occurs when a bone moves away from the midline of the body. Bringing the bone toward the midline of the body is called adduction of the joint.
- **Circumduction**—Circumduction is a circular movement that combines flexion, abduction, extension, and adduction. This type of movement occurs at ball-and-socket joints.
- **Elevation and depression**—Typically, elevation is produced by shrugging the shoulders upward (scapular elevation), whereas depression is produced by lowering the shoulders below anatomical position (scapular depression).
- **Medial and lateral rotation**—To rotate a joint, the moving bone is turned about its axis or centre. Rotation toward the midline of the body is called medial (or internal) rotation. Rotation away from the midline of the body is called lateral (or external) rotation.
- **Supination and pronation**—These movements occur primarily at the forearms. External movement, or movement away from the midline of the body, is called supination (e.g., turning the forearm externally so that the palm faces up). Internal movement, or movement toward the midline of the body, is called pronation (e.g., turning the forearm internally so that the palm faces backwards from anatomical position).

TABLE 5.3   Summary of Movements Allowed by Major Joints

Joint	Movements
Shoulder girdle (scapula, clavicle)	Elevation–depression
	Abduction (protraction)–adduction (retraction)
	Upward rotation–downward rotation
Shoulder joint	Flexion–extension
	Abduction–adduction
	Medial rotation–lateral rotation
	Transverse flexion or horizontal adduction–transverse extension or horizontal abduction (flexion or extension along the transverse plane)
	Circumduction
Elbow joint	Flexion–extension
Radioulnar joint	Pronation–supination
Wrist joint	Flexion–extension
	Radial flexion (deviation)–ulnar flexion (deviation)
Vertebral column Spine	Flexion–extension
	Lateral flexion
	Rotation
Lumbosacral joint	Flexion–extension (anterior pelvic tilt–posterior pelvic tilt)
Hip joint	Flexion–extension
	Abduction–adduction
	Medial–lateral rotation
	Circumduction
Knee joint	Flexion–extension
	Rotation (only at 90° flexion)
Ankle joint	Plantar flexion–dorsiflexion
	Eversion–inversion

- **Inversion and eversion** (sometimes referred to as supination and pronation)—These movements occur at the ankle joint. Turning the medial, or inner, side of the foot off the ground toward the midline is called inversion. Turning the outer side off the ground away from the midline is called eversion.

The movements of each joint and the muscles that work to create those movements are discussed in detail in chapter 6. Familiarize yourself with table 5.3, and refer to it as you read chapter 6, to build your understanding of the movements of muscles and joints throughout the body.

- **Dorsiflexion and plantar flexion**—These movements also occur at the ankle joint. Flexing the foot upward so that the toes point toward the head is called dorsiflexion. Flexing the foot so that the toes point downward is called plantar flexion.

Program Design for Bone Health

When designing exercise programs for your clients, you want to keep in mind the ways in which physical activity relates to the overall health of their bones and joints. Two particular considerations are your clients' bone density and back health. Bone density is maintained through weight-bearing activities, which are especially important for older adults or those at risk of developing osteoporosis. This topic is covered in detail in training guidelines for the older adult population. Back pain, however, is something that you may often encounter with clients, regardless of age. The remainder of this section outlines possible causes of back pain and general guidelines that you can share with your clients to help prevent or reduce its occurrence.

Back Health

The spine consists of four major sections: the cervical spine (neck), thoracic spine (upper back), lumbar spine (lower back), and sacral spine (bottom of the spine). At the very bottom of the spine is an additional section, the coccygeal spine, which is typically referred to as the tailbone (figure 5.4). Given that the spine is a commonly injured part of the skeletal system, Personal Training Specialists need to take care to protect it when planning and coaching exercise sessions. Key to protecting the spine is understanding the role of the core muscles in all movement. The core of the body spans the rib cage to the pelvis. The core is important in load carriage and spinal nerve root protection, and it provides the foundation from which forces are transmitted from the lower body to the upper body and vice versa. Proper functioning of the core is provided through various stabilization mechanisms, and the term *core stability* is often used. Core stability can be thought of as having passive, active, and control subsystems. The passive subsystem involves the bones and ligaments within the **spinal column**, whereas the active subsystem is related to the muscles that act on the spine. The control subsystem is managed by the nervous system. All three components of this **spinal stabilization system** must work in unison for proper function and lower back health (figure 5.5).

Lower Back Pain

Lower back pain is defined as pain localized between the rib cage and the buttocks, commonly occurring in the lower lumbar area. At some point in their lifetime, at least three-quarters of the population will experience lower back pain to a level that prevents them from performing some of their daily tasks. In fact, lower back pain is one of the most frequent chronic concerns seen by family

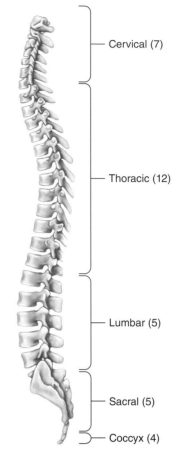

FIGURE 5.4 Anatomy of the spine, showing the cervical, thoracic, lumbar, sacral, and coccygeal vertebrae.

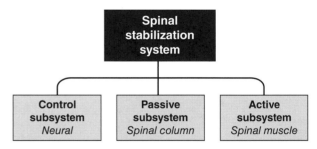

FIGURE 5.5 Spinal stabilization subsystems.

physicians and one of the most common reasons for surgical procedures in North America. The direct treatment cost for lower back pain exceeds $100 billion annually in North America, and the loss of time from work and reduced productivity (indirect costs) are in excess of $35 billion. Lower back pain is not only a personal health concern but also an economic burden to society, so it is an important area for Personal Training Specialists to understand when working with clients.

The causes of lower back pain are usually documented as strain, overexertion, and irregular or unsafe performance of movements such as lifting, twisting, turning, bending, pushing, and pulling. These examples reflect dysfunction in both the active (muscular) subsystem and the passive subsystem (joints). The most common causes of back pain that originate from the passive stabilization subsystem include herniated disks, disk degeneration, facet joint inflammation, and ligament damage. Throughout the course of daily activity, the low back system is subjected to loading from external forces (such as gravity and loads we carry) and from forces produced by the internal tissues that create movement and maintain posture. The **intervertebral discs** are the major weight-bearing component of forces through the trunk. When damaged, they can bulge and apply pressure on a spinal nerve (causing referred pain). The most common area where your clients may experience pain from a protruding disc is the lower lumbar spine, which results in pain radiating down the sciatic nerve (sciatica). Depending on whether the protrusion is in the anterior or posterior direction, either forward flexion or extension could cause increased pain.

More than three-quarters of the people who experience lower back pain have no specific diagnosis for the origin of their pain, so it is difficult to provide generic training programs for back health for those who already have pain. Each person may have different movements that exacerbate the pain, so no specific exercises are good for all potential causes of lower back pain. As a Personal Training Specialist, you should refer your clients to a reha-bilitative, medical, or appropriately qualified fitness professional if they are experiencing back pain that prevents them from completing the exercises you have selected for them. In this way, you can get specific instructions on what will be best for your clients' individualized exercise programs.

General Precautions

Even when working with clients who do not currently have lower back pain, you can help prevent its future occurrence by paying close attention to their posture, alignment, and form during each exercise and by including activities that help them strengthen the spinal stabilization system. Good posture involves a balance between flexion and extension. In this balanced position, the discs, spinal facet joints, ligaments, and muscles are under the least amount of stress. In contrast, excessive flexion puts continuous stress on the disc, leading to chronic repetitive trauma that ends in damage. Extreme extension increases the wear and tear of the facet joints.

Several activities that your clients perform daily can put their lower backs at risk. Simple behavioural changes may protect general back health during workouts and in the activities of daily life. For example, when standing, work should be kept at a proper height. Work that is too low increases disc loading, and work that is too high can strain the joints in the back. During prolonged standing, placing one foot on a bar or low stool occasionally and changing position can relieve possible strain on the back. For lifting, the low back should be in slight extension and the load should be close to the body to distribute it equally between disc and facet joint in a balanced way. Doing this may be easier with the knees slightly bent. Many health professionals believe that the combination of twisting with flexion is harmful to both facet and disc. Pivoting is preferable to twisting, and sudden jerky movements should be avoided. These guidelines are important to consider during your training sessions and in your clients' daily life. Additional recommendations for general maintenance of back health are given in table 5.4.

No general exercises can be recommended for all clients who experience back pain. A training program for a client with back pain must be individualized to avoid exacerbating the pain. The program should be coordinated as appropriate with rehabilitative, medical, or otherwise qualified exercise professionals.

TABLE 5.4   General Back Health Recommendations

Activity	Do	Do not
Sitting	• Avoid prolonged static posture by taking frequent minibreaks by standing up or walking • Sit with the lower back in either a neutral or slightly flexed position • Sit fully back in the chair using the back support • Relax the leg muscles and allow the chair to support the weight of the legs	• Sit forward on the edge of the chair • Place a pillow or rolled towel in the lumbar spine • Cross the legs at thigh level while sitting
Walking	• Keep the hips as level as possible • Move the feet to turn the body rather than twist the trunk	• Swing the hips from side to side • Bring the arms across the body when walking • Lean forward or back
Forward bending	• Contract the abdominals to support the spine in a neutral or slightly flexed alignment • Flex and extend at the hip, not the lumbar spine	• Arch the lower back when returning to the upright position
Overhead and cross-body reaching	• Contract the abdominals to support the spine in neutral alignment when moving the arms • Whenever possible, stand directly in front of an item before reaching to reduce the combination of effort and twisting	• Arch the lower back when reaching overhead • Twist the lower back when reaching across body

Summary of Main Points

1. Bones protect the internal organs and provide the body with structure and the ability to move.

2. Bones are divided into four classifications: long, short, flat, and irregular.

3. In the anatomical position, the body is erect, the arms are at the sides, and the palms are facing forward.

4. The axial skeleton consists of the head, trunk, and vertebrae. The appendicular skeleton consists of the appendages (i.e., upper and lower limbs) and the pelvis.

5. Joints are classified by the amount of movement they allow. The three types of joints (fibrous, cartilaginous, and synovial) differ in the amount of movement they can create.

6. The three most common types of synovial joints referred to in fitness are the hinge, condyloid, and ball-and-socket joints.

7. Ligaments connect bone to bone within a joint.

8. Various terms are used to describe body position and joint movement.

9. The big picture of human movement is described by the possible movements that can occur at each joint and the muscles that produce those movements.

10. Lower back pain is a common condition, but the causes may be diverse and difficult to determine. Prevention of lower back pain starts with good posture and safe movement habits.

Key Concepts for Study

Axial skeleton	Plantar	Protraction
Anatomical position	Distal	Retraction
Appendicular skeleton	Proximal	Circumduction
Synovial joints	Supine	Elevation
Flexibility	Prone	Depression
Anterior	Supination	Medial rotation
Posterior	Pronation	Lateral rotation
Medial	Flexion	Inversion
Lateral	Extension	Eversion
Inferior	Hyperextension	Dorsiflexion
Superior	Abduction	Plantar flexion
Dorsal	Adduction	Spinal stabilization system

Review Questions

1. List the four classifications of bones and give an example of each classification.

2. Define the following anatomical terms and provide the term used to identify the opposite: anterior, medial, inferior, distal, supine, supination, flexion, abduction.

3. The skeleton provides all the following essential functions *except*

   a. protection of the vital organs and soft tissue

   b. production of red blood cells

   c. storage for minerals (calcium and phosphate)

   d. attachments for organs and blood vessels

4. The adult human body contains approximately _____ bones, most of which are found in the _____ skeleton.

   a. 270; appendicular

   b. 206; appendicular

   c. 175; axial

   d. 230; axial

5. What are the three categories of joints?

   a. fibrous, cartilaginous, and synovial

   b. fibrous, synovial, and condyloid

   c. cartilaginous, synovial, and syndesmoses

   d. cartilaginous, synovial, and hinge

6. True or false: Ligaments are bands of connective tissue that connect muscles to bones to allow movement of the skeletal joints.

   a. true

   b. false

7. What components are involved in the spinal stabilization system?

   a. active subsystem and control subsystem

   b. control subsystem, passive subsystem, active subsystem

   c. active subsystem, passive subsystem, central subsystem

   d. passive subsystem and central subsystem

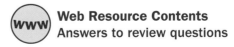

Web Resource Contents
Answers to review questions

Muscular Anatomy

Gregory S. Anderson, PhD

LEARNING OUTCOMES

After completing this chapter, you will be able to

1. identify the major muscles;

2. identify the origins and insertions of the major muscles;

3. list and locate major muscle pairs;

4. describe the structure of skeletal muscle;

5. describe the sliding filament theory of muscular contraction;

6. define types of muscle fibers and list their characteristics;

7. differentiate among types of muscle contractions;

8. describe the basic organization of the nervous system and its role in muscular contraction;

9. name the muscles that produce all possible movements in the major joints;

10. understand the role of the core muscles in the body; and

11. identify basic differences in developing resistance training programs based on clients' activity level and program goals.

The scientific study of the muscular system and muscle tissue is known as **myology**. Muscle tissue is a highly specialized grouping of cells that has four unique characteristics: excitability, contractility, extensibility, and **elasticity**.

- Excitability is the ability of the muscle tissue to carry an electrical impulse called an action potential, which initiates the muscle contraction.
- Contractility refers to the response of the muscle cell to the electrical impulse. The muscle cell responds by shortening, pulling the two ends of the muscle toward each other.
- Extensibility allows the muscle to be lengthened without damaging the tissue.
- Elasticity allows the muscle to return to its resting length after being either shortened or lengthened.

The human body contains three distinct types of muscle tissue: skeletal muscle, cardiac muscle, and smooth muscle. Each type exhibits the four characteristics of muscle outlined earlier, but each also has a unique structure and function (table 6.1). Skeletal muscle is typically connected to the skeletal system by being attached to two bones across a joint. These muscles produce the forces required for human movement. Each muscle cell has to be stimulated to contract separately, so skeletal muscles are highly controlled. Cardiac muscle cells are interconnected so that when one cell is stimulated to contract, they all contract in a predictable sequence, allowing the heart to pump blood to the tissues. Smooth muscle is found in hollow organs of the digestive, urinary, and circulatory systems. The smooth muscle cells may work as a collective or independently, but their structure does not allow much force to be generated when contracting.

Of these three types of muscle tissue, skeletal muscle is the focus of this chapter. It carries out voluntary movements and is the primary type of muscle you will have your clients train with resistance exercises.

Structure and Function of Skeletal Muscle

The human body contains over 600 individual skeletal muscles, making up about 23% of a woman's body weight and about 40% of a man's body weight. In fact, skeletal muscle is the most abundant tissue in the body.

Skeletal muscle functions to provide the force for human movement, to maintain upright posture, and to generate heat used to maintain constant body temperature. All these functions are related to the ability of the muscular system to convert chemical energy (ATP) into mechanical energy to generate force, perform work, and produce movement.

Muscle cells are primarily water (73%), a well-organized set of proteins (24%), and a limited amount of inorganic salts (such as sodium, potassium, calcium, and chloride). Each skeletal muscle consists of thousands of elongated, rod-shaped cells called **muscle fibers**. Muscle fibers are grouped into bundles of 10 to 150 fibers. A bundle is referred to as a fascicle and is held together by another connective tissue layer called the perimysium. Groups of fasci-

TABLE 6.1   Three Types of Muscle Tissue

Characteristic	Skeletal	Cardiac	Smooth
Location	Attached to bones	Walls of the heart	Walls of the hollow organs such as the stomach, intestines, bladder, and blood vessels
Cell shape and appearance	Single long cylindrical cells with a striated or banded appearance	Branched chains of cylindrical cells with striations or bands	Irregularly shaped, thin cells with no striations or bands
Regulation of contraction	Voluntary (can be consciously controlled)	Involuntary (cannot be consciously controlled)	Involuntary (cannot be consciously controlled)
Arrangement of contractile proteins	Regular, in parallel	Regular, in parallel	Irregular, random
Force production	Along the length of the cell	Along the length of the cell	In all directions equally

cles that make up an entire muscle are held together by the epimysium, which is the shiny outer layer of connective tissue surrounding the muscle (figure 6.1a). All these layers of connective tissue amalgamate at the ends of the muscle and form the tendon of the muscle, which attaches to the bone. The tendons and connective tissue within and around the muscles that lead into them are components of the overall fascial tissue of the body. This fascial tissue is a large contributor to your clients' flexibility.

Each muscle fiber is surrounded by a thin elastic membrane called the sarcolemma that encloses the contents of the fiber. Within the sarcolemma are contractile protein, enzymes, fat and glycogen particles, the nuclei, and various specialized cell organelles. Covering the sarcolemma is a fine sheath of connec-

tive tissue known as the endomysium, which wraps individual fibers, separating them from the adjacent muscle cells. This covering allows each fiber to be independent from adjacent ones and not influenced by the contraction of adjacent muscle cells. Figure 6.1 shows the structures within a skeletal muscle and within an individual muscle fiber.

Each muscle fiber is packed full of thinner fibers called myofibrils, a smaller structural component that runs the length of the muscle. Each myofibril is composed of a long series of **sarcomeres**, which are the basic unit of muscle contraction. Each sarcomere comprises two types of protein: a thin filament called actin and a thick filament called myosin (figure 6.1c). These protein filaments slide along each other when a muscle contracts.

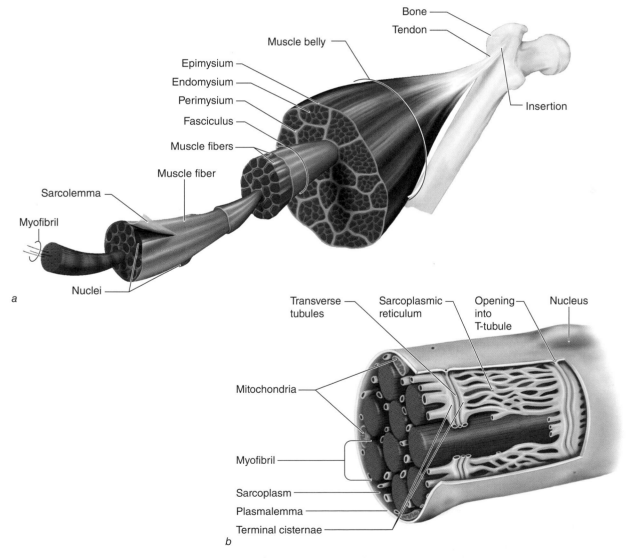

FIGURE 6.1   Levels of organization within a skeletal muscle: *(a)* skeletal muscle, *(b)* muscle fiber, and *(c)* sarcomere.

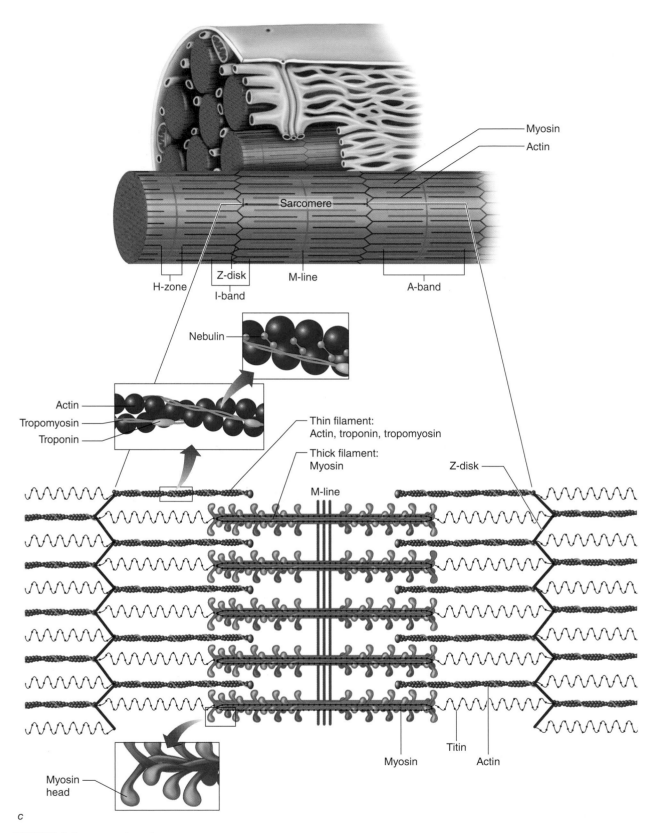

FIGURE 6.1 > *continued*

Muscle Contraction

As explained earlier, each muscle cell contains organized packages of contractile protein known as myofibrils. The individual myofilament protein strands within the myofibrils (such as actin and myosin) are organized longitudinally along the length of the muscle cell and interact to allow muscle contraction.

In a relaxed muscle, myosin and actin myofilaments have some overlap so that they can interact. When the muscle cell is stimulated by a nerve impulse, the thick filaments (myosin) pull on thin filaments (actin), causing them to slide past each other until they completely overlap, pulling the ends of the sarcomere closer together. This process is known as the sliding filament theory of muscle contraction. As the cell shortens, the muscle contracts but the contractile proteins do not change in size or shape. The force of this contraction is transmitted directly from the muscle to the tendon and on to the bone. For the muscle to shorten, its cells must convert energy (ATP) into mechanical work (contraction). Relaxation of the muscle tissue occurs when the myosin and actin return to their unbound state. Figure 6.2 demonstrates the movement of the actin over the myosin during contraction.

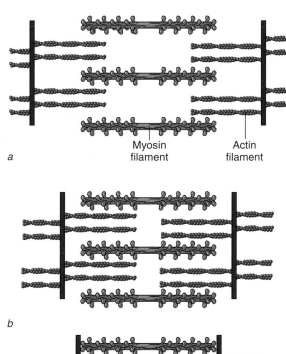

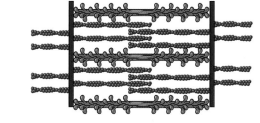

FIGURE 6.2 Sliding filament theory with a muscle fiber *(a)* relaxed, *(b)* contracting, and *(c)* fully contracted.

Types of Muscle Contractions

When muscles produce movement, they contract and relax. The term used to describe contraction in which the muscle shortens is **concentric contraction**, and the term used to describe a force exerted by a muscle as it lengthens is **eccentric contraction**. A third term used is isometric action, in which the muscle stays contracted at the joint angle where the client stops moving. The resulting movements are based on the response of the muscle, as described in table 6.2.

Basic Organization of the Nervous System

Skeletal muscle contractions are controlled by the nervous system, requiring neural input from the brain to initiate a contraction. For this reason, skeletal muscle is classed as voluntary muscle, typically contracting only in response to a conscious decision

TABLE 6.2   Three Types of Muscle Contractions

Type of action	Description	Examples
Isotonic—concentric	Movement occurs when the muscle contracts with enough force to shorten.	Lifting phase of a biceps curl
Isotonic—eccentric	The muscle generates tension as it lengthens (e.g., like a braking mechanism).	Lowering phase of a biceps curl
Isometric	In this static contraction, the muscle exerts force to counteract an opposing force; no change in muscle length occurs.	Holding the arm at a fixed angle of 90° with resistance in the hand

to initiate a contraction. This decision from the brain is passed into the peripheral nervous system, moving through a single neuron from the level of the spinal cord to the muscle fiber itself.

The nervous system is divided into two parts: the **central nervous system** (CNS) and the **peripheral nervous system** (PNS). The CNS is composed of the brain and spinal cord and is enclosed by the skull and spinal column. It is the control centre of the nervous system because it receives information from the PNS and develops an appropriate response. The PNS is made up of nerves that connect the extremities to the CNS. It continuously delivers information about all body parts to the brain for processing.

Nerve signals are transported in the body by neurons, or nerve cells. There are two kinds of neurons: sensory and motor. Sensory neurons carry information and sensations from the body and environment to the CNS. Motor neurons carry information from the CNS back to the muscles to create a response or movement.

Each muscle has several neurons that lie within the body of the muscle. Some of these motor neurons activate only a few muscle fibers (e.g., in the muscles of the hands where fine motor control and dexterity are required), whereas other motor neurons may activate hundreds of fibers (e.g., in muscles of the thigh where the movements are larger and less refined). A single neuron together with the fibers that it commands is called a **motor unit** (figure 6.3). When the neuron is stimulated, all the associated muscle fibers create tension (the all-or-none law). Thus, motor units consisting of many muscle fibers produce strong contractions, and motor units with only a few muscle fibers produce weaker contractions.

Proprioceptors are specialized sensory receptors found in joints, muscles, and tendons. They are sensitive to pressure and tension and are responsible for sending messages to the CNS to maintain muscle tone and perform coordinated movements. **Muscle spindles** are a type of proprioceptor that consists of several modified muscle fibers enclosed in a blanket of connective tissue. These spindles provide information about the length of a muscle fiber and the rate of change in its length. Spindles tell the muscle how much it needs to contract to overcome a given stretch.

Golgi tendon organs (GTO) are proprioceptors located within tendons. GTOs are activated when

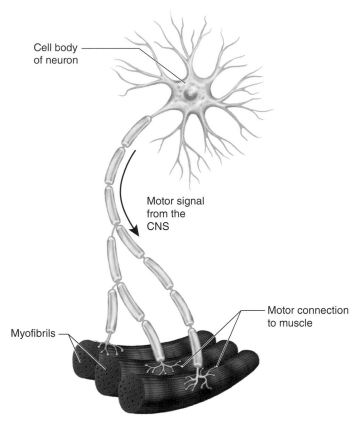

FIGURE 6.3   A motor unit, consisting of a motor neuron and the muscle fibers it innervates.

the tendon attached to an active muscle is stretched. They function similarly to the muscle spindles in that they also measure changes in the muscle. But whereas the muscle spindle is active even while the muscle is at rest, the GTO becomes activated only when the muscle contracts. Further, GTOs are concerned not with changes in muscle length but with the increased tension of the muscle because of a change in its length. GTOs are high-threshold, slow-adapting receptors and apparently serve, at least in part, to prevent excessive stresses at joints. If the strain on the muscle and tendon becomes excessive, the GTO sends an impulse to the CNS, causing the muscle to relax, theoretically preventing injury.

Muscle Fiber Types

Motor units are classified according to the physiological and mechanical properties of the muscle cells innervated, including their twitch speed, resistance to fatigue, and maximum amount of tension created during a contraction. Although all fibers within a motor unit function in a similar manner, there are differences among motor units related to the types of muscle fiber being recruited.

Skeletal muscle can be classified according to its fiber type. In basic terms, fibers can be distinguished as either **slow twitch** or **fast twitch**. Slow-twitch fibers are best suited for endurance work because they have greater ability to use oxygen and resist fatigue. Slow-twitch fibers have the following characteristics:

- Contain a higher amount of mitochondria compared with fast-twitch fibers
- Contract slowly and produce a smaller amount of force than fast-twitch fibers but are resistant to fatigue
- Work aerobically, for the most part

In contrast, exercise that requires short, intense bursts of activity uses fast-twitch fibers. Fast-twitch fibers have the following characteristics:

- Have the ability to produce and use ATP more quickly
- Contract quickly and produce a great deal of force but fatigue quickly
- Work anaerobically, for the most part

All muscles have a combination of these fiber types, but the percentage of fiber types in each muscle varies according to the function of the muscle, training, and genetics. During exercise, the nervous system generally recruits slow-twitch fibers first. As muscle contractions become more intense, fast-twitch fibers are added.

Factors Related to Strength

Strength is not as simple as the idea that bigger muscles are stronger muscles. Several factors play a role in the ability of a muscle or muscle group to generate force (strength):

- **Muscle size**—The force that a muscle can generate is related to its size.
- **Muscle length**—A muscle has the potential to generate its greatest force when it is at its resting length because the actin and myosin filaments lie next to each other and all potential cross-bridges are exposed. As the muscle shortens and filaments slide past each other, some of the cross-bridges become fully covered, reducing the amount of additional force that the muscle can generate.

- **Speed of contraction**—For concentric muscle actions, maximal force can be achieved with slower contractions, whereas eccentric muscle actions produce more force with faster movements.
- **Neural control**—Muscle force is generally greater when
  - more motor units are involved in a contraction,
  - the motor units are bigger in size, and
  - the rate at which the motor units fire is faster.

Personal Training Specialists should note that most of the gains made in the first few weeks of a resistance training program can be attributed to neuromuscular adaptation as the brain learns how to tell the muscles to generate more force. As clients continue to train consistently, the rate at which their neuromuscular gains occur will slowly diminish, but hypertrophic gains (increase in the size of the muscle) will contribute to their strength gains. The amount of increased strength will depend on multiple factors, including frequency of training and recovery, nutrition, and genetic potential.

 Muscle size is not the only factor in strength. Position and type of movement, as well as neural control of the muscle, also affect strength. In beginning exercisers, most of the early strength gains are the result of improved activation of muscle by the nervous system.

Muscles and Muscle Groups

We have examined the different muscle fiber types, the way that a muscle produces a contraction, and the role that the nervous system plays in coordinated movement. Now we can move back to the macroscopic level and look closer at how muscles and muscle groups work together to produce movement. To understand how to produce and perfect human movement, we study the science of anatomy in action, also known as *kinesiology*.

Movement occurs when muscles, bones, and joints work together to set the body (or a body part) in motion. Skeletal muscles produce movement by exerting force on tendons, which then pull on bones to cause motion at the joint. Most muscles cross a joint and attach to the articulating bones that form the joint. The attachment of the muscle tendon to the stationary bone is called the *origin* of the muscle. The attachment of the muscle tendon to the moving bone is called the *insertion* of the muscle. In limbs, the origin is usually on the proximal bone and the insertion is usually on the more distal bone. When a muscle contracts, it pulls its insertion toward its origin. The fleshy portion of the muscle between the origin and insertion is referred to as the *muscle belly.*

As mentioned earlier, the human body has some 600 muscles, many of which are located in the head, hands, and feet where fine motor control is required. These muscles generally work together in functional groups to accomplish tasks.

When muscles work in a coordinated fashion with other muscles, they are synergists (helpers). The muscle that provides most of the tension is referred to as the **prime mover**, or agonist. The muscle that performs the opposite movement to the agonist, generally located on the opposite side of the limb, is called the **antagonist**. When a prime mover is active, the antagonist muscle is relaxed, yielding to the movement of the prime mover. Antagonists can also help regulate the action of the prime mover by partially contracting to provide some resistance or to slow or stop the action. Many muscles work in opposition to each other; one muscle produces movement in one direction and its partner produces movement in the opposite direction. As an example, during elbow flexion, the biceps brachii is the agonist and the triceps brachii is the antagonist. The following list identifies a few common muscle pairs that Personal Training Specialists should be familiar with.

Rectus abdominis	Erector spinae
Biceps brachii	Triceps brachii
Quadriceps	Hamstrings
Anterior tibialis	Gastrocnemius and soleus

Synergists are muscles that perform two functions in the context of the action of a muscle or muscles. First, synergists may act as contributors to the agonist to make the movement easier. They are not the primary muscle working to create movement, but because of their anatomical placement, they may be contributors. In the example of a biceps curl, the brachioradialis contributes to elbow

flexion, but the prime movers are the brachialis and biceps brachii. Second, synergists may play the role of stabilizers, thereby making the movement more efficient and maintaining proper alignment. In the example of a biceps curl, the deltoid, rhomboids, erector spinae, and pectoralis major all work as synergists, among others, to maintain proper posture and ensure correct technique.

Depending on the movement, muscles can act as prime movers, antagonists, or synergists at any one time. Figure 6.4 illustrates the concepts of agonist, antagonist, and synergist muscle groups during a biceps curl movement.

In the following sections, the major muscles of the body are described based on anatomical location, and their movements are described using the terminology introduced in chapter 5. For simplicity and ease of learning, the origin and insertion points for these muscles are labeled as approximate anatomical positions only.

Shoulder and Shoulder Girdle

The shoulder girdle, an articulation between the scapula and the clavicle, is the set of bones that connect the upper limbs with the axial skeleton. It is considered a group of floating bones because the bones are secured only by muscles. The floating nature of this joint makes the area unstable but allows a large ROM. Multiple bones and joints make up what we commonly call the shoulder. In this text we discuss the shoulder girdle (i.e., the scapula and clavicle, moving together as a unit) and the shoulder (i.e., the glenohumeral joint, where the scapula and humerus articulate to allow movement of the upper limb). See figure 6.5.

Figure 6.6 shows the posterior and anterior views of the shoulder and shoulder girdle muscles. Note that on the right-hand side of each diagram, the superficial muscles (trapezius, pectoralis, and deltoid) are removed to show the deep muscles that lie below. On the anterior view, the pectoralis and deltoid muscles are removed to show the deeper musculature.

Shoulder Girdle

As mentioned earlier, the shoulder girdle region is considered a floating joint because it is stabilized primarily by muscles. To generate maximum force and optimal contraction of upper-body muscles,

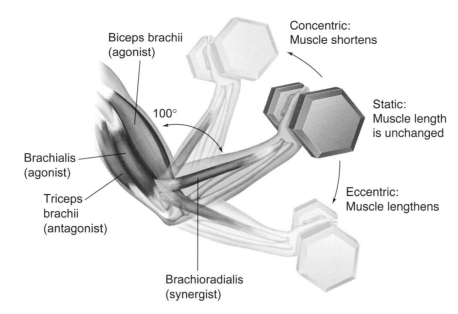

FIGURE 6.4 The actions of agonistic, antagonistic, and synergistic muscles during elbow flexion.

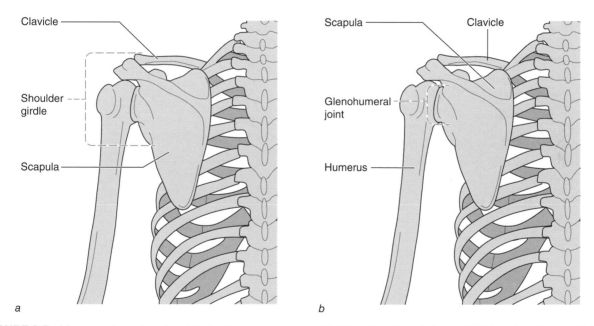

FIGURE 6.5 Movements at the shoulder include movements of (*a*) the shoulder girdle and (*b*) the glenohumeral joint.

the shoulder girdle must be stable (not moving) before contraction. The best way to cue clients to stabilize the shoulder girdle is to ask them to lift the shoulder blades (elevation), pull the shoulder blades back (retraction), and pull them down (depression) (see figure 6.7 and table 6.3). This is called the *set position*. When the shoulder girdle is in the set position, it is stable. To enhance muscle contraction

while maintaining stability (and therefore safety) of the shoulder during exercise, Personal Training Specialists should cue the set position before clients perform any upper-body movements.

Shoulder

The shoulder (glenohumeral) joint is an articulation between the humerus bone (upper arm) and the

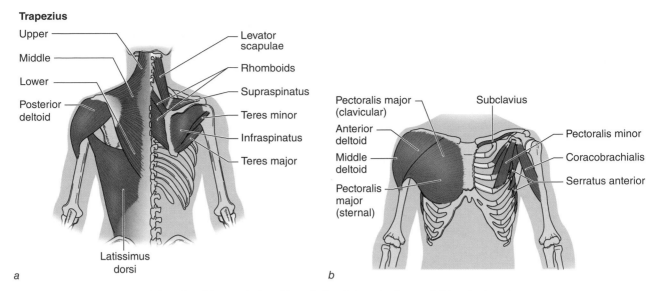

FIGURE 6.6 Muscles of the shoulder and shoulder girdle: *(a)* posterior and *(b)* anterior views.

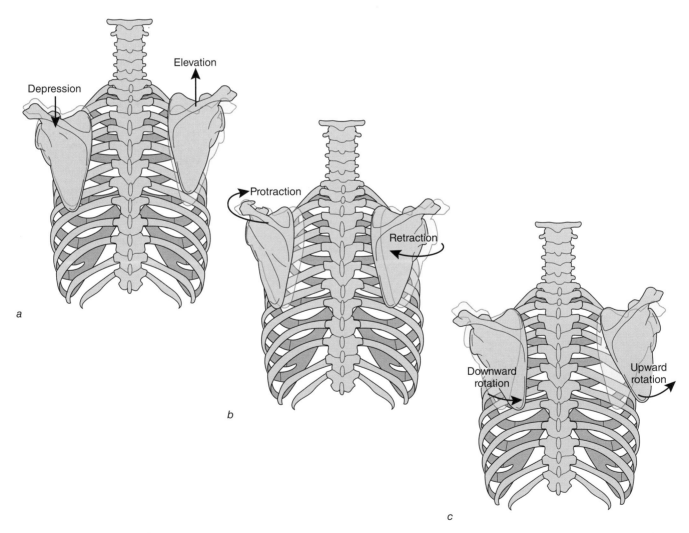

FIGURE 6.7 Movements of the scapula (posterior view): *(a)* elevation and depression, *(b)* retraction and protraction, and *(c)* upward and downward rotation.

TABLE 6.3   Muscles and Movements of the Shoulder Girdle

Muscle	Origin	Insertion	Function
Trapezius 1. Upper fibers 2. Middle fibers 3. Lower fibers	Base of skull Vertebrae C1–T12	Clavicle Scapula (upper medial and medial surface)	1. Elevation 2. Adduction or retraction 3. Depression and upward rotation and stability of scapula
Levator scapulae	Vertebrae C1–C4	Scapula (upper medial surface)	Elevation of scapula
Rhomboids Major Minor	Vertebrae C7–T5	Scapula (medial surface)	Adduction or retraction of scapula
Pectoralis minor	Ribs 3–5	Scapula (coracoid process)	Depression and abduction or protraction of scapula
Serratus anterior	Ribs 1–8	Scapula (anterior medial surface)	Abduction or protraction and upward rotation of scapula Moving scapula anteriorly against chest wall

scapula. It is a synovial ball-and-socket joint that has a large ROM in all three planes of movement. This large ROM is difficult to stabilize, leading to a large amount of instability. Thus, the muscles of the rotator cuff are essential for joint integrity in this area.

The rotator cuff muscles are also known as the SITS (i.e., supraspinatus, infraspinatus, teres minor, and subscapularis) muscles (figure 6.8). The SITS allow rotation of the humerus in the scapula and stabilize the shoulder joint (i.e., they keep the ball in the socket), allowing it to produce power and movement through its full range of motion. Three of these muscles lie as a group on the posterior surface (supraspinatus, infraspinatus, and teres minor) of the scapula, and one muscle lies on the anterior surface of the scapula (subscapularis).

The largest muscles acting on the shoulder include the deltoid, latissimus dorsi, and pectoralis major (figure 6.6). These large, strong muscles often overpower the smaller rotator cuff muscles, at times leading to injury if the rotator cuff muscles are not strong enough to stabilize the shoulder under the resistance used to train these larger muscle groups. Movements of the shoulder are described in table 6.4 and illustrated in figure 6.9.

Elbow

The forearm has two distinct joints. The first joint is the elbow, and the second is the articulation between the radius and ulna bones called the *radioulnar joint*. The elbow joint is an articulation between the humerus bone (upper arm) and the radius and ulna bones (forearm). It is a hinge joint, and its range of motion is limited because of the bone structure. Note, however, that movement occurs between the radius and the ulna at the radioulnar joint. Figure 6.10*a* shows the elbow and forearm with the palm rotated forward from the anatomical position, showing the inside surface of the arm. Figure 6.10*b* shows the elbow joint muscles of the back of the arm. Movements of the elbow are further described in table 6.5 and illustrated in figure 6.11.

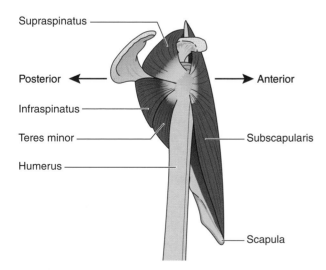

FIGURE 6.8   Lateral view of the muscles of the rotator cuff.

TABLE 6.4 Muscles and Movements of the Shoulder

Muscle	Origin	Insertion	Function
Pectoralis major Clavicular (upper) Sternal (lower)	Clavicle, sternum, upper six ribs	Upper humerus	Flexion, adduction, internal rotation, horizontal adduction
Deltoid Anterior Medial Posterior	Clavicle, scapula (spine of scapula)	Upper humerus	Abduction, external rotation; assists in flexion, extension, horizontal abduction
Coracobrachialis	Scapula (coracoid process)	Middle of humerus	Flexion, adduction
Teres major	Scapula (lateral surface)	Upper humerus	Adduction, extension, internal rotation
Latissimus dorsi	Vertebrae T6–S5	Upper humerus	Extension, adduction, internal rotation
Triceps brachii (long head)	Upper humerus, scapula	Ulna	Extension
Biceps brachii (short head)	Scapula	Radius	Flexion

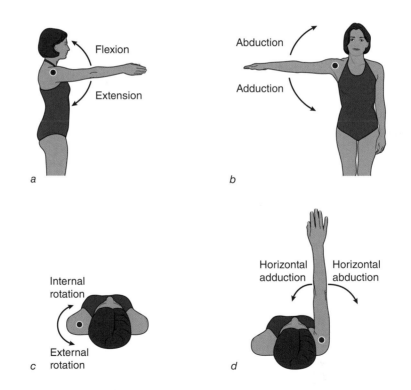

FIGURE 6.9 Glenohumeral (shoulder) movements: *(a)* flexion and extension, *(b)* abduction and adduction, *(c)* internal (medial) and external (lateral) rotation, and *(d)* horizontal abduction and adduction.

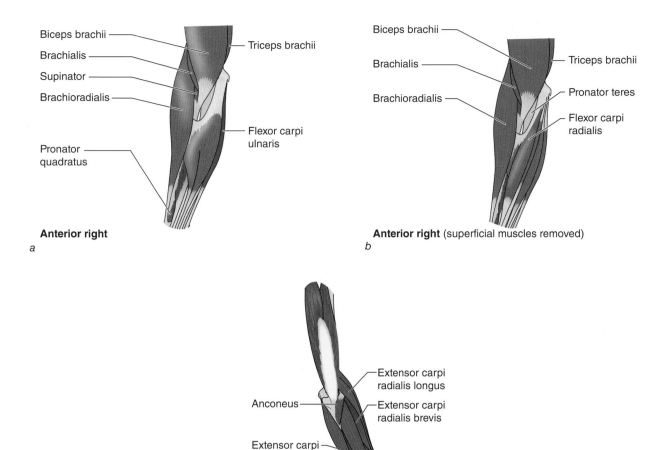

FIGURE 6.10 Muscles of the elbow: *(a)* anterior right (palm forward) view, *(b)* anterior right view (with superficial muscles removed), and *(c)* posterior right view.

TABLE 6.5 Muscles and Movements of the Elbow

Muscle	Origin	Insertion	Function
Biceps brachii Long head Short head	Scapula	Radius	Elbow flexion, supination of forearm
Brachialis	Humerus	Ulna	Flexion
Pronator teres	Humerus	Radius	Pronation of forearm (weak elbow flexion)
Brachioradialis	Humerus	Radius	Elbow flexion Pronation and supination of the forearm
Triceps brachii	Upper humerus, scapula	Ulna	Elbow extension
Anconeus	Humerus	Ulna	Elbow extension
Supinator	Humerus/Ulna	Radius	Supination of forearm

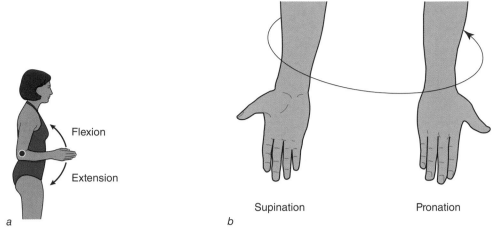

FIGURE 6.11 Movements of the elbow: *(a)* extension and flexion and *(b)* supination and pronation.

Wrist

The wrist joint is an articulation between the radius and ulna bones and the proximal carpal bones of the hand (called the scaphoid, lunate, and triquetrum). Joints are also located between the carpal bones in the hand and between the metacarpals and the phalanges (fingers). This large number of bones allows us to create fine movements with our hands, fingers, and thumbs. Figure 6.12 shows the forearm and wrist in anatomical position. In the anterior view the palms are turned forward, showing the inside of the wrist and palm. This view illustrates the muscles that flex (bend) the wrist. The tendons of these muscles

come together at the wrist and are bound together by a fibrous sheath called the flexor retinaculum, creating what is known as the carpal tunnel. The posterior view shows the back of the hand and the muscles that extend (straighten) the wrist. Although many muscles act on the forearm, wrist, and fingers, the important point to understand is which muscles are flexors and which are extensors, rather than the minute details of each of these muscles. Further study will accentuate your knowledge as a Personal Training Specialist. Movements of the wrist are described in table 6.6 and figure 6.13.

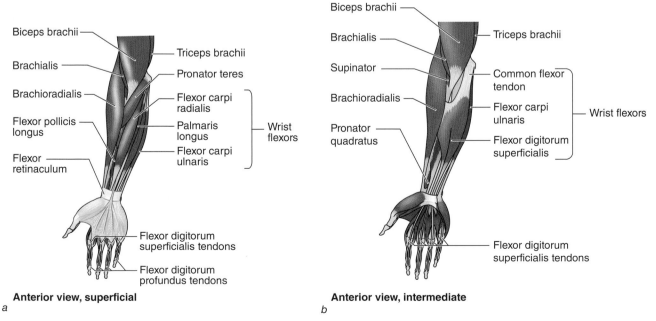

Anterior view, superficial

a

Anterior view, intermediate

b

FIGURE 6.12 Muscles of the wrist (right): anterior view of the *(a)* superficial, *(b)* intermediate, and *(c)* deep layers, and *(d)* posterior view.

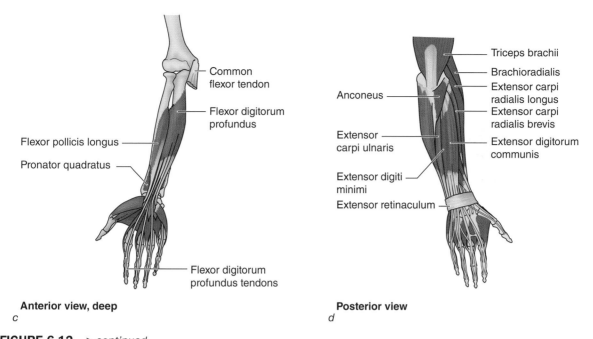

Anterior view, deep
c

Posterior view
d

FIGURE 6.12 > *continued*

TABLE 6.6   Muscles and Movements of the Wrist

Muscle	Origin	Insertion	Function
Flexors of the wrist Flexor carpi radialis Flexor carpi ulnaris Palmaris longus Flexor digitorum superficialis	Medial surface of lower humerus	Carpals, metacarpals, fingers	**Wrist flexion** Radial deviation Ulnar deviation
Extensors of the wrist Extensor carpi radialis longus Extensor carpi radialis brevis Extensor digitorum Extensor carpi ulnaris Adductor pollicis longus Extensor indicis Extensor pollicis brevis Extensor retinaculum Interossei	Lateral surface of humerus	Carpals, metacarpals, fingers	**Wrist extension** Radial deviation Ulnar deviation

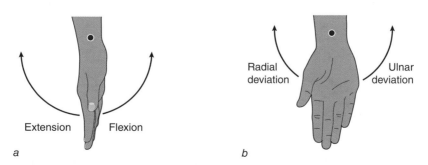

FIGURE 6.13   Movements of the wrist: *(a)* flexion and extension and *(b)* radial and ulnar deviation.

Hip

The articulation of the femur bone with the base of the pelvis forms the hip joint. Several ligaments help support this synovial ball-and-socket joint. The hip joint has great ROM and a large amount of muscle surrounding it. Like the shoulder joint, the hip joint has a number of deep muscles that allow stability and rotation. Figure 6.14 illustrates the anterior and the posterior muscles of the hip area.

The hip joint gains stability from deep ligaments and deep muscles that create rotation and hold the ball in the socket. Movements of the hip are described in table 6.7 and illustrated in figure 6.15.

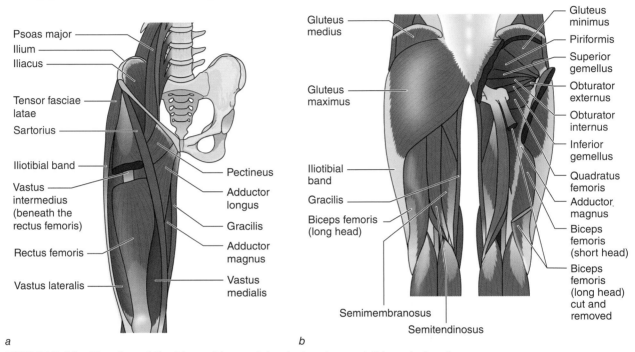

FIGURE 6.14 Muscles of the hip and knee: *(a)* anterior view and *(b)* posterior view.

TABLE 6.7 Muscles and Movements of the Hip

Muscle	Origin	Insertion	Function
Psoas major	Thoracic (bottom few) and lumbar vertebrae	Femur	Hip flexion
Iliacus	Pelvis (iliac crest)	Femur	Hip flexion
Adductor group Adductor longus Adductor magnus Adductor brevis Gracilis Pectineus	Base of pelvis	Length of femur (medial edge)	Adduction
Tensor fasciae latae	Pelvis (iliac crest), IT band (lies in the middle of the muscle)	Lateral tibia, head of fibula (via the IT Band)	Hip flexion, abduction, medial rotation
Rectus femoris	Pelvis (iliac spine)	Patella and patellar ligament (to the tibia)	Hip flexion
Sartorius	Pelvis (iliac spine)	Tibia (medial edge)	Hip flexion, lateral rotation
Gluteus medius	Pelvis (iliac spine)	Upper femur	Hip extension, abduction
Gluteus maximus	Pelvis (sacrum and iliac crest)	Upper femur	Hip extension
Hamstrings Biceps femoris Semitendinosus Semimembranosus	Base of pelvis	Upper tibia, fibula	Hip extension

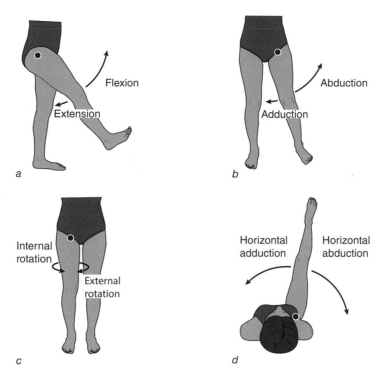

FIGURE 6.15 Movements of the hip: *(a)* flexion and extension; *(b)* abduction and adduction; *(c)* internal and external rotation; and *(d)* horizontal abduction and adduction.

Knee

The knee joint is the articulation between the femur bone of the thigh, the tibia of the lower leg, and the patella. The knee joint provides limited ROM, but it is important for weight bearing and for many major lower-body movements. Because of its construction, the joint itself is not very stable (i.e., the bones do not fit together well); therefore, the knee requires additional support from a collection of ligaments. The medial and lateral collateral ligaments (MCL and LCL) provide lateral stability for the knee to prevent excessive side-to-side motion. The anterior and posterior cruciate ligaments (ACL and PCL) cross inside the knee joint, providing internal stability and preventing displacement of the tibia and femur forward or backward (figure 6.16). The primary movements at the knee joint are flexion and extension, although some rotation is possible with the knee in a flexed position. See figure 6.17 and table 6.8. Figure 6.14 shows the muscles that move the knee joint, and figure 6.18 in the next section shows the muscles that attach below the knee joint and assist in moving the knee.

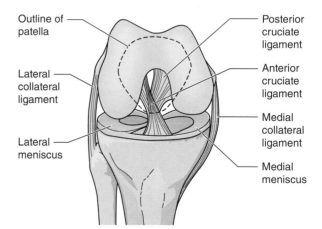

FIGURE 6.16 Anterior view of the ligaments that support the knee joint.

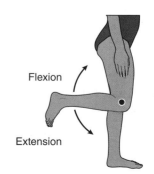

FIGURE 6.17 Movements of the knee.

TABLE 6.8   Muscles and Movements of the Knee

Muscle	Origin	Insertion	Function
Quadriceps Rectus femoris Vastus lateralis Vastus medialis Vastus intermedius	Pelvis (rectus femoris only), upper femur (all others)	Patella and patellar tendon (to tibia)	Knee extension
Hamstrings Biceps femoris Semitendinosus Semimembranosus	Base of pelvis	Upper tibia, fibula	Knee flexion
Plantaris	Lower femur	Heel	Knee flexion
Popliteus	Lower femur	Medial tibia	Knee flexion
Gastrocnemius	Base of femur	Heel (Achilles tendon)	Knee flexion

Ankle

The ankle joint is a synovial joint formed by the articulation of the tibia and fibula bones and the foot (talus bone). A synovial condyloid joint provides the ability to move the foot upward and downward (in dorsiflexion and plantar flexion) as well as side to side (in inversion and eversion). Because of weight bearing and gravity, the ankle joints endure a great deal of stress. They gain stability from a number of ligaments that prevent excessive forward, backward, and sideways motion. To identify the muscles important to this joint, we will examine the ankle and foot from an anterior view, a lateral view, and a posterior view in figure 6.18. The movements of the ankle joint are listed in table 6.9 and shown in figure 6.19.

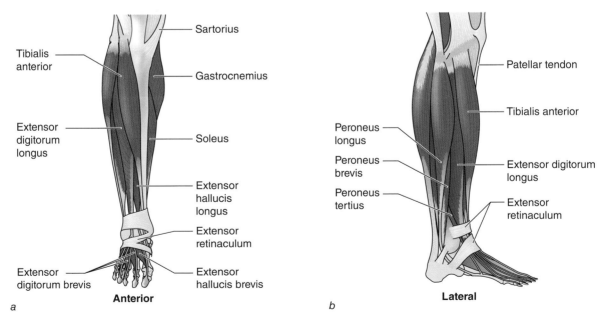

FIGURE 6.18   Muscles and structures of the ankle joint (right leg): *(a)* anterior, *(b)* lateral, *(c)* superficial posterior, *(d)* intermediate posterior, and *(e)* deep posterior views.

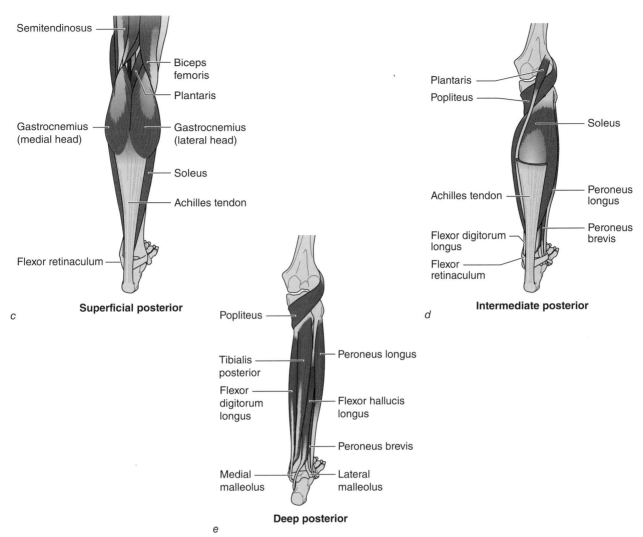

Superficial posterior

c

Semitendinosus
Biceps femoris
Plantaris
Gastrocnemius (medial head)
Gastrocnemius (lateral head)
Soleus
Achilles tendon
Flexor retinaculum

Intermediate posterior

d

Plantaris
Popliteus
Soleus
Achilles tendon
Peroneus longus
Flexor digitorum longus
Peroneus brevis
Flexor retinaculum

Deep posterior

e

Popliteus
Tibialis posterior
Flexor digitorum longus
Peroneus longus
Flexor hallucis longus
Peroneus brevis
Medial malleolus
Lateral malleolus

FIGURE 6.18 > *continued*

TABLE 6.9 Muscles and Movements of the Ankle

Muscle	Origin	Insertion	Function
Tibialis anterior	Proximal two-thirds of tibia	Metatarsal	Dorsiflexion, inversion
Extensor digitorum longus	Anterior tibia, fibula	Top of second through fifth toes	Dorsiflexion, eversion
Extensor hallucis longus	Anterior fibula	Big toe	Dorsiflexion, inversion
Peroneus tertius	Anterior fibula	Metatarsal	Dorsiflexion, eversion
Gastrocnemius	Base of femur	Heel (Achilles tendon)	Plantar flexion
Soleus	Proximal posterior tibia, fibula	Heel (Achilles tendon)	Plantar flexion
Tibialis posterior	Posterior tibia, fibula	Bones in foot, second through fourth toes	Plantar flexion, inversion
Flexor digitorum longus	Posterior tibia	Bottom of second through fifth toes	Plantar flexion, inversion
Flexor hallucis longus	Distal posterior tibia	Bottom of big toe	Plantar flexion, eversion
Peroneus Longus Brevis	Lateral fibula	Side of foot and fifth toe	Plantar flexion, eversion

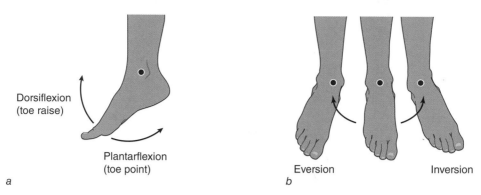

a *b*

FIGURE 6.19   Movements of the ankle: *(a)* dorsiflexion and plantar flexion, and *(b)* eversion and inversion.

Core Muscles

The core of the body spans the entire trunk extending from the rib cage and diaphragm on the superior border to the pelvis inferiorly. Muscles of the core (the active subsystem of spinal stabilization) have been described by function as stabilizers or mobilizers since the late 1960s.

Movement of the torso occurs at two primary joint locations—at the spine and at the pelvis.

Spinal movement occurs at the intervertebral joints (the joints between the vertebrae of the spine). An articulation between the fifth lumbar vertebra and the sacrum of the pelvis allows the pelvis to tilt. The core or torso area is best illustrated by viewing the torso from both the front (anterior view) and the back (posterior view) as seen in figure 6.20. The muscles and movements of the torso are listed in table 6.10 and illustrated in figure 6.21.

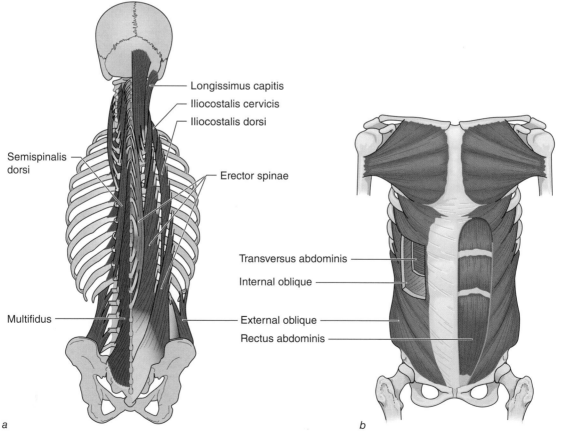

a *b*

FIGURE 6.20   Muscles of the core: *(a)* posterior and *(b)* anterior views showing abdominal and back core muscles and *(c)* deep muscles of the lower spine and pelvis.

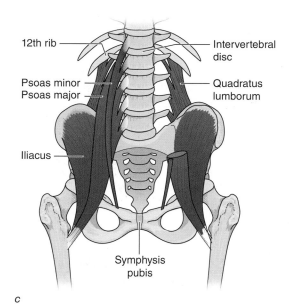

FIGURE 6.20 > continued

TABLE 6.10   Muscles and Movements of the Core

Muscle	Origin	Insertion	Function
Rectus abdominis	Pubis	Ribs 5 through 7, sternum	Spinal flexion, posterior pelvic tilt
Internal oblique	Pelvis	Lower ribs	Spinal rotation, lateral flexion, posterior pelvic tilt
External oblique	Lower 8 ribs	Pelvis	Spinal rotation, lateral flexion, posterior pelvic tilt
Transversus abdominis	Lateral torso	Linea alba, pelvis	Internal stability
Erector spinae	Lower thoracic vertebrae, lumbar spine	Cervical and thoracic vertebrae, ribs, base of skull	Spinal extension
Quadratus lumborum	Pelvis (iliac crest)	Rib 12, lumbar vertebrae	Lateral flexion
Multifidus	Posterior sacrum	Spinous processes of the vertebrae	Spinal extension and stabilization of spinal column

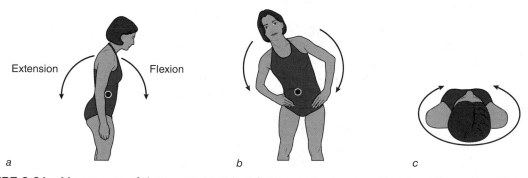

FIGURE 6.21   Movements of the torso: *(a)* spinal flexion and extension, *(b)* lateral flexion, and *(c)* rotation.

Stabilizers are deep, shorter muscles (such as the transversus abdominis, multifidus, and intervertebral muscles) that function primarily to stabilize adjoining vertebrae and the sacroiliac joint. Stabilizers help control movement of the spine during motion and facilitate the action of the mobilizer muscles. These stabilizing muscles are composed primarily of slow-twitch muscle fibers that produce continuous force with little or no shortening or resultant range of motion. The mobilizer muscles are longer and possess large lever arms that allow them to produce large amounts of torque and movement across a greater range of motion.

Both the stabilizer and mobilizer muscle systems work together to control neutral spine. People with existing anterior or posterior tilt of the pelvis present dysfunction and imbalances between these systems. These imbalances are caused by tightness and weakness in the stabilizing and mobilizing muscles. Anterior tilt occurs when the front of the pelvis tilts forward, thus increasing the curve in the lumbar spine. People with anterior tilt typically have tight erector spinae, iliopsoas, and rectus femoris muscles and weak transversus abdominis, hamstrings, external oblique, and gluteus maximus muscles. In cases of posterior pelvic tilt, the lumbar curve is reduced because the back of the pelvis tilts posteriorly. People with a posterior pelvic tilt typically have tight hamstring, rectus femoris, and tensor fasciae latae and weak iliopsoas, erector spinae, and multifidus muscles. Both anterior and posterior pelvic tilt can increase lower back pain.

Besides helping in the management of low back pain, core stability increases the ability of the body to produce power from the appendages (arms and legs). A stable core provides the arms and legs with a solid anchor to produce force and movement. Clients with strong core muscles experience better body control, balance, and coordination. Optimal function of the core requires integration of its anterior and posterior musculature. This is done through the thoracolumbar fascia (TLF), which is the sheath of connective tissue that covers key muscles in the centre of the trunk and low back. It is through this fascial system that forces are transferred from the upper extremities to the lower extremities through the lumbar spine and vice versa.

Multifidus Muscles

The multifidus muscles span the entire length of the spine, attaching one vertebra to another. The lumbar portion of the multifidus is the most developed part of the muscle group. In this region, the muscle travels superiorly and medially from the posterior surface of the sacrum (origin) to attach to the spinous processes of the lumbar and sacral vertebrae (insertion). The multifidus acts both as a prime mover in lumbar extension and as a stabilizer of the lumbar spine. But because most of its fibers are slow twitch, the multifidus acts primarily in its stabilizing role, preparing the spine for movement, preventing spinal injury, and increasing stability of the sacroiliac joint. This muscle appears to atrophy in people with lower back pain and may compound lower back pain issues.

Transversus Abdominis Muscles

The transversus abdominis, the deepest layer of the abdominal muscles, is located beneath the internal oblique. Its fibers run in the transverse plane (i.e., side to side), and it wraps around from the posterior to anterior aspect of the torso. The origin of the transversus abdominis is on the iliac crest and thoracolumbar fascia, and its insertion is at the midline of the abdominal muscles (the linea alba). Because it runs around the abdominal region like a thick belt, the transversus abdominis is often referred to as the body's natural corset. Its main function is to stabilize the pelvis and spine, and compress the internal organs. Because of the orientation of the fibers, transversus abdominis compresses the sacrum between the two hip bones (ilia) to maintain stability and decrease laxity of the sacroiliac joint.

Because of the segmental stabilizing effects of both the multifidus and the transversus abdominis, several specific exercise techniques focus on the cocontraction of both muscles independently of the other trunk muscles.

Internal and External Oblique Muscles

The internal and external oblique muscles also assist in the stabilization of the lumbar spine. The internal oblique not only pulls on the thoracolumbar fascia to increase lumbar stability but also works contralaterally with the opposite external oblique to create rotation in one direction and prevent rotation in the other and vice versa. For that reason, twisting exercises aimed at strengthening the obliques are often felt on both sides of the torso simultaneously.

Erector Spinae: Superficial and Deep Muscles

The erector spinae is a muscle group that runs vertically along the spinal column throughout the sacral, lumbar, thoracic, and cervical regions. As a muscle group (and not a specific muscle), it varies in size, structure, and function at different levels within the vertebral column. The muscle mass is most pronounced in the lumbar region and becomes smaller as the muscle ascends.

The function of the superficial erector spinae is to contract concentrically to produce lumbar extension, eccentrically to control lumbar flexion, and isometrically to control the position of the lower thorax with respect to the pelvis during functional movement. The erector spinae group is made up primarily of slow-twitch muscle fibers and is therefore less susceptible to injury induced by eccentric contraction. Personal Training Specialists should consider this point when structuring exercise programs because many people who suffer from lower back pain experience the deconditioning syndrome in which the superficial erector spinae is atrophied and lacks endurance and strength. Recruitment of the erector spinae is maximized through 70° of hyperextension. Therefore, hyperextension exercises have been suggested to address erector spinae deconditioning.

The deep erector spinae muscles originate from the ilium and travel superiorly, anteriorly, and medially to insert onto the lumbar transverse processes. The attachment of the deep erector spinae to the lumbar transverse processes indicates that its function is not lumbar extension or controlling lumbar flexion as the superficial fibers do, but to compress the lumbar spine on to the sacrum, providing a stabilizing role.

Iliopsoas: Psoas Major and Iliacus Muscles

Both the iliacus and psoas major muscles are normally considered together, using the term *iliopsoas*. The iliopsoas acts along with the rectus femoris as a hip flexor and external rotator of the femur. If either the iliopsoas or rectus femoris becomes tight, anterior tilt of the pelvis occurs, causing an increased curve in the lumbar spine (lordosis), which increases the compression and stress on the lumbosacral joint. This condition increases the likelihood of lower back pain. If only one side of the hip flexors is tight, rotation of the pelvis will also occur and may affect the function of the quadratus lumborum.

Quadratus Lumborum

The quadratus lumborum is located in the lower back. It functions concentrically and eccentrically to control the rate of descent in side bending. A tight quadratus lumborum causes a lateral tilt of the pelvis and may cause tension and dysfunction in other muscles that contribute to lower back pain.

Benefits of Resistance Training

Muscle is an adaptable tissue. With proper training, muscles grow stronger and larger (**hypertrophy**), which enables us to perform everyday activities more easily. Conversely, muscles can also become smaller and weaker (**atrophy**) if they are not used on a regular basis. Therefore, some form of resistance training should be part of every client's exercise program.

When we impose demands on our muscles to perform physical work that is greater than usual, they get stronger. This rise in strength results from increases in

- muscle fiber size,
- muscle contractile strength,
- coordination among muscle groups,
- muscle fiber recruitment,
- tendon and ligament contractile strength, and
- bone strength.

Positive changes in the muscular system have a large effect on our everyday lives (table 6.11). Personal Training Specialists need to help clients identify reasons why they should be involved in regular resistance training as it relates to their individual goals, health, and everyday life.

TABLE 6.11   Physical Improvements and Benefits as a Result of Resistance Training

Improvements	Benefits
Increases muscular strength, power, and endurance	Makes everyday activities easier
	Improves sport performance
	Improves strength for cardiorespiratory exercise
Increases core strength	Improves posture
Increases muscles mass	Complements the maintenance of a healthy body weight
	Reduces loss of muscle mass due to inactivity and aging
Improves bone density and connective tissue strength	Helps prevent osteoporosis
	Reduces the incidence of joint and muscle overuse injury

Resistance training can improve muscular strength, power, and endurance. Personal Training Specialists should understand the differences between these terms. **Muscular strength** is the maximum amount of force that a muscle or muscle group can generate. **Muscular power** is the explosive aspect of strength. It is the product of strength and speed of movement: power = (force × distance) / time. **Muscular endurance** is the ability of a muscle to exert force repeatedly over time.

Muscular strength and endurance are related; an increase in strength can lead to improvements in endurance. A reasonable amount of strength and endurance may help clients be more efficient in daily tasks and reduce their chances of having pain and dysfunction in everyday life. Power is a key component for most athletic performances.

Program Design for Resistance Training

When planning a resistance training program, Personal Training Specialists need to understand and apply the FITT formula (frequency, intensity, time, and type; see chapter 2) to their workouts to achieve optimal results and greater physical fitness benefits.

Frequency

canfitpro's *Recommendations on Physical Activity, Nutrition, and Positive Mindset for Optimal Health* recommends three or more resistance workouts per week. Muscle building and recovery varies among people, and adequate rest is required between resistance training workouts to facilitate the muscle-building process. Generally, about 48 hours between workouts is needed to avoid overtraining, injury, and poor results. For most clients, more

rest is better than not enough rest, especially when beginning a training program. The sidebar highlights factors that have an effect on the frequency of resistance training.

Considerations for Resistance Training Frequency

When planning a resistance training program, consider the following when determining frequency:

- **Client's goals for resistance training**—Clients who are working toward muscular endurance can train every other day. Clients who train for muscle strength, hypertrophy (growth), or power may require a recovery period longer than 48 hours for optimal results.
- **Intensity of the workout**—Clients who train at a lower intensity require less recovery between workouts compared with those who train at higher intensity.

Intensity

Intensity in resistance training is based on repetitions, sets, and loads. The sidebar lists factors that have an effect on exercise intensity.

When determining repetition range, be aware of the inverse relationship between number of repetitions and load or amount of resistance. Typically, the higher the number of reps is, the lower the load should be. Choose a number of repetitions that the client can complete with proper technique and safety, keeping in mind the goals: strength, power, hypertrophy, or endurance. This concept can be illustrated with an intensity continuum (see figure 6.22).

Considerations for Resistance Training Intensity

When planning a resistance training program, consider the following when determining intensity:

- **Client's experience**—Resistance training design is based on the client's experience. Beginners should train at reduced intensity and focus on developing technique before increasing intensity.
- **Client's current fitness level**—Clients with higher levels of muscular strength, endurance, and power can train at intensities higher than 70% of their 1 repetition maximum (1RM), which is the maximum load that they could lift, pull, or push in a single rep. Clients who are less conditioned should train with loads that are less than 70% of their 1RM.
- **Client's goals for resistance training**—Clients have different goals with respect to resistance training. Common goals include muscle growth (hypertrophy), muscle definition, and overall improved strength or endurance. Intensity varies based on these goals.

The decision to perform more than one set of an exercise is based on clients' goals and the amount of time they have to spend training. Performing multiple sets has several purposes:

- Helps the client learn the correct technique—practice makes perfect.
- Increases fatigue of the muscle fibers, which encourages greater muscle growth during the recovery stage. (Many clients do not lift a load heavy enough to promote muscle failure in a single set. To encourage growth, use multiple sets of each exercise.)

Workout intensity significantly affects the results of resistance training. In the first six to eight weeks of a resistance training program, beginners experience significant results because of improvements in motor unit recruitment (mentioned earlier in this chapter) of previously underused muscle fibers. Seeing changes early in the program helps motivate beginners, but the rate of change in muscle recruitment slows significantly after the first eight weeks. For this reason, Personal Training Specialists need to modify each client's program regularly to increase intensity progressively, prevent plateauing, and ensure continued improvements toward the client's overall goals.

The force output of a muscle can vary widely. The more muscle fibers that are activated during exercise, the more force will be produced. If an activity requires near-maximal performance (i.e., close to the client's 1RM), more muscle fibers are recruited (see figure 6.23).

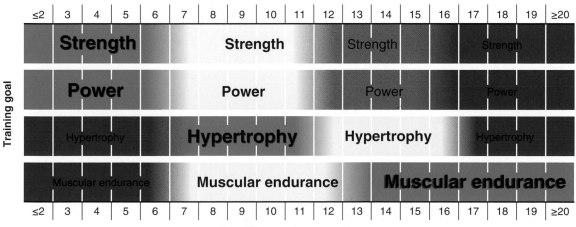

FIGURE 6.22 Intensity continuum.

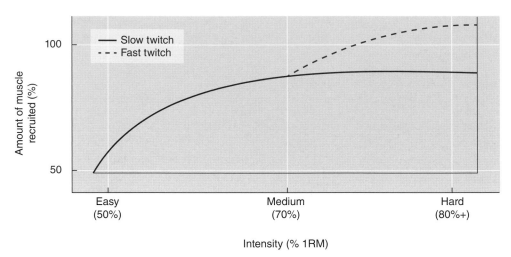

FIGURE 6.23   Muscle fiber recruitment.

Time

The duration of a resistance training session depends on clients' personal goals, experience, and the duration of their rest between sets and exercises. The sidebar lists factors that have an effect on exercise time.

Considerations for Resistance Exercise Duration

When planning a resistance training program, consider the following to determine exercise time:

- **Client's experience**—When they begin a resistance training routine, beginner clients may have low fitness or lack confidence. Begin resistance training for a short duration (20 to 30 minutes) until the client develops proper technique, form, and confidence.

- **Client's goals for resistance training**—As the client's goals become more serious and focused on developing muscle mass, time spent on resistance training should increase. To fatigue and develop muscles properly, clients should complete multiple sets at high intensity. The harder the workload is, the longer the rest between sets should be. More sets and more rest result in longer total workout time.

To make workouts more time efficient, you can modify routines for clients by using split programs, which are explained in the program design section of this text (chapters 11 through 13).

Type

This area allows a considerable amount of variety and imagination. Consider the type of muscle contraction (isometric, isotonic, or isokinetic), the type of equipment (constant versus variable resistance), and the exercises most appropriate for the client. The sidebar lists factors that have an effect on exercise type.

Resistance training programs use isometric, isotonic (with and without variable resistance), and isokinetic protocols.

Isometric Training

Isometric training involves static muscle contraction in which the length of the muscle does not change when force is applied against a fixed resistance (e.g., static plank, wall sit, yoga postures). Isometric training has certain limitations. One major criticism is that it does not require the limbs to move. As a result, strength gains occur only at the specific joint angle at which the exercise takes place rather than through a full ROM.

Isotonic Training

Isotonic training involves both concentric and eccentric muscle contractions. In a concentric contraction, the muscle shortens as the joint moves against the force of resistance. In an eccentric con-

Considerations for Resistance Exercise Type

When planning a resistance training program, consider the following to determine exercise type:

- **Client's experience**—Beginner clients can have major safety and confidence problems when getting started. In these cases, the general recommendation is to use weight machines that put them in a fixed position and allow muscle isolation. As clients become more experienced, they can begin to use equipment that provides less structure and control, such as free weights and pulleys.

- **Client's goals for resistance training**—Clients who work toward general muscular strength and endurance could benefit from resistance machines. Clients who want functional strength and muscle growth should use a combination of equipment, including (but not limited to) free weights, pulleys, and machines. Exercise type is limited only by the client's level of fitness and the Personal Training Specialist's enthusiasm to teach new techniques and add program variety.

traction, the muscle lengthens as the joint moves back toward its starting point.

Isotonic training includes either constant or variable resistance. An arm curl with a dumbbell is an example of an isotonic exercise that uses constant resistance because the load stays constant through the entire ROM. The lifter experiences changes in exercise intensity because of changes in the length of the lever arm at various stages of the lift. In contrast, variable (or accommodating) resistance equipment requires the lifter to exert maximum effort throughout the entire ROM. Theoretically, this equipment provides more resistance at the joint angles where the lifter is stronger and less resistance at weaker positions; in other words, it accommodates the lifter's leverage or strength. This mechanical change is achieved through **cams**, which change the direction of the force (e.g., Nautilus equipment), and leverage, which varies the length of the moment arm of the resistance (e.g., Universal equipment).

Isokinetic Training

Isokinetic training is done on specialized equipment that controls the speed of movement through the ROM. This equipment offers variable resistance and accommodates changes in mechanical advantage (i.e., the resistance matches the strength of the muscle at each point in the ROM and alters the amount of load when it senses that the contraction is changing in speed).

Putting It All Together

Clients of all ages and fitness levels can benefit from building muscular capacity. Most people understand that they should perform resistance training, but they are often unsure about what exercises they should do and how to perform them safely. Thus, the demand for more information and instruction on resistance training has increased the demand for knowledgeable Personal Training Specialists.

One of your roles as a Personal Training Specialist is to introduce clients to various exercises and alleviate their intimidation about being in a weight room. Personal Training Specialists must have experience and a solid knowledge base about a range of exercises, mechanically correct technique, and results of various approaches to resistance training. The best way to learn how to train others is first to train yourself.

Errors in program design can be costly, because an improper resistance training program can lead to

1. injury,
2. dissatisfaction or lack of enjoyment,
3. lack of results, and
4. loss of clients.

Personal Training Specialists should always make informed and educated choices when creating exercise programs for clients. In this way, you can provide each client with a program that is safe, results oriented, and enjoyable.

Table 6.12 summarizes basic resistance training guidelines, offering a basic introduction to guidelines, techniques, and exercise choices for resistance

TABLE 6.12   Resistance Training Guidelines

Client type		Physical activity profile	Possible program focus	Frequency	Exercise type	Routine choices
Nonexerciser	No habitual activity and extremely deconditioned	Sedentary	Learning proper technique Learning correct exercises	2–3 workouts per week	Simple movements requiring minimal challenge to balance, stability, and coordination and involving fewer muscle groups (e.g., weight machines, stability ball, simple body-weight exercises, closed kinetic chain movements)	Total-body workout Balanced workout Basic circuits
Occasional exerciser	Minimal current exercise and moderately to highly deconditioned	Minimal activity	Developing core strength Gaining muscular endurance			
Recreational exerciser	Suboptimal exercise frequency - mildly to moderately deconditioned	Sporadic physical activity	Exercise variety Refining proper technique Learning new exercises Developing core strength Gaining muscular endurance Gaining muscular strength	3–4 workouts per week	Any of the preceding plus Moderately complex movements involving some challenge to balance, stability, and coordination, involving one or more muscle groups (e.g., intermediate-level exercises with weight machines, stability ball, body weight, free weights; basic exercises with pulleys, kettle bells, suspension straps, and so on)	Total-body or split program Intermediate circuits
Committed exerciser or athlete	Regular moderate to vigorous activity	Habitual physical activity	Exercise variety Maximizing core strength Maximizing training time Gaining muscular endurance Gaining muscular strength Increasing muscular size	4–6 workouts per week	Any of the preceding plus Complex movements that challenge balance, stability, coordination, and involve multiple muscle groups (e.g., advanced exercises with weight machines, stability balls, body weight, free weights, pulleys, kettle bells, suspension straps, medicine balls, specialty equipment, open kinetic chain movements, and so on)	Total-body or split programs Advanced set performance Sport-specific training Advanced circuits (Many possible modifications)
Dedicated exerciser or elite athlete	Regular vigorous activity	High amounts of physical activity				

Note: Exercise characteristics, rather than equipment type alone, dictate the complexity and challenge of a given exercise. Thus, a skilled Personal Training Specialist may choose to use a variety of equipment options for any level of exerciser. The important points are to ensure that the client maintains proper form and technique and to match the intensity of the challenge to the particular client's ability and goals.

training. Table 6.13 provides more details based on the goals of the resistance training program.

Appendix A contains over 100 exercises that are the basis for most resistance training programs. This list of possible exercises is not complete, but it will show you how to teach and spot basic resistance training exercises. The focus here is on developing your knowledge and building your comfort level with teaching standard resistance exercises that most clients would begin with before you attempt more advanced training methods. After you master teaching these standard exercises, you can choose more advanced movements, equipment, and routines for your clients.

TABLE 6.13   Resistance Training Guidelines for Specific Training Results

Desired training result	Intensity (% of 1RM)	TIME		
		# of reps	# of sets	Rest between sets
Muscular endurance	Less than 70% of 1RM	12–15	1–3*	30 sec–1 min
Muscular strength and hypertrophy	70–80% of 1RM	8–12	1–4	30 sec–2 min
Muscular power and maximal strength	80–100% of 1RM	1–8	1–6	>2 min

*Additional sets may be performed at the Personal Training Specialist's discretion, if the client maintains proper form and technique throughout the recommended number of repetitions.

Summary of Main Points

1. Skeletal muscle comprises many muscle fibers that are made up of myofibrils. Myofibrils contain protein filaments called *actin* and *myosin.*

2. The sliding filament theory explains how a muscle contracts.

3. The three types of muscle contractions are concentric (in which the muscle shortens and lengthens), eccentric (in which the muscle produces force with no change in muscle length), and isometric (in which the muscle exerts force to counteract an opposing force with no change in muscle length).

4. Several factors determine the force of a muscle contraction, including the neural stimuli for contraction, size and length of the muscle, joint angle, and speed of the contraction.

5. The two primary muscle fiber types are fast twitch for hard, short-duration exercise and slow twitch for moderate, long-duration exercise.

6. The origin of a muscle is usually closer to the midline of the body (proximal), and the insertion is usually away from the midline of the body (distal).

7. Muscles of the core (the active subsystem of spinal stabilization) have been described by function as stabilizers or mobilizers. Both systems work together to maintain neutral spine.

8. Resistance training is an essential component of a balanced and effective training program.

9. Regular resistance training increases muscle fiber size, contractile strength, bone strength, and ligament strength.

10. Clients experience many positive health benefits from resistance training, including improved body composition, reduced injury, better posture, improved daily activities, improved sport performance, and better body awareness.

11. To develop a sound resistance training program, consider principles such as exercise selection, muscle balance, exercise order, rest, breathing, speed, technique, and loading.

12. The FITT formula for resistance training is based on a client's goals and experience. In general, the higher the total load lifted, the harder the workout is and the more muscle mass the client builds.

13. You can vary a client's exercise routine in many ways using new exercises and programs. Variety is essential to success and adherence.

Key Concepts for Study

Muscle fiber

Sarcomere

Concentric contraction

Eccentric contraction

Central nervous system (CNS)

Peripheral nervous system (PNS)

Proprioceptors

Motor unit

Fast-twitch muscle fiber

Slow-twitch muscle fiber

Prime mover

Antagonist

Muscular strength

Muscular power

Muscular endurance

Cams

Review Questions

1. List and describe the three types of muscle tissue.

2. Briefly describe the significance of the core.

3. What type of muscular contraction is responsible for elbow flexion during a biceps curl exercise?
   a. eccentric
   b. concentric
   c. isometric
   d. none of the above

4. People with anterior tilt typically have tight _____, _____, and _____ muscles.
   a. external oblique, illiopsoas, gluteus maximus
   b. erector spinae, hamstrings, external oblique
   c. gluteus maximus, hamstrings, rectus femoris
   d. erector spinae, iliopsoas, rectus femoris

5. The rotator cuff is described by the acronym SITS, which stands for
   a. supraspinatus, interosseous, teres minor, and sartorius
   b. subscapularis, interosseous, trapezius, and serratus anterior
   c. supraspinatus, infraspinatus, teres minor, and subscapularis
   d. supraspinatus, infraspinatus, trapezius, and subscapularis

6. The stabilizing muscles are composed primarily of
   a. a mixture of fast- and slow-twitch muscles
   b. fast-twitch muscles
   c. slow-twitch muscles
   d. none of the above

7. Seeing changes happen quickly can provide great motivation to beginners, but the rate of change in muscle recruitment tends to slow significantly after the first
   a. 2 weeks
   b. 4 weeks
   c. 8 weeks
   d. 10 weeks

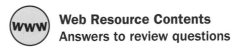

Web Resource Contents
Answers to review questions

Flexibility and Mobility Concepts

Chris Frederick, B.PT

LEARNING OUTCOMES

After completing this chapter, you will be able to

1. define flexibility and mobility and explain their relationship to fitness;

2. identify the mechanical properties of myofascia and explain how stretching promotes flexibility;

3. identify the purpose of flexibility training;

4. describe the changes that occur as a result of regular flexibility training;

5. determine appropriate parameters for flexibility training; and

6. identify basic guidelines for flexibility training.

Flexibility is recognized as one of the elements of fitness needed to achieve and maintain optimal health, yet it is also one of the least understood aspects of fitness. Controversy continues about when (and even if) stretching is an appropriate means to improve flexibility. Some of these conflicting views may result in part from increasing evidence that each client needs an individualized approach to stretching that is related to accurate assessment of personal movement patterns, in both training and stretching positions. Discussion of these issues and others will give you confidence and success when assessing and training flexibility.

More than being a goal itself, adequate flexibility enables clients to get better results from exercise. Table 7.1 lists benefits of improved flexibility.

This chapter discusses the preceding concepts to help you improve fitness outcomes and achieve the goals set by you and your clients.

Definition of Flexibility

Flexibility can be defined as more than just range of motion; it is having the ability to adapt successfully to challenges to motor control, strength, balance, coordination, endurance, and mental and emotional focus. For our purposes, flexibility refers to the absolute range of motion, or relative range of motion, of a joint as a result of muscles that cross the joint. Although we have standards by which to assess a client's flexibility, there will still be aspects that vary for all joints, movements, and activities. For example, people commonly think that someone who can do the splits on the floor is flexible. However some people who can do the splits cannot squat in a low position and keep their heels on the ground. These people are not flexible for squats, yet they are quite flexible for the splits. Another example is someone who has flexible hamstrings but has restricted ankles or shoulders.

Given that no general benchmark measures overall flexibility, each client's general and specific movements must be assessed accurately to see exactly where she or he is restricted in mobility. As a Personal Training Specialist, you need to identify the joints or muscles that may be contributing to these restrictions (or recognize that you only need to teach the client good form and technique) and then design an appropriate flexibility program for that person.

Relationship of Flexibility to Overall Fitness

A client's flexibility can affect his or her ability to generate strong muscular contractions. In simple terms, when a person activates one muscle as the prime mover (agonist), its antagonist will be inhibited to allow the desired movement of the joint that they both cross. This action is called reciprocal inhibition. In some cases, a muscle may be inhibited because of overactivation of its antagonist. A common example is found in clients who sit all day at work. Their hip flexors get short, tight, and overactivated, which reciprocally inhibits and weakens the gluteal muscles. Stretching of the hip flexors during flexibility training allows the gluteals to contract with more strength and power in any exercise that challenges them. Knowing how appropriate stretching of inhibited muscles can lead to increases in strength will help you develop effective training programs for your clients.

TABLE 7.1   Physical Improvements and Benefits as a Result of Flexibility Training

Improvements	Benefits
Improves overall body mobility	Removes imbalances that restrict muscle contraction
	Improves posture
	Improves blood flow
Improves range of motion (ROM) of joints	Improves balance
	Removes barriers to speed and agility
	Reduces feelings of stiffness
Improves ability of muscles and connective tissues to lengthen	Increases efficiency of movement
	Improves the ability to relax and recover from training
	Decreases trigger point formation

Balance is another component of fitness that is related to muscular capacity and flexibility as well as to other systems of the body. In the case of flexibility, tight joints (most notably the hips) can contribute to decreased balance and may prevent clients from progressing to training on unstable surfaces. Tight joints are referred to as hypomobile, meaning that have restricted range of motion. This condition is often related to tightness in soft tissue (i.e., muscles and fascia).

Although clients will not stretch their joints directly, stretching any muscle that crosses or attaches near a tight joint can help increase the joint's ROM. With tight hips, for example, taking clients through a flexibility program that includes stretching tight adductors, flexors, and rotators tends to improve balance. Assessing balance before and after stretching will confirm whether balance improves and whether poor balance was in fact caused by one or more tight joints.

By helping clients increase the ROM of tight joints and muscles, you are also helping to remove soft-tissue resistance to movement that could otherwise reduce clients' speed and agility. Although some clients (especially athletes) can power through the resistance caused by soft-tissue tightness, this action is inefficient and wastes the body's precious energy systems. After stretching, your tight clients will experience noticeable improvements in speed as well as improved agility, coordination, and quickness as their training program progresses.

Mobility and Fascia

Mobility simply means to be capable of moving, and it is closely related to the concept of motor control. To move effectively, clients need adequate passive and active mobility in addition to stability. They also need the ability to move with or through resistance.

Clients need mobility not only in the joints but in all soft tissues. As mentioned in chapter 6, **fascia** is the word we use for all the connective tissue that wraps around and between muscles, tendons, and ligaments. It also binds other tissues, every organ, and all systems together in the body. Besides providing structural connections, fascia is innervated with sensory receptors that provide the brain, the rest of the nervous system, the skeletal muscle system, and the rest of the body with constant information about the state of kinesthesia and pro-

prioception (the body's sense of movement and its location in space).

Fascia, like most biological tissues, has qualities of mobility and stability, which are called viscoelasticity and stiffness. Viscoelasticity is a combination of elastic and plastic properties, which allows soft tissues in the body to return to their original shape after stretching (elasticity) and to adapt to sustained periods of stretch (plasticity). Elasticity in the human body allows us to build or lose muscle tissue, absorb collision and other forces, and perform dynamic stretches or active stretches without permanently changing tissue length. Plastic properties allow the body to change in response to sustained periods of lengthening, such as performing a static stretch of 30 seconds. Note that if a stretch is performed at excessive intensity or is held too long, soft tissues can be permanently damaged. In general, muscle tends to be more elastic, whereas fascia is usually more plastic.

 Stretching at excessive intensity or for too long can injure fascia or muscles, resulting in permanent deformation (i.e., tears) in the tissues. As a Personal Training Specialist, it is important that you incorporate the FITT guidelines described in this chapter, to ensure each client can safely perform each stretch at optimal intensity.

Stiffness is a quality in fascia that is necessary for stability, and it allows better mobility. An optimal amount of stiffness will prevent hypermobility and instability. If tissue in the area of a joint is not stiff enough, then the arm, leg, or other body part may move excessively and be weak because of lack of stability. Note, however, that excessive stiffness will inhibit mobility. If the tissue is too stiff, a person may not be able to move across the full ROM expected of a particular joint or muscle.

Muscle and fascia, together called myofascia, are completely integrated and always function together passively, actively, and under load or resistance. Fascia gives muscle a flexible and strong structure from which it can function, owing in part to the structural design of myofascia. As discussed in chapter 6 (see figure 6.1 on pp. 97-98), the structure of a muscle from the outer layer of fascia to the inner layer is as follows:

- Epimysium
- Perimysium
- Endomysium
- Sarcolemma
- Myofibril

Because the brain and nervous system are also part of this fascial connection, crucial information about body position (kinesthesia) is affected by the flexibility and mobility of fascia. Fascia covers all muscles and connects them to each other, so anything that restricts the mobility of fascia will negatively affect muscle mobility and function. The following is a list of circumstances that can restrict mobility of fascia and thereby prevent optimal muscle function (Alter, 2004):

- Insufficient hydration
- Immobility (e.g., sitting all day without frequent movement)
- Excessive fitness training
- Excessive physical labor
- Daily emotional stress
- Insufficient sleep
- Inability to relax
- Anxiety
- Poor diet

Any of the preceding will contribute to a negative change in the structure and function (physiology) of the myofascia and can lead to the following conditions:

- Tight muscles and fascia
- Poor posture
- Pain
- Stiff joints
- Scar tissue

- Restricted ROM
- Restricted general mobility
- Decreased strength
- Decreased balance
- Decreased speed

To lead clients through safe and effective exercise programs, Personal Training Specialists need to apply their knowledge of anatomy in a practical sense. For this reason, you must begin to consider the body as a whole and gain an understanding of how the mobility of one joint can affect other areas of your client's body. This interconnectivity of joints, muscles, and fascia is explained through the concept of **myofascial slings**, which was made popular by researchers such as Tom Myers and Andry Vleeming. These connective tissue pathways, also referred to as myofascial lines, trains, chains, or systems, allow us to trace the characteristic patterns of tension within the body. When looking at a certain movement, any weakness, tightness, or other restriction of any of the myofascia within that particular sling can cause a significant effect on the stability and mobility of other joints and tissues along the same chain. An understanding of myofascial connections will help you create individualized exercise programs that increase your client's activity performance while minimizing the occurrence of overuse injuries.

Although the study of myofascial chains and slings is expansive, we will focus our attention on those that closely relate to the assessment protocols and programming choices discussed within this text. The list that follows is intended to introduce you to some of the myofascial pathways that you should be aware of as you begin to work with personal training clients. Although many structures are involved in each line or sling, we focus on muscles and bones you have already learned about in chapters 5 and 6.

Anterior Superficial (Superficial Front Line)

Pathway—Runs from the top of the toes, up the shin and anterior thigh. Travels up the abdominals and chest into the neck.

Significant muscles and structures—Extensors of the toes, tibialis anterior, patellar tendon, rectus femoris, rectus abdominis, and muscles of the neck and scalp.

Functional relevance—Helps the body maintain posture and offers balance to the superficial back line. Responsible for flexing the trunk and the cervical spine, extending the knee, and dorsiflexing the ankle. Can affect many functions of the body—especially breathing.

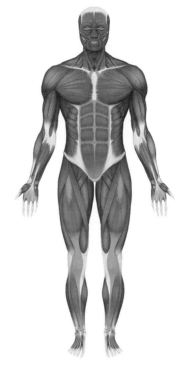

Anterior superficial line

Posterior Superficial (Superficial Back Line)

Pathway—Runs from the bottom of the foot, up through the calves, hamstrings, and lower back and then along the spinal extensor muscles to the fascia of the scalp and forehead.

Significant muscles and structures—Plantar fascia, gastrocnemius, ischial tuberosity, hamstrings, thoracolumbar fascia, erector spinae, and fascia of the scalp and forehead.

Functional relevance—Helps the body maintain posture and generates movements of extension or hyperextension. Tension in this line can restrict forward bending movements or cause locking in the knees or compression of the lumbar spine.

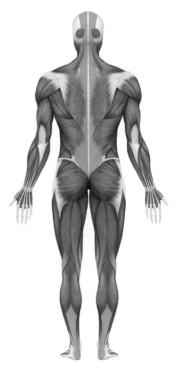

Posterior superficial line

Posterior Longitudinal Sling (Deep Longitudinal System)

Pathway—Runs up from the hamstrings, through the pelvis, and along the muscles of the back.

Significant muscles and structures—Erector spinae, multifidus, thoracolumbar fascia, and biceps femoris.

Functional relevance—Activated during forward flexion, particularly through the trunk, assisting in bringing the trunk back to a neutral position. Involved in actions such as jumping, kettlebell swings, and the top half of the deadlift.

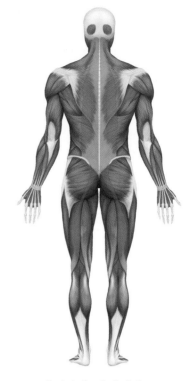

Posterior longitudinal sling

Lateral Line

Pathway—Runs from the bottom of the foot, up the side of the leg and thigh, crisscrossing up the side of the torso, and into the muscles of the neck.

Significant muscles and structures—Peroneal muscles (which evert and plantar flex the ankle), IT band, gluteus maximus, tensor fasciae latae, iliac crest, oblique abdominal muscles, intercostals (muscles that run between the ribs and assist in breathing), and muscles of the neck.

Functional relevance—Stabilizes the body through lateral or rotational movements and provides stability to the pelvis and hips during standing, walking, twisting, and so on.

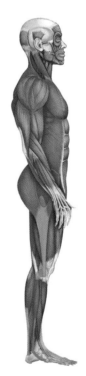

Lateral line

Lateral Sling

Pathway—Runs up the lateral thigh, across the pelvis, and into the lower back muscles on the contralateral side. Supported by the ipsilateral adductors.

Significant muscles and structures—Gluteus medius, gluteus minimus, tensor fasciae latae, iliotibial band, adductor muscles, and quadratus lumborum.

Functional relevance—Helps control sideways movement of the pelvis, especially in single-leg activities. Assists in bringing the pelvis back to a neutral position during movements such as walking, running, and rotation.

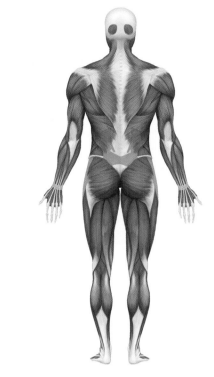

Lateral sling

Spiral Line

Pathway—Runs down from the side of the skull, across the neck, and under the shoulder to the front of the torso. Crosses through the navel to the opposite hip and then down the lateral thigh, across the shin, and under the foot. Travels back up through the lateral leg and then crosses to the lateral hamstrings and up the back, finishing at the skull, where it started.

Significant muscles and structures—Posterior neck muscles, rhomboids, serratus anterior, internal and external obliques, tensor fasciae latae, IT band, tibialis anterior, biceps femoris, and erector spinae.

Functional relevance—Controls and stabilizes rotational movements in the body, helping the body maintain balance in all planes.

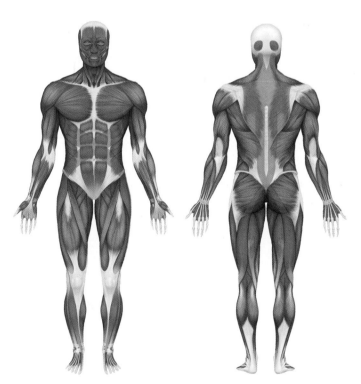

Spiral line

Arm Lines

These four lines connect the axial skeleton to the upper limbs, beginning at the chest, upper back, or neck and ending at the palm, dorsum (back) of hand, thumb, or little finger. They allow the shoulder to support the many intricate movements of the arm, hand, and fingers.

Superficial Front Arm Line

Pathway—Runs from the chest and latissimus dorsi, through the front of the arm, and into the palm of the hand.

Significant muscles and structures—Pectoralis major, latissimus dorsi, humerus, sternum, ribs, forearm flexors, and palm.

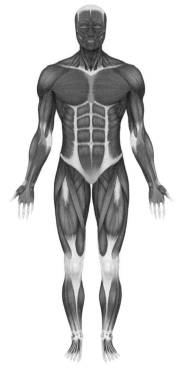

Superficial front arm line

Deep Front Arm Line

Pathway—Runs through the deep chest muscles down the front of the forearm to the thumb.

Significant muscles and structures—Pectoralis minor, subclavius ribs, biceps brachii, radius, and thumb.

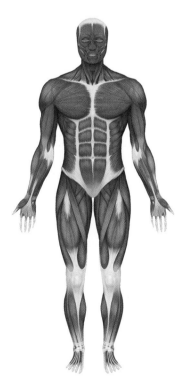

Deep front arm line

Superficial Back Arm Line

Pathway—Runs from the neck and middle back through the shoulder to the outside of the arm and the back of the hand.

Significant muscles and structures—Superficial trapezius, deltoid, forearm extensors, and dorsum of hand and fingers.

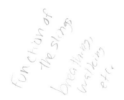

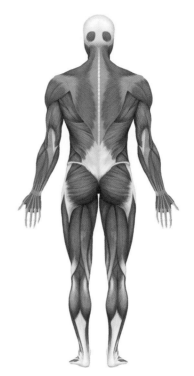

Superficial back arm line

Deep Back Arm Line

Pathway—Runs from the neck and upper back, through the deep muscles of the shoulder, and along the posterior aspect of the arm to the little finger.

Significant muscles and structures—Levator scapulae, rhomboids, infraspinatus, teres minor, triceps brachii, ulna, and fifth digit (i.e., little finger).

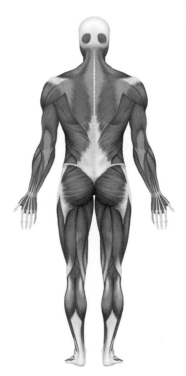

Deep back arm line

Anterior Functional Line (Front Functional Line)

Pathway—Runs from chest, down the abdominal muscles, and then across to the opposite thigh.

Significant muscles and structures—Pectoralis major, rectus abdominis, pubis, adductor longus, and femur.

Functional relevance—Involved in many functional movements because it connects the upper limb and rib cage with the opposite side of the pelvis and thigh and joins the front arm lines to the abdomen.

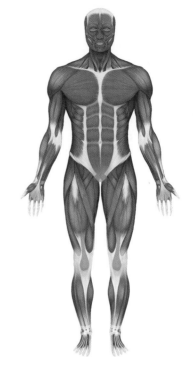

Anterior functional line

Anterior Oblique Sling

Pathway—Runs from the external obliques on one side to the internal obliques and adductors on the other side.

Significant muscles and structures—External obliques, transversus abdominis, internal obliques, and adductors.

Functional relevance—Involved in powerful rotational movements such as pushing, striking, and throwing patterns. Stabilizes the spine and torso during rotation and weight transfer. Closely related to the anterior functional line.

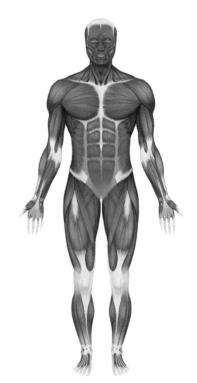

Anterior oblique sling

Posterior Functional Line (Back Functional Line)

Pathway—Runs from one shoulder, diagonally down across the back, and then down the front, back, and side of the thigh.

Significant muscles and structures:—Latissimus dorsi, thoracolumbar fascia, gluteus maximus, vastus lateralis, and subpatellar tendon.

Functional relevance—Connects the movements of one shoulder to the opposite lower limb. Often involved in the initial windup then deceleration of throwing activities.

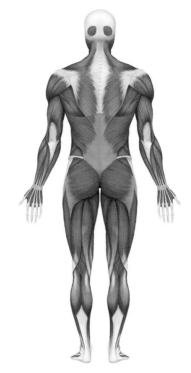

Posterior functional line

Posterior Oblique Sling

Pathway—Runs from the back, across the midline, to the back of the opposite thigh.

Significant muscles and structures—Latissimus dorsi, gluteus maximus, and biceps femoris.

Functional relevance—Provides stability and power during rotational motions, connecting movements of the lower and upper limbs. Closely related to the posterior functional line.

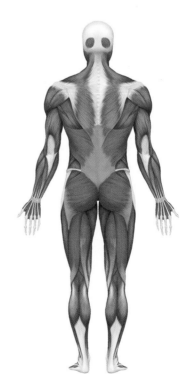

Posterior oblique sling

Deep Front Line

Pathway—Runs from the sole of the foot, along the inside of the leg, across the anterior hip, up the anterior spine, and through the thoracic cavity to the skull.

Significant muscles and structures—Flexors of the toes, tibialis posterior, popliteus, adductors, pelvic floor, iliacus, psoas, quadratus lumborum, diaphragm, vertebrae, sternum, and muscles of the neck.

Functional relevance—The deepest identified myofascial line. Maintains core alignment and stability. Connects core stabilization to breath.

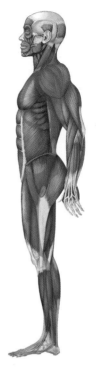

Deep front line

As evidenced by the preceding lists, healthy muscle and fascia are essential for optimal movement. Myofascia that is dehydrated, deconditioned, tight, and stiff will become dry, hard, dense, and immobile (Schleip et al., 2012). Many clients will come to you in this state wanting to start an exercise program with various goals in mind. If they are inhibited in their mobility, then well-planned flexibility training must be part of the training program if it is to achieve optimal results.

When assessing a client's mobility, you should first use full-body movement patterns that mimic the training exercise but use little to no load. If no mobility problems are evident, then slowly progress by adding load as planned. If you see a faulty movement pattern that looks like a mobility restriction, then you must confirm it with a specific ROM assessment (see pp. 137-141). Before adding heavy loads to your client's training program, you need to improve her or his range of motion and limit mobility restrictions.

For example, if one shoulder does not reach the full extended position to do a proper overhead squat (described in chapter 10), then assess all movements of the restricted shoulder first without

 Before beginning any training program, you must assess the client's mobility and identify any flexibility restrictions that might prevent the person from performing the exercises safely and effectively. These restrictions should be addressed before load is added. Specific flexibility and ROM assessments can be found later in this chapter, as well as in chapters 9 and 10.

load, and then compare with the other one. If the client reports tightness or stiffness, then having him or her do one to three stretches to remove the restriction is appropriate. Often, stretching allows the client to continue training after the restriction is removed. You should include stretches for this area in your client's regular pre- and post-training flexibility programming. If the client has pain or persistent restrictions in movement, refer him or her to a physician or qualified health professional for further assessment. Other regions of the body that do not have mobility restrictions may be loaded and trained as long as the training session is balanced.

Range of Motion and Joint Mechanics

Range of motion (ROM) refers to the amount of movement around a particular joint, measured in units of degrees using a device called a goniometer. Most trainers do not use a goniometer and simply perform an eyeball measurement to make an educated estimate of the degrees of motion. For example, a result of 45 degrees of hip flexion in the straight-leg raise indicates poor hip ROM, possibly as a result of tightness in the hamstrings. If the client is relaxed and doesn't help the trainer lift the leg, the movement is called passive ROM, or PROM. If the client actively lifts the leg with no assistance, the movement is called active ROM, or AROM.

PROM in any joint is normally greater than AROM because the client is relaxed and doesn't need to activate stabilizing or postural muscles. In contrast, AROM is normally less than PROM because stabilizer and synergist muscles are helping the body achieve and maintain the position of stretch. This action of stabilization before mobilization has the effect of transferring stiffness, resulting in decreased AROM compared with PROM (see figure 7.1). A relatively small difference of 5° to 15° is normal. A value greater than that may indicate excessive effort from the client to stabilize for weakness or inhibition that needs to be addressed.

Joint mechanics (i.e., how joints move) are greatly affected by whether a client is standing and bearing weight through the joint or lying on the floor with no weight being transferred through joints. For example, a client may be able to do a body-weight squat only halfway before stopping, making it appear that the back, hip, knee, or ankle has mobility restrictions (figure 7.2). Yet when the person gets on hands and knees and squats all the way down on the haunches, no restrictions are evident. In this case, the increased tension from muscle and fascia activation in the standing position may be restricting joint mobility. Flexibility training can help with this type of restriction.

Joint mechanics can also be affected by excessive mobility, also called **hypermobility**. An example is seen in old ankle sprains that have overstretched ligaments, resulting in an ankle that is less stable than normal. Personal Training Specialists need to be cautious with a client who has this history

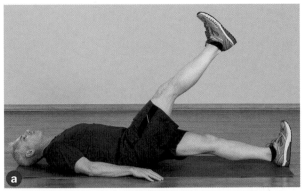
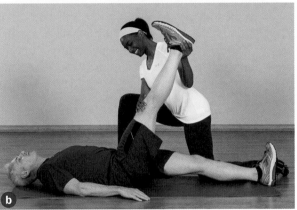

FIGURE 7.1 Difference between *(a)* active and *(b)* passive range of motion in straight-leg raise.

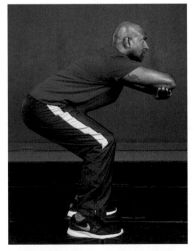

FIGURE 7.2 Excessive forward lean because of decreased ankle mobility.

(which is common) and should focus on stability exercises for the affected ankle and entire leg. At the same time, tight hips and back often occur as compensation for loose ankles. Therefore, adding stretches to the client's program to address those tight regions would be appropriate. Any joint that appears unstable during movement (i.e., wobbles, shakes, moves out of alignment, or appears unsteady) requires stabilization. In these cases, the client will need specific training to improve strength in the weak areas.

Hypermobility may increase injury risk as much as limited mobility. Clients with hypermobile joints should do stabilization training to improve strength and stability.

Although tables that outline PROM of all major joints of the body exist, they do not reflect the fact that ROM is function specific. For example, a gymnast or dancer has a functional need to be able to perform the splits passively and actively, whereas a middle-aged businessperson typically does not. By closely observing performance of the movements that are part of the training plan, a Personal Training Specialist can identify the places in the range of motion where better flexibility is needed. To do this, you should look for symmetry in all three planes of movement. The following are specific steps to use in assessing and correcting common ROM problems:

1. Observe whether your client can move into an exercise or maintain an exercise position.
2. Feedback: note whether your client complains of tightness or stiffness that correlates with mobility restrictions.
3. Assess ROM of any specific region that is asymmetrical or restricted and compare with the other side.
4. Mobilize and stretch what is restricted to match the other side, unless the other side is hypermobile.
5. Reassess exercise movement to see whether the problem has been corrected.

When evaluating your client's performance of an exercise, you should observe side-to-side differences in symmetrical training exercises in all three planes of the movement (sagittal, frontal, transverse). The following are some common examples of faulty movement patterns you may observe during a squat exercise, common regions of discomfort that might result, flexibility tests to use in those instances, and appropriate mobility exercises to help correct the observed issues.

Example 1

Movement plane—Sagittal

Issue—Excessive forward lean during squat

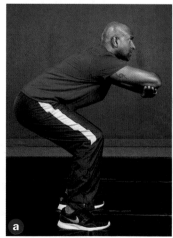

Observation: excessive forward lean

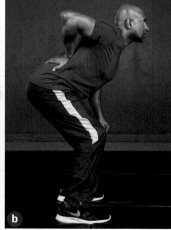

Feedback: low back strain from forward lean

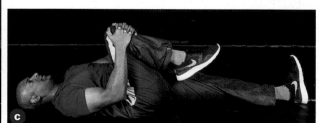

Assessment: Check passive hip flexion in spine.

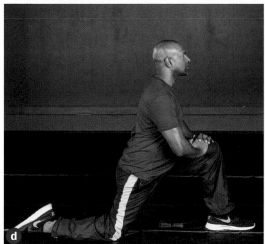

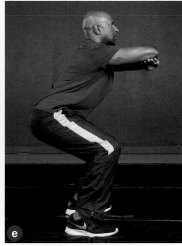

Mobilization: Mobilize and then stretch hip flexors.

Reassess: Is forward lean or other problem gone, better, or no change?

Example 2

Movement plane—Frontal

Issue—Hip shift during squat

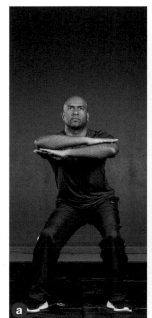

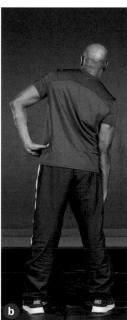

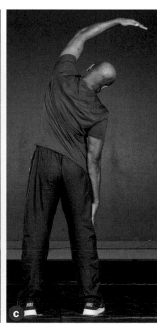

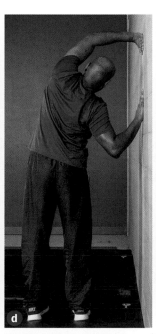

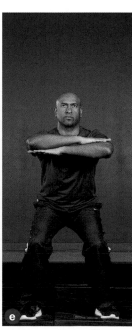

Observation: hip shift

Feedback: hip strain from hip shift

Assessment: Check range of motion in full-body side bending.

Mobilization: Mobilize and then stretch entire lateral line of body.

Reassess: Is hip shift, knee rotation, and pronation gone, better, or no change?

Example 3

Movement plane—Transverse

Issue—Foot pronation and knee rotation during squat

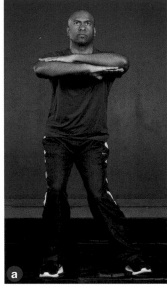

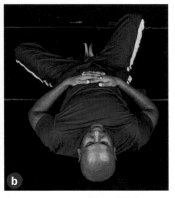

**Observation: foot prona-
tion with knee rotation**

**Feedback: knee strain
from rotation and prona-
tion**

**Assessment: Check hip
rotation and abduction in
supine.**

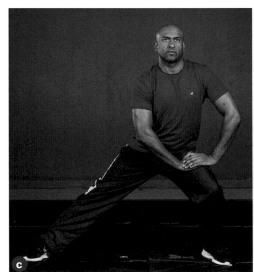

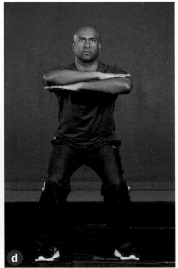

**Mobilization: Mobilize and then
stretch hip adductors.**

**Reassess: Is hip shift, knee
rotation, and pronation
gone, better, or no change?**

If after your assessment and efforts to stretch and mobilize the problem area, the problem only partially corrects, do the following:

- Repeat the stretch with slightly more intensity and longer duration, but no pain.
- Reassess other regions above and below the restricted area to check for other restrictions. If you find restrictions, stretch and reassess.

Movement, Mobilization, and Flexibility Training

Personal Training Specialists and fitness consumers often misuse the terms *movement*, *mobilization*, and *flexibility training*. To clarify the differences, we provide clear definitions and examples of how each one is incorporated into personal training.

Movement

Any activity of daily living or training exercise is a movement. Examples are walking, washing dishes, and doing squats. Faulty movement that does not involve a lot of load commonly indicates either a technique problem or a mobility problem. For example, if resolving a client's restricted dorsiflexion does not correct his squat technique (as shown in figure 7.2), you as the Personal Training Specialist must first assess AROM to compare both sides and then give that client a mobility or stretch exercise to correct the problem in the movement.

Mobilization

When used for physical activity, the terms *mobilization* and *mobility exercises* mean the same thing. Mobility exercises are dynamic movements that are either the same movement that the client will perform in the workout or, when the client has significant mobility problems, are a series of various movements that prepares him or her for the exercise. An example of a mobility exercise to prepare a client for a squat workout is to perform body-weight squats and then squats with only a barbell before performing the first squat set with added load. To prepare for the body-weight squat, clients can perform these exercises to mobilize the hips and ankles:

- Front lunges
- Side lunges
- Back lunges

Mobilization and mobility exercises offer several benefits:

- General warm-up of joints, muscles, and fascia for all types of training
- Specific warm-up of body regions that will be the focus of a training session
- Preparation for stretching areas of the body that need more mobility

When a client demonstrates restricted movement patterns even after doing a sufficient number of preparatory mobility exercises, she or he must be given specific stretching exercises.

Flexibility Training

Flexibility training can be defined as lengthening myofascia to increase general mobility or specific joint ROM. As we learned earlier, muscle and fascia are integrated structurally and always function together, so stretching muscle will also stretch fascia. Because fascia connects all individual muscles and groups of muscles to each other, a stretch cannot be isolated to only one muscle. Therefore, keep in mind that although you may intend to focus on one muscle, other muscles, both proximal and distal, will be affected by the stretch.

In your physical screening, you will notice that clients come with a large variety of issues that may affect their overall flexibility and specific mobility, such as the following:

- Scar tissue from surgery or injury
- Chronic muscle tightness from stress
- Joint stiffness from aging or past surgery or injury
- Poor posture

Because of the variety of individual life histories, clients often feel the same stretch in different places. For example, while performing a hamstring stretch, one client may feel it in the middle of the hamstrings while another feels it in the back of the knee. Both responses are normal because the hamstring is anatomically located in both locations. One client is simply tighter in one location than the other client is. So when clients ask, "Where am I supposed to feel the stretch?" the answer is, "Wherever you are tightest." As regions of tightness become mobile and change with training, clients may begin to feel the stretch in another appropriate location. Reassure clients that this variation does not mean that they are performing the stretch incorrectly.

Flexibility training can be done actively, such as when a client lies on his or her back and contracts the quadriceps to stretch the hamstrings. Or it may be done passively, such as when a client uses a band to pull the leg up and stretch the hamstrings or when another person holds the leg in the stretch position. Whether done actively or passively, flexibility training may be static or dynamic. When performing **static stretching**, the client gets into a position that lengthens one or more muscles and holds that stretch for a specified time. Commonly, static stretches are held for up to 30 seconds and repeated two or three times. **Dynamic stretching** can be described as moving into and out of positions that mobilize soft tissues first and then stretching them. Positions are not held as they would be in static stretching; instead, joints, muscles, and fascia are moved through their normal range of motion and then eased through tension or resistance to optimize ROM (as long as the movements remain pain free). The tempo of these movements may vary from slow dynamic stretches to faster dynamic stretches, depending on how you intend the client to move during the training session.

 Another stretching technique used by some Personal Training Specialists is proprioceptive neuromuscular facilitation (PNF), which operates on the neurological principle of reciprocal inhibition. PNF is used in static stretching only, and it consists of a one- to two-second contraction of the tight muscle, followed by a static stretch of the same muscle. An example would be a client contracting the hamstrings and then performing a stretch of the hamstrings. PNF is an advanced stretching technique, which requires additional training and qualifications beyond the scope of this text.

Tissue Changes With Flexibility Training

Research shows that human soft tissues, like muscle and fascia, have several biomechanical properties that are essential to their proper function (Alter, 2004). Although these topics are complex, only the basics as they pertain to flexibility training will be discussed here.

As author Alter states, "Biological tissues are neither perfectly elastic nor perfectly plastic" (Alter, 2004). Instead, they exhibit a combination of properties, together referred to as viscoelasticity. These properties include elasticity, plasticity, and creep.

Elasticity describes the ability of the tissue to adapt quickly and stretch into different shapes and directions. **Plasticity** refers to the way in which tissue structure and function can adapt in response to various demands and environmental conditions. The mechanical property called *creep* helps to prevent overstretching and thus reduces the risk of myofascial injury.

At low loads, myofascial tissues exhibit elastic behaviour. Specific dynamic stretches will improve the elasticity of muscle for function only within the limits of movements required for that workout (i.e., no permanent lengthening or deformation of tissue occurs). At higher loads, the tissues exhibit more plastic behaviour. Specific static stretching (or very slow dynamic stretching) will increase the plasticity of muscle and allow more permanent lengthening of the tissue. The result is increased mobility, up to or beyond what may be functionally required (but not so far as to cause pain). Plasticity in response to stretching also allows restoration of the ROM that may have been lost throughout the training session. But if tissue is stretched too hard (intensity), too long (duration), or too often (frequency), it can tear and be injured. Pain during flexibility training indicates that tissue could possibly be injured, so it must be avoided. To minimize the risk of injury and maximize the positive effects of flexibility exercises, Personal Training Specialists should have their clients stretch in the elastic zone before or during training and in the plastic zone after training.

 As a Personal Training Specialist, you should always ensure that clients move only through a range that is comfortable and pain free. Take care to have them move only within the natural ROM of a joint during flexibility training.

Fortunately, creep also helps to protect the tissue from injury that could be caused by overstretching. Creep is the property of continued lengthening of tissue when stretching without requiring further effort or intensity. As noted earlier, this kind of stretching works best under low loads or low intensity.

If clients are stretching correctly, each repetition is rewarded with more gains in ROM without extra work or effort. After a certain number of repetitions of a stretch, clients will achieve no further gains in ROM, which is the sign to stop that stretching exercise.

Last, desensitization of muscle spindles may be related to the mechanical properties discussed earlier. Spindles are the primary stretch receptors and proprioceptors in muscle, and they help the body detect the speed and length of stretch. If a stretch is detected as too fast or lengthens tissue too much, then the spindle sends feedback to the muscle to contract (called a **stretch reflex**) to protect the area from injury. Nerves that detect pain also respond. A simple example of muscle spindle activity is the well-known knee-jerk reflex (when a health professional taps your patella tendon with a hammer and your knee extends involuntarily in response). Research suggests that a slackening effect produced from stretching the muscle spindles may cause a reduction, slowing, or even elimination of the stretch reflex (Alter, 2004). Clients therefore may be able to tolerate more stretching over time as their sensitivity to the tension decreases. Note, however, that if the client overstretches, the stretch reflex may not operate effectively, which can serve as a warning to stop the stretch. As a Personal Training Specialist, the instruction you provide your clients about how to perform stretching exercises safely will minimize the risk of overstretching and help prevent injury.

Contraindications and Precautions in Flexibility Training

When introducing a flexibility program for your clients, you need to consider any conditions they may have that would prevent them from being able to perform stretching exercises safely. In some cases absolute contraindications will be present, and in others you will simply need to be cautious as you proceed.

The following list explains contraindications and precautions that Personal Training Specialists should consider when training clients for flexibility:

- **Recent injury or surgery**—In general, you should avoid stretching areas of the body that have recently undergone medical procedures. Note, however, that although you need clearance from your client's qualified health professional about when stretching may be resumed in these areas, stretching other regions of the body that do not strain or stress the injured or surgical region may still be conducted.

- **Inflammation or infection**—These conditions are most often also accompanied by colour changes and pain, but not always. In this situation, you need to be sure that the client has received clearance from a qualified health professional before resuming flexibility training in the affected area.

- **Diseases that affect tissues to be stretched**—Down syndrome, rheumatoid arthritis, and many other diseases result in changes to the properties of connective tissue (myofascia), leading to changes in joint integrity and stability. Therefore, in the case of diseases that you are not familiar with, you must educate yourself and check with your client's qualified health professional before having her or him do any stretching. (Note that these conditions would be screened for during the PAR-Q+ assessment process.)

- **Excessive pain or other negative reactions to flexibility training**—These occurrences may indicate a tear of myofascial tissue, infection, or other condition not appropriate for stretching.

- **Lack of joint stability**—Stretching anywhere immediately around an unstable joint may increase instability. If this prevents training progression, consider referring your client to a physician or other qualified health professional.

 If a client has any of the contraindications listed earlier, the Personal Training Specialist should ensure that she or he receives clearance through the PAR-Q+ or from a qualified health professional before starting any flexibility training program.

Program Design for Flexibility Training

When designing either a static or dynamic flexibility training program for your client, you should follow a progression of sequential elements to produce the best outcomes:

- Start with the gluteal muscles, hip flexors, quadratus lumborum, latissimus dorsi (i.e., the Core Four, described later in this chapter) because these muscles affect all movements from the core to the extremities.
- Add muscles that cross one joint (e.g., bent-knee hamstring stretch).
- Progress to muscles that cross multiple joints (e.g., straight-leg hamstring stretch).
- Use multiple planes of movement (e.g., stretch medial and lateral hamstrings by taking the leg out and in at different angles).
- Increase ROM progressively without causing pain.
- Stretch fascia, not just muscles. In addition, target the areas where individual muscles connect to each other. For example, fascia connects the hamstrings to the adductors and iliotibial band (ITB), which is also stretched using multiple planes of hamstring-targeted stretches.
- Change flexibility training parameters (frequency, intensity, time, and type) based on the goals for the session. For example, use faster tempos for dynamic pre-training stretches and much slower tempos (or static stretching) for post-workout flexibility training.

General Parameters for Stretching

Before considering the frequency, intensity, and duration (time) of stretching, you should recognize the guidelines that are common to both static and dynamic stretching:

- Both static and dynamic stretching should be done to the body regions that are the focus of a specific training session.
- Avoid pain to prevent injury.
- Inhale to prepare to stretch and then exhale while stretching (several inhalations and exhalations occur with long-duration static stretching, whereas only exhalations occur during the stretch phase with short-duration dynamic stretching).
- Progressively increase ROM with each subsequent rep until no more gain occurs in ROM.
- Tighter regions or limbs may need more repetitions.
- When the end of ROM is met with no further gains, stop stretching because no further benefit can be gained.

Both static (post-training) and dynamic stretching have the following parameters that can be adjusted to create an individualized flexibility prescription for each client's personal training program.

Frequency

Frequency of stretching may be described in terms of the number of times it is done within a week, a day, or even within a single training session. When designing a flexibility program, note that the optimal frequency of any stretch may vary from person to person (and from one part of a client's body to the other).

The recommended frequency for clients who are particularly tight, immobile, or previously sedentary is four to seven days per week. These clients can benefit from stretching in the morning, during the day, within their training sessions, and before bed. For more flexible and mobile clients, the minimum frequency should be three days per week, but they may also find benefit from daily stretching at various points throughout the day, depending on their individual need for flexibility (specific to their training or activities of daily living).

Within a single training session, clients who are experiencing limited mobility or high levels of muscle tension may benefit from pre-training flexibility exercises to prepare the body regions that will be trained. During the actual workout, if clients are demonstrating movement restrictions while performing a particular exercise, they should stop that exercise and use a dynamic stretch that targets the body regions involved in the restriction. For example, tight hip flexors can restrict the performance of a squat, so stretching them dynamically during the session may lead to immediate improvements in squat technique.

After a workout is complete, all clients can benefit from static or very slow dynamic stretching to target the specific body regions that have been trained, as well as any muscles that tend to tighten at cool-down.

Considerations for Flexibility Training Frequency

When planning a flexibility training program, consider the following when determining frequency:

- **Client's current training demands—** Flexibility exercises should be included post-training on every workout day and as needed on nontraining days. Additionally, clients who require a certain level of mobility to perform their prescribed workouts may find it helpful to include dynamic flexibility exercises pre-training as part of their warm-up and during training if restricted ROM is preventing use of proper form or technique of another exercise.

- **Client's goals for flexibility training**—Clients who are working toward improved mobility and flexibility can perform stretches every day, and they may even choose to do certain stretches multiple times in the same day. Clients who are mobile and flexible should perform flexibility exercises at least three days per week on training days, but they may also choose to stretch outside their training sessions, depending on their personal goals and daily life activities.

Some clients need more stretching, whereas others need less. Your initial assessment of multiple movement patterns, as described in chapters 9 and 10 (along with continued observation of your client during workouts) will help you determine an appropriate prescription for flexibility exercises. The more restrictions to movement that you see that do not result from poor technique, injury, or instability, the more stretching you should recommend to your client before, during, and after training as well as at home. As the client performs movements better, you can reduce the frequency of a specific stretch or eliminate certain stretches one at a time (if the stretches are no longer providing improvements in ROM and mobility).

Decreasing the frequency of particular stretches as flexibility and mobility improve can occur within a single session or as a reduction in the total number of times the stretch is repeated over the course of a week. Within a session, you may choose to decrease the number of repetitions if a larger number is no longer needed to get the same effects on ROM and movement improvement. Within the week, you can decrease the number of times the same stretch is performed outside the post-training flexibility program.

After frequency has been decreased, you may also choose to eliminate any stretch that no longer gives the client the desired gains in ROM or improvements in mobility that used to result from the same stretch. This process of elimination commonly results in a set of key stretches remaining, which the client must still perform for optimal pre- and post-training effect. Many factors may be involved here, including a genetic propensity to being tight in specific body regions, history of scar tissue that decreases elasticity and plasticity of myofascia, chronic suboptimal hydration and nutrition issues, sleep deprivation or mental stress, and other factors that have not been studied or researched.

Intensity

Performing a stretch at the appropriate intensity creates a sensation of lengthening in the target body region, but not to the point that the client feels pain. The challenge for many clients is to interpret the subjective sensations they feel when stretching. Some clients cannot easily distinguish between pain and an awareness of tissue lengthening. Individual response and interpretation of pain varies widely. Therefore, as a Personal Training Specialist, you need to help clients understand that every part of the body has an initial barrier of stretch and that when they start to feel this barrier, they should stop pushing farther and either hold a static stretch or move up to release before easing back into a dynamic stretch. This approach will ensure a proper and safe intensity for most stretching activities.

As a demonstration of what appropriate stretch intensity feels like, you can use this simple technique:

- Ask the client to push one finger backward into extension (toward the back of the hand) until the person just starts to feel tension or resistance that starts to slow down the movement (but before any pain occurs).
- Then have the client push the finger back farther until slight discomfort is felt, but not pain.

This point of mild discomfort (but not pain) is the maximum range of stretch recommended. Understanding that pushing the finger beyond this level

Considerations for Flexibility Training Intensity

When planning a flexibility training program, consider the following when determining intensity:

- **Client's experience level**—When working with clients who have limited experience with flexibility training, you need to educate them on the difference between mild discomfort and pain. With these clients you may want to use an intensity that is slightly less than you would use with someone who is more mobile or is familiar with the sensation of flexibility training. In all cases, the stretch intensity you recommend should not push clients beyond the point of mild discomfort, and the intensity should always be in a pain-free zone.

- **Timing of flexibility exercises during training session**—When using pre-training dynamic stretches, the intensity should be less than that used post-exercise. Have clients move through ROM gently and progressively push through mild tension (but not pain) until no further gain is made in ROM. Avoid overstretching that could occur if they push too hard through tension.

During post-training stretches (static or slow dynamic), clients have more mobility, so they can move more deeply through ROM and tension as long as the stretch continues to be pain free. Remember that the intensity of each stretch may vary from one part of a client's body to another.

of stretch could cause pain or injury gives the client an experiential example of what optimal stretch intensity is for other areas of the body.

Coaching breathing can also help ease clients into the desired intensity of stretch. The general guideline is to inhale to prepare for a stretch, exhale while going into (or holding a stretch), and then inhale again when coming out of it. Breathing in this way produces better results and outcomes because it helps clients avoid the common tendencies to struggle, strain, or otherwise not relax when stretching.

Time

Flexibility timing can be described in terms of the duration (i.e., how long clients hold a stretch), the number of repetitions, or the pace at which they move into and then out of a stretch. In the instance of pre-training dynamic stretching, the duration is short and is limited to going through the ROM up to the barrier of resistance (which gives a mild to moderate stretch) and then immediately returning to the starting position. The timing may be breath guided, such that exhalation occurs on the stretch and inhalation occurs coming out of (or preparing for) the stretch. Alternatively, a count of one or two seconds can be used while in the stretch.

For post-training stretching (either static or very slow dynamic), the duration is much longer and is guided by deep breaths. The client remains at the point of the initial barrier of resistance for 30 seconds or until he or she notices no further gain in ROM. The timing here may be breath guided. Deep, prolonged exhalation occurs on the stretch, and deep, prolonged inhalation occurs as the client comes out of the stretch.

As your client performs repetitions of a particular stretch, at some point additional reps of that stretch will give no further gain in ROM. The optimal number of reps of a particular stretch can be determined by counting to the last rep that gives your client a noticeable gain in ROM.

In some instances, the frequency of repetitions will change if one side of the body is significantly different from the other. For example, if your client's left hamstring is tighter than the right, the flexibility program could start with the stretch on the left side because it is tighter, move to a stretch for the right hamstring (for the same amount of time), and then

Considerations for Flexibility Training Duration

When planning a flexibility training program, consider the following when determining duration:

- **Timing of flexibility exercises during training session**—Pre-training flexibility exercises can be done with a shorter duration than post-training exercises. The faster pace of dynamic pre-training stretching keeps each rep short (1 to 2 seconds) and total stretch time short (i.e., a few minutes during the warm-up). Take care that your client does not move so quickly that the stretches become ballistic.

  Post-training stretches should be slower paced and longer in duration. Clients should use either static stretches (30 seconds) or slow dynamic movements (4 to 6 seconds).

- **Client's goals for flexibility training**—If the client is using flexibility exercises to help warm up and prepare for exercise, the focus is on preparing for the workout. These dynamic stretches should be short in duration and limited to going through the ROM to mild or moderate stretch. The client should then immediately return to the starting position. Take care that the client does not move so slowly that the heart rate decreases and she or he begins to relax. The pace should be just quick enough to keep the client alert, engaged, and ready to train.

  To maximize the recovery effects of post-workout flexibility training, these stretches should be longer in duration and guided by deep, prolonged breaths that also help slow the heart rate and get the client to relax. At this point, the client can explore various angles in the stretch to reach all muscle fibers. The best effects from post-training stretching occur if it is done within 15 minutes of ending the training session or before the client reports feeling that he or she has started cooling off.

repeat again on the left side (giving a 2:1 ratio). Over time, the tighter side will usually start to feel and move like the other side. At that point the client can stop using the 2:1 ratio and continue to stretch both areas evenly, as needed.

Type

As mentioned earlier in the chapter, flexibility and mobility exercises can be described as either static or dynamic. Each type of stretching has specific guidelines and parameters, which are described in detail in the next sections.

Static Stretching

Traditionally, static stretches are performed in positions that clients hold for a stated period while breathing into the stretch. Another option that may be more comfortable and effective is having the client perform very slow movements that involve slightly coming out of the static stretch while inhaling and then gently going back into the stretch while exhaling. The client can progress ROM without pain in either case.

Current research shows that static stretching increases ROM but also temporarily reduces power and strength (Page, 2012). Because of these outcomes, static stretching should be avoided pre-training, but it may be used post-training to aid in recovery and to regain lost ROM (Page, 2012).

Dynamic Stretching

When using dynamic stretches, the client moves through ROM first without resistance before gradually moving through resistance with a moderate to fast tempo. Progressive increases in amplitude occur as tolerated. Examples of common dynamic stretches are leg swings and trunk rotations. In any dynamic stretch sequence, movement through tension or resistance should always be done progressively with multiple repetitions until no further gains in ROM are achieved.

Because of its shorter duration and higher tempo of movement and breathing, dynamic stretching can be done pre-training to prepare a client for a workout or before a specific exercise within a training session. After the client has warmed up and achieved the desired general mobility or specific ROM required, she or he is ready to continue the rest of the training program.

At the end of the training session, very slow dynamic stretching is an alternative technique to static stretching. In this case, instead of holding a position of stretching for a long duration, the client performs micromovements by moving slowly a few degrees into and out of the stretch, as well as side-to-side (or any other small movement of the body region that the stretch allows). As a Personal Training Specialist, you may find many clients who respond better to slow dynamic stretching than to static stretching. You should use this information to design individualized flexibility programming.

Table 7.2 summarizes recommendations for stretching before and after a workout.

Note: Although the previous sections mention pre- and post-training stretching, having a client stretch during the personal training session is appropriate if a particular area feels stiff, tight, or restricted. Taking a minute or two to perform a few reps of dynamic stretching usually corrects the problem so that the client is able to finish the workout.

Putting It All Together

People today find themselves in a state of chronic tightness as a result of the modern lifestyle. By the time they reach out to a Personal Training Specialist for assistance, their tightness has progressed to cause limitations in mobility and therefore functional movements. The flexibility and mobility of each client needs to be addressed prior to beginning any exercise program to minimize the risk of injury and maximize program effectiveness. Table 7.3 summarizes canfitpro's position on flexibility training, drawing in all components of the FITT model for different types of clients.

Considerations for Flexibility Training Type

When planning a flexibility training program, consider the following when determining training type:

- **Client's current training demands**—Clients who require a certain level of mobility to perform their workouts may find it helpful to include dynamic stretches before or during their sessions. If the focus is on using stretching as a form of recovery from training, then either static or slow dynamic stretches should be used.

- **Timing of flexibility exercises during training session**—Because static stretching temporarily reduces power and strength, it is best to use dynamic stretching during the warm-up and save static stretching for the end of a workout. Flexibility exercises that are performed pre-training or during a workout should be dynamic. Post-workout stretching may be either static or slow dynamic (or a combination of both).

The following section presents Core Four on the Floor, an excellent self-stretch program that you can start with almost all clients who have restricted mobility or decreased ROM. This program can be done as a pre-training mobility warm-up and as a post-training mobility restoration and recovery exercise. You can also give it to your clients as a home program so that they can progress more quickly in their training program with you.

TABLE 7.2   Stretching Recommendations

Stretching parameters	Intensity	Duration	Reps	Sets	Notes
Pre-training (dynamic)	Light to moderate	Short 2 to 3 counts	3*	1	Add an extra rep if needed to get full ROM. Add an extra set to the tighter side.
Post-training (static)	Moderate to deep	Long 30 sec	1	1 to 3	See above. Adjust reps and sets to what the body needs that day.
Post-training (slow dynamic)	Moderate to deep	Long 4 to 6 counts	3–6*	1 to 3	

*Suggested number of reps is approximate and should be based on the client's gains in ROM.

TABLE 7.3 Flexibility Training Guidelines

Client type		Physical activity profile	Possible program focus	Frequency	Intensity	Time	Type
Nonexerciser	No habitual activity and extremely deconditioned	Sedentary	Increase mobility	4 to 7 days per week and multiple times per day	Light tension and pain free	Dynamic pre-workout: 1 to 2 sec	Pre-workout: dynamic
Occasional exerciser	Minimal current exercise and moderately to highly deconditioned	Minimal activity			Light to moderate tension and pain free	Static post-workout: 30 sec	Post-workout: static or slow dynamic
Recreational exerciser	Suboptimal exercise frequency and mildly to moderately deconditioned	Sporadic physical activity	Increase or maintain mobility			Dynamic post-workout: 4 to 6 sec	
Committed exerciser or athlete	Regular moderate to vigorous activity	Habitual physical activity	Maintain optimal mobility	Minimum 4 days per week (possibly multiple times per day)			
Dedicated exerciser or elite athlete	Regular vigorous activity	High amounts of physical activity			Moderate to deep tension and pain free		

CORE FOUR ON THE FLOOR

1. Glutes

1. Sit more on one glute and place the front foot on the back knee. Make adjustments for comfort.
2. Lengthen the whole spine out from the top of your head as you inhale. Exhale, moving out, down, and forward into the stretch, keeping the spine long.
3. Flex, rolling up through spine to the beginning erect position. Repeat, taking the torso forward over the front of the knee at various angles, targeting the various gluteal fibers.

Tips—Breathe, waving into and out of the stretch until you feel your tissues release. Drop your body down closer to the floor and move from side to side.

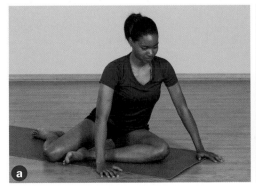
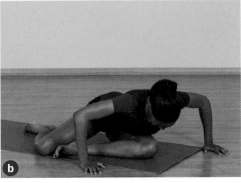

2. Quadratus lumborum (QL)

1. From the glute stretch, start walking the hands back until you feel a slight stretch in the back, hips, or legs.
2. Keeping the hands still, lean to the front hand and inhale.
3. Exhale as you lean into the back hand, slightly bending the elbow.

Tips—Walk the hands slightly farther with each rep to progress the stretch.

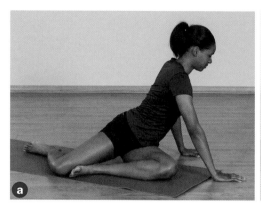 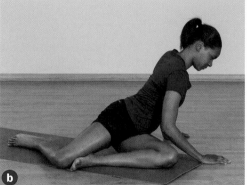

3. Hip flexors

1. From the last position, place the back forearm on the ground and find a stable position to balance on that arm with your full weight.
2. Lean slightly forward on both hands and inhale.
3. Exhale while leaning back, looking up to the ceiling. Repeat.

Tips—Lean farther back to progress the stretch. Turn your chest toward the floor and then to the ceiling to stretch different angles.

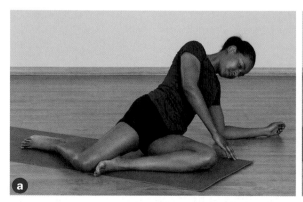 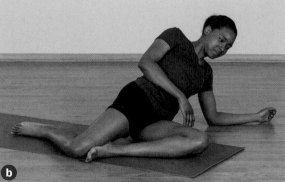

4. Latissimus dorsi (lats)

1. Moving from the last position, inhale and then reach your arm overhead.
2. Extend the arm out from the hip as you reach up and overhead.
3. Exhale as you rotate your chest toward the floor, reaching your arm out.
4. Circle your arm down and back up overhead to repeat.

Tips—Keep reaching your arm throughout the stretch for maximal effect. Try to get your chest closer to parallel to the floor with each rep.

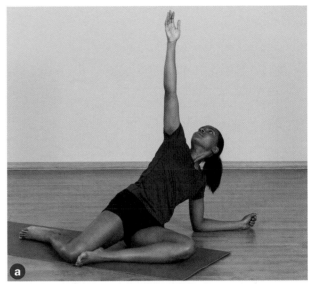

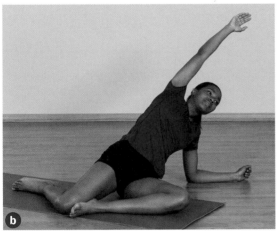

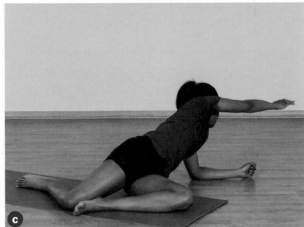

Central core stability and strength are needed not only for good posture but also for effective mobility. Core stability is one of the foundations of any good training program, but it should be paired and complemented by a core flexibility program for a complete, balanced approach to training. Tight muscles can affect neighbouring muscles in their respective myofascial chains. Those muscles can also become tight to help the body function with imbalances. An example is a flexibility imbalance in one of the four core muscles that affect one side of the body. If the left quadratus lumborum (QL) is significantly tighter than the right, the client may exhibit a shorter left leg, a hip shift, a lower shoulder, and more. Naturally, many more muscles than just the QL can become tight and restrict motion. Any

tightness can increase stress on the body, increase risk of injury, and negatively affect the squat, deadlift, and other exercises. Coaching your client to improve technique will fail because the client has a core muscle flexibility imbalance that needs to be specifically addressed. Stretching not only the key muscle (e.g., QL) but also some or all of the muscles in the same myofascial chain can often correct these imbalances so that training can progress safely and immediately.

The stretch matrix diagram (figure 7.3) can help you rapidly identify the muscle chain connections so that you can assess and train the whole person. In the centre of the diagram are the four core muscle groups that lie in the centre of the body. From the centre are branches of myofascial chains, running from head to foot and overlaying a faint figure of a human. This figure is referenced to locate the specific areas of the body represented in the matrix diagram:

- **Head**—Spine and paraspinal muscles.
- **(R) arm**—Front of the upper body, generally flexors from the abdominals to the front of the shoulder, arm, and hand.
- **(L) arm**—Back of the upper body, generally the erector spinae to the back of the shoulder, arm, and hand.
- **(R) abducted leg**—Back of the hip, thigh, and leg and bottom of the foot.
- **(L) abducted leg**—Front of the hip, thigh, and leg and top of the foot.
- **(R) standing leg**—Outside of the hip, thigh, leg, and foot.

- **(L) standing leg**—Inside of the hip, thigh, leg, and foot.

The stretch matrix can give Personal Training Specialists a basic idea of what myofascial regions to stretch in each client, beginning with the Core Four stretches and adding other stretches in a logical way. To use the stretch matrix in conjunction with the Core Four stretches:

- Use the Core Four movements to complement your other assessments of posture and movement to identify the key muscles that are tight.
- If a key muscle is tight, use the diagram to note where the muscle sits within a myofascial chain.
- Begin a stretch program with the Core Four stretches to address core imbalances first. Use the Core Four before you attempt stretching

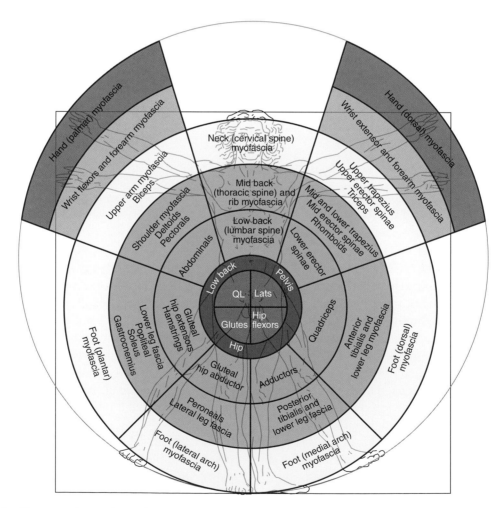

FIGURE 7.3 The stretch matrix can be used to determine target areas for your flexibility training program.

Reprinted, by permission, from A. Frederick and C. Frederick, 2006, *Stretch to win* (Champaign, IL: Human Kinetics), 115.

other muscle groups because those muscles usually release more and are easier to stretch after the Core Four stretches have been done.

- If the four core muscles do not lengthen or have a poor response after three sessions of focused stretching both in training sessions and on the client's own time, stretching needs to be progressed to include additional muscles found in the same chain.

For example, if the quadratus lumborum (QL) is identified as tight and stretches for that area do not seem to correct the problem, follow the myofascial chain down the leg to the next muscle groups in the diagram—the hip abductors (gluteus medius and so on), IT band, peroneals (fibularis), and lateral ankle and foot. Stretching of those muscles and tissues may help improve the client's overall mobility and flexibility.

Summary of Main Points

1. Flexibility is recognized as one of the elements needed to achieve and maintain optimal fitness because it enables clients to get even better results from their exercise programs.

2. Flexibility can be defined as more than just range of motion; it is having the ability to adapt successfully to challenges to motor control, strength, balance, coordination, endurance, and mental and emotional focus.

3. General flexibility is associated with the ability to perform any full- or partial-body movements required during normal daily activities without experiencing pain. Specific flexibility is associated with the ability to perform any specific movement required to progress toward specific goals.

4. Motor control, as an aspect of flexibility, is achieved through stability and mobility. Joints and soft tissue must have sufficient mobility for efficient movement.

5. Clients need mobility not only in the joints but also in all soft tissues. Fascia is the connective tissue that wraps around and between muscles, tendons, and ligaments.

6. Fascia is more than just connective tissue; it provides sensory information to the brain and the rest of the body that is used for body sense and position.

7. Fascia has qualities of mobility and stability, as well as viscoelasticity, meaning that it has mechanical properties of elasticity and plasticity. Regarding stretching, elasticity yields shorter gains in ROM, whereas plasticity yields longer gains.

8. Together, muscle and fascia are called myofascia. Restricted myofascia negatively affects muscle mobility and function and is associated with poor posture, decreased speed, decreased balance, and decreased strength, among other things.

9. PROM is always greater than AROM because muscles aren't being actively contracted unless the client is not relaxed.

10. Mobilization and flexibility training are used to improve faulty patterns or poor mobility in movement exercises.

11. Static and dynamic stretching can be done actively or passively. Dynamic stretching is recommended before, during, or after training. Static stretching should be done only after training. It is not recommended before or during training because it can reduce power and weaken muscles. Stretching should be performed with a faster tempo before training and a slower tempo after training.

12. Flexibility training should not be done when the client feels pain, has recently had surgery or been injured, or has unstable ligaments.

13. When designing a stretch program, start with a program like the Core Four, which begins with the core or centre of the body. Start stretching shorter muscles that cross one joint and progress to longer muscles that cross many joints.

Key Concepts for Study

Flexibility

Mobility

Fascia

Static stretching

Dynamic stretching

Planes of movement

Sagittal plane

Frontal plane

Transverse plane

ROM

Hypermobility

Review Questions

1. Define flexibility and describe the benefits of including it as part of a personal training program.

2. Briefly describe how weak muscles can be made stronger through flexibility training.

3. What kind of flexibility training is not recommended before or during training because it can reduce power and weaken muscle?

   a. passive stretching

   b. dynamic stretching

   c. static stretching

   d. active stretching

4. Flexibility is

   a. joint specific

   b. specific to an exercise

   c. individual specific

   d. all of the above

5. The physiological property that allows tissues in the body to return to their original state after stretching is called

   a. mobility

   b. plasticity

   c. elasticity

   d. flexibility

6. The interconnectivity of joints, muscles, and fascia can be described using

   a. myofascial slings

   b. myofascial systems

   c. myofascial chains

   d. all of the above

7. Assessment of mobility and flexibility can include the performance of

   a. daily movement activities

   b. the Core Four movements

   c. a specific exercise movement (e.g., squat)

   d. all of the above

 Web Resource Contents
Answers to review questions

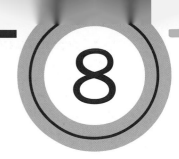

Foundational Movement Sequences

Mark Stone, BSc
Rod Macdonald, BEd

LEARNING OUTCOMES

After completing this chapter you will be able to

1. describe the difference between functional and performance-based movement;

2. highlight the importance of integrating functional and performance movement;

3. understand postural stability, reflexes, and open and closed chain movements;

4. identify how biomotor abilities relate to foundational movement sequences;

5. discuss the classifications of foundational movement sequences; and

6. understand how to apply regression and progression exercises to a program.

Successful Personal Training

Specialists blend their knowledge of the components of the body with an understanding of how the body is meant to move, for both function (i.e., movement for the necessities of everyday life) and performance (e.g., exercise and sport). Whether for function or performance, all your clients will want to progress from wherever they start toward improved health and fitness. To assist clients in doing this safely and effectively, you need to understand the foundational movement sequences that all humans should ideally be able to perform and know how to incorporate those movement patterns into a training program.

For most of our evolution, before we began to succumb to the detrimental aspects of modern living, foundational movement sequences were the basic movements required by the human body to survive. The ability to perform pushing, pulling, squatting, and lifting movements, as well as to run, climb, and throw could be taken for granted. But reduced physical activity and poor food choices have resulted in a marked deterioration of the abilities of many people to function at even a basic level, let alone at a high level of performance. Because of the modern lifestyle, many people find their way to a Personal Training Specialist in a state of chronic limitation, which, if left untreated, may result in injury or even disease. For this reason, Personal Training Specialists need to be able to identify shortcomings in foundational movement sequences and develop programs to address clients' needs while preventing injury.

What Is Functional Training?

Functional training is an approach to training in which the primary goal is to improve the daily function of clients. For example, people need the ability to go to and from work, do housework, and otherwise enjoy the activities of daily life, pain free. This kind of training is different from **performance training**, which has the goal of improving performance regardless of whether daily function is improved. For example, a person may train enough to run a marathon in under four hours but have difficulty washing dishes due to a lack of mobility in the lower back.

The paradox of functional training and performance training may seem confusing at first, given the fact that several otherwise reputable sources often discuss the benefits of functional training as they relate to sport performance (or the functional benefits of participating in certain sports). This notion might suggest that they are one in the same, but Personal Training Specialists should understand them in their correct context. True functional training stems from physiotherapy, whereby therapists attempt to return injured people to normal function by retraining the ability to go about their daily lives without impediment. Although a crossover of benefits from one training approach to the other will likely occur, these approaches should be seen as unique and important, but only so far as they align with the client's goals.

Defining daily function is important when working with a specific client to ensure that she or he is getting the desired results in a safe and effective way. For example, one client's daily function might simply be getting up, going to work, and returning home each day, whereas another's daily function might include delivering parcels as a courier. You can imagine that these two clients have differing functional needs, although neither is attempting to increase performance in a sport environment.

As a Personal Training Specialist, you must always consider the client's functional needs, even if he or she has a performance-related goal. Observing this policy will help you design programs that avoid the possibility of a deterioration of function for the benefit of performance.

The foundational movement sequences introduced later in this chapter should be understood as the common ground between functional training and performance training. These movements can be embraced as functional, although when they are combined and properly progressed, they will eventually go beyond functional application and apply readily to performance training. For example, walking and running are functional by nature, but when they are combined with pushing and pulling and progressed to higher intensity, you can see how they might better apply to a football player than to the average person.

When assessing function, especially in deconditioned clients, you should establish a baseline understanding of what they can and cannot do by performing the assessments found in chapters 9 and 10 of this text.

The basic ability to remain functional as well as to improve performance requires an integrated approach to both understanding movement and designing programs. When developing programs for clients, particularly deconditioned clients, Personal Training Specialists should do the following (Chek, 2001):

1. Evaluate the client's static and dynamic postural stability and plan to develop balance skills as needed.

2. Understand the righting and equilibrium reflexes and what they require to function properly.

3. Identify when the training program should include open chain versus closed chain movements.

4. Evaluate the client's biomotor abilities and adapt the training program to develop them as needed.

5. Incorporate foundational movement sequences.

6. Regress or progress the basic movement sequences as appropriate.

Postural Stability and Balance

During all movement, the ability to stabilize posture statically and dynamically using muscle strength and reflexes optimizes the efficiency of movement while reducing the risk of injury. These optimized strategies create more efficient movements for function and performance.

The simple everyday process of lowering an object to the floor requires the body to bend forward. This motion loads the extensors of the hips and spine eccentrically in flexion of the hips and spine. The process of picking up the object requires the same joints and muscles to contract concentrically to stand again without injury or loss of balance during extension of the hips and spine. At the same time the body must continually monitor the effects of gravity and make adjustments to compensate and avoid falling over.

What is often taken for granted in this movement and other seemingly simple everyday tasks is the role that **postural stability** plays in the home, exercise, or sport environment.

Static and Dynamic Stability

In picking up an object from the floor, **static postural stability** is the process needed to keep the angle of the spine straight during the lowering and raising of the body to and from the floor. **Dynamic postural stability** is the process needed to maintain alignment of the actively moving knees and hips to ensure optimal alignment, therefore increasing efficiency of movement and reducing the risk of injury from repetitive stress overload to the involved joints.

Both static and dynamic postural stabilization require the recruitment of stabilizing muscles as well as major muscle groups to complete each task. These simultaneous processes have the additional outcome of maintaining the body's centre of gravity of the body over its base of support (e.g., when running), or returning it there (e.g., when recovering from jumping and reaching to catch a ball). Whether participating in a sport, exercising in the gym, or performing daily household duties, the body is always changing its position relative to the force of gravity. Every movement, whether performed during sitting, standing, walking, or running, involves the management of the body's centre of gravity. When we are successful in this task, we are able to maintain our balance whether we are resistance training, ice skating, jogging, or walking. When we are unsuccessful, we lose our balance either momentarily or completely (e.g., slipping while walking on ice or performing an exercise on a stability ball). The addition of sports equipment and other external loading (e.g., weights, carrying a child) challenges the body's ability to maintain its centre of gravity over its base of support.

Righting and Equilibrium Reflexes

Performing routine movements of daily life requires the nervous system to practice the process of stabilization continuously, which allows us to function in the earth's field of gravity. These nervous system processes, known as reflexes, allow the body to maintain or regain balance when we feel as if we might fall (e.g., by maintaining a position of stillness when sitting on a stability ball). In situations when the body cannot maintain an upright position through a change in its base of support, reflexes allow us to catch ourselves by extending an arm to break the fall (which may result in injury).

The body uses two classes of reflexes—righting and equilibrium. **Righting reflexes** are reactions that are expressed when the body attempts to move or maintain a position on a stable or fixed surface (such as a gym floor, sidewalk, or artificial surface like a dry soccer field).

Equilibrium reflexes are primarily used when the body attempts to move or maintain a position on a surface that is unsteady or moves underneath the point of contact (typically the feet or hands), such as when riding in an elevator, walking up or down an escalator, or skating across the surface of an ice rink.

Stability and Balance in the Training Program

The initial phase of a well-planned, functional exercise program requires the client to demonstrate mastery in the ability to maintain her or his centre of gravity over the base of support during body-weight exercises. After successfully managing this phase, the client may progress to exercises involving minimal loading and challenging changes of position in the various planes of movement. Ultimately, the client may be challenged with moderate to heavy loads and rapid changes of tempo, taking care to maintain proper form and technique and being sure not to compromise joint stability.

Four key components influence the successful recruitment of both static and dynamic postural stabilizers. The development of efficient strategies to maintain the centre of gravity over the base of support and the development of adaptive reflex profiles depend on these components:

1. The design of a comprehensive flexibility assessment and flexibility training program. As discussed in chapter 7, limited flexibility may compromise the ability of the body to perform movements with proper alignment.

2. The practice of a program that develops the strength of the stabilizing muscles.

3. The appropriate progression into resistance exercises that mimic the client's functional and performance needs.

4. The use of tempo to increase neuromuscular recruitment and enhance power output in the client's program.

Each client must progress through these steps under the watchful eye of the Personal Training Spe-cialist to achieve the goals of the program. Failure to respect the client's optimal pace of progress could result in reduced improvement or injury.

Open Chain and Closed Chain Movement

Our understanding of biomechanics and its importance in fitness has advanced significantly in the field of exercise science. Applying the concepts of open and closed kinetic chain exercise is necessary when designing safe and effective programs. Arthur Steindler, who popularized the kinetic chain concept, defined an open kinetic chain system as "successively arranged joints in which the terminal segment can move freely". This simply means that, during the execution of an exercise, the hand (upper body exercise) or foot (lower body exercise) is free to move. **Open kinetic chain exercises** usually develop skills specific to sport or performance, whereas closed chain exercises generally have more benefits to **functional movements**. An example of an open chain lower-body exercise that has little functional application is a seated knee extension machine, in which the feet are free to move in space. An example of an open chain upper-body exercise is a standing barbell or dumbbell arm curl in which the biceps are recruited to flex the elbow joint.

A **closed kinetic chain exercise** is characterized by successively arranged joints in which the terminal segment (hand or foot) cannot be moved freely. An example of a closed kinetic chain exercise for the lower body is body-weight or loaded squats, in which the body pushes itself away from the immovable surface of the floor. When applying the principle of closed kinetic chain exercise to the upper body, the body-weight push-up from the floor can be used to recruit the entire shoulder girdle and core.

When attempting to maximize the results of an exercise program, you, as a Personal Training Spe-cialist, should choose exercises that most closely resemble the applicable environment of the client. If the client lacks functional ability as determined in an assessment, then closed kinetic chain system exercises should be the focus of the program. Similarly, if the client or athlete is involved in a throwing or striking sport, open kinetic chain system exercises that focus on prime movers and stabilizers of the shoulder girdle should be a focus of the program. When selecting exercises for any client, you should always begin with an assessment and then proceed to design the program based on your client's unique needs, taking into account where the client is currently and with an eye on where he or she wants to go. Although you should typically use closed kinetic chain exercises for most clients (because they are functional and often lend benefit to performance as well), you must also respect the individuality of your clients as you make choices about their programs. In some cases, you may even choose to begin with easy-to-teach open kinetic chain exercises for deconditioned clients or clients with specific needs or limitations. If you have a client who presents with severe limitations, you should consult with the appropriate qualified health professional to ensure that your approach is correct for the situation.

Biomotor Abilities

Another key component that must be considered as it relates to foundational movement and function is the characteristic of **biomotor ability** (Bompa, 2009). In the study of human movement, a distinction is made between abilities and skills. Ability refers to a genetically derived talent to perform a physical skill or movement without practice or rehearsal. Ability may be considered the movement skill set that a person is born with, and the person needs little instruction to maintain or advance its efficiency. People with high levels of biomotor ability are those who we typically consider natural-born athletes, fast learners, or those who "just get it" when it comes to understanding posture, stability, and movement. In addition, these people tend to progress through ascending sequences of movement more quickly than the average personal training client does.

The term *skill* describes the learned ability to carry out a task with pre-determined results, often within a given amount of time, intensity, or volume. Skill is something that clients develop over the course of their exercise-training programs. Clients with limited movement skills may be more likely to be injured by using a program that is too complex for their level of expertise. As a result, such clients must be provided less complex movements until their level of skill adapts to progressively more challenging movements and programs.

The following aspects have been identified as biomotor abilities:

- Agility
- Flexibility
- Coordination
- Balance
- Strength
- Power
- Endurance
- Speed

When programming foundational movement and function into a client's program or enhancing the way in which an athlete or client moves, remember that the sequences of movement being developed all contain essential components of each of these biomotor abilities, when practiced in their optimal environment. A client's abilities may improve as flexibility, strength, and coordination respond to training.

 You may notice that many of the biomotor abilities listed here are also secondary components of fitness as discussed in chapter 2. Although clients will vary in their level of innate biomotor ability in each of these areas, most clients will see relative improvement with training.

The development of the client's biomotor abilities is essential when considering exercise selection in the context of the function and skill being trained. In addition, you need to consider the client's skill, movement ability, and physical ability.

You should assess the physical ability of the client before designing a program and continually watch for improvement or decline during the teaching and execution of new exercises. Physical ability defines the person's current orthopedic status, which may interfere with meeting the challenges of a new program. For example, a client who lacks the physical ability to squat properly will usually, through assessment, be found to have limited range of motion at the hip, knee, and ankle joints. These issues must be resolved if the client is expected to learn and perform the exercise correctly. See chapter 10 for an in-depth discussion about how to use dynamic assessments to evaluate your clients' movement ability.

Foundational Movement Sequences

Certain foundational movement sequences and accompanying exercises should be incorporated into most, if not all, programs. These sequences serve as the templates of movement on which successful physical performance is practiced in the activities of daily life, work, and sport. Through safe and effective programming, your client will acquire these sequences, upon which more complex strategies can then be built.

The foundational movement sequences can be trained with varying levels of simplicity or complexity, depending on the individual needs of your clients. Each sequence possesses a baseline standard of performance, the successful execution of which requires the integration of multiple joint functions as well as the creation of strategies necessary to both move and stabilize the involved joint structures. Incorporating these movements into the client's exercise program will contribute to motor skill development and further enhance the client's abilities in the work and sport environment.

We have classified the foundational movement sequences into three categories:

- Passive sequences (positions from which movement is typically performed)

- Active sequences (primarily compound sequences that create movement)

- Complex sequences (the combination of active sequences that contribute to most sport performances)

The use of foundational movement sequences in program design ensures that the client will learn to integrate all the key components of optimal stabilization through the use of movements that recruit multiple joint functions. In situations in which the client cannot successfully integrate all the key joint functions of a foundational movement sequence, it may be necessary to strengthen the accessory movements of the knee, hip, or shoulder using isolation exercises.

Passive Sequences

Three passive movement sequences provide the foundation for any activity that your client may perform in daily life, work, or sport. The ability to lie down, sit, or stand comfortably will need to be established before you add active movement sequences and more complex exercises. Table 8.1 describes possible regressions and progressions of each passive sequence.

Development of the spinal stabilization system and core musculature (discussed in chapters 5 and 6) will help your clients perform each successive level of the passive movement sequences.

Active Sequences

Active sequences are the foundational movements that the body uses to perform most exercises and activities of daily life (ADLs). They include pushing, pulling, squatting, lunging, lifting, and twisting. Assuming that the client can perform the

TABLE 8.1   Passive Movement Sequences

Regression 2	Regression 1	Passive sequences	Progression 1	Progression 2
Lying with knees, low back, and neck supported	Lying with knees supported	**Lying comfortably (unsupported)**	Lifting one or both hands Lifting one or both legs	Like progression 1, on an unstable device or otherwise decreasing stability
Sitting with low back and upper back supported	Sitting with low back supported	**Sitting comfortably (unsupported)**	Lifting one or both hands Lifting one or both legs	Like progression 1, on an unstable device or otherwise decreasing stability
Standing with low back supported	Standing with one leg elevated for support	**Standing comfortably (unsupported)**	Lifting one or both hands Lifting one or both legs	Like progression 1, on an unstable device or otherwise decreasing stability

passive sequences of lying, sitting, and standing comfortably, the active movement sequences can be added to create various training exercises. If the client cannot perform these foundational movements without restriction or discomfort, then regression is appropriate, even to the point of performing the movement with no external resistance. Table 8.2 describes the active sequences and some possible modifications to progress or regress each movement.

An Example of Progression and Regression in Active Movement Sequences: The Squat

As an example of training active sequences, consider teaching the squat exercise. After addressing any flexibility issues from short and tight muscles, the Personal Training Specialist may need to regress the squat sequence and identify the joint functions that may appear to be weak or lack coordination between muscle groups. In cases of severe lack of conditioning, the program may need to include an exercise or series of exercises that primarily recruits and reinforces the accessory movements of knee flexion and extension with hip flexion and extension in a supine position, without the demands of spinal stabilization required by standing erect against the pull of gravity. In this case, the Personal Training Specialist may use an exercise such as hip bridging on the floor or a stability ball to decrease the demands placed on the client's spinal stabilization system. After mastering the regressed sequences of the squat and developing the stabilization needed to support the pelvis and spine in a supine position, the client may progress to performing the squat in the traditional standing position.

For all the sequences, reducing resistance, speed, and range of motion will also regress the movement. Note that the need for certain regressions may also suggest that the client requires expertise that falls beyond your *Standards of Practice* as a Personal Training Specialist. You may need to consult with a qualified health professional to provide recommendations for a client who cannot perform the foundational sequences. When moving beyond the foundational sequences, progression 1 movements can be additionally modified by adding a source of external resistance (dumbbell, barbell, tubing, cable, and so on) or by increasing speed or range of motion. Personal Training Specialists need to understand that by increasing speed, resistance, instability, or other challenges (i.e., progression 2 in table 8.3), risk of injury increases substantially. Always keep in mind that progressions are not appropriate for clients who have not yet mastered the foundational sequences.

Complex Sequences

Complex sequences go beyond the typical movements that you will use with your clients and delve into the realm of sport coaching because many of the movements would be sport specific. Table 8.3 describes the complex sequences of walking and running, climbing, and throwing, giving examples of progression and regression for each movement.

TABLE 8.2   Active Movement Sequences

Regression 2 (isolation)	Regression 1	Active sequences	Progression 1	Progression 2
Pec deck Triceps extension	Machine chest press	**Pushing**	Bench press	Standing cable press
Scapular retraction Biceps curl	Seated row	**Pulling**	Bent-over row	Standing cable pull
Leg extension Leg curl	Leg press	**Squatting**	Squat	Single leg squat or jump squat
Leg extension Leg curl	Static lunge	**Lunging**	Walking lunge	Jumping alternating lunge
Lying back extension	Back extension machine	**Lifting**	Deadlift	Kettlebell swing
Unweighted, seated twist	Oblique machine	**Twisting**	Standing cable twist	Back-to-back medicine ball pass

TABLE 8.3   Complex Movement Sequences

Regression 2	Regression 1	Complex sequences	Progression 1	Progression 2
Slow walking	Brisk walking	**Walking and running**	Running	Trail running
Pulling movements Squatting and lunging movements	Patterned climbing (e.g., Versa Climber or Jacob's ladder machine)	**Climbing**	Indoor wall climbing or bouldering	Free climbing
Underhand throw	Standing throw	**Throwing**	Step and throw	Throwing while running

 The in-depth analysis of complex sequences goes beyond the *Standards of Practice* of the Personal Training Specialist certification because of the complexity and multivariable factors involved in their execution. If assessing these sequences interests you, we recommend seeking educational opportunities specific to those activities.

Regression of Movement Sequences

In the event of a preexisting, unresolved injury or deconditioned state, the baseline standard of a foundational movement sequence may prove too difficult or unsafe to perform without loss of form or risk of injury. In this situation, a regressed version of the sequence should be used to allow the client to perform the joint functions and stability strategies needed to complete and master the sequence successfully. The tables provided give you just some of the possible regressions and progressions that a Personal Training Specialist might use. You may

choose to regress or progress slightly differently to suit your client's individual needs. Returning to our squat example, if a client does not require as much regression as indicated in table 8.2, other possible variations could include the following:

1. Squat with one dowel rod in each hand, touching the floor and positioned vertically like ski poles for stability assistance (regression 1)

2. Squat with one centralized dowel rod for stability assistance (regression 2)

3. Stability ball wall-assisted squat (regression 3)

4. Stability ball supine hip extension and bridging (regression 4)

5. Floor hip extension and bridging (regression 5)

Figures 8.1 and 8.2 show two example regressions for this movement sequence.

Although safety is of primary importance, as a Personal Training Specialist you need to also take

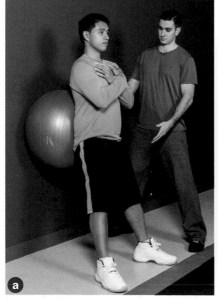
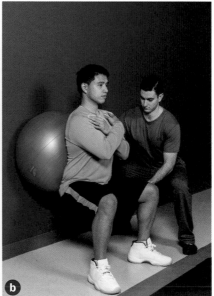

FIGURE 8.1   Stability ball wall-assisted squat.

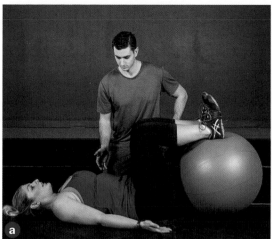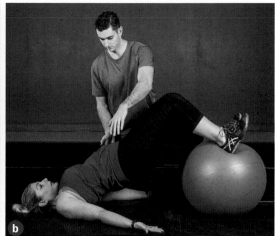

FIGURE 8.2   Stability ball supine hip extension (bridging).

special care in choosing a regression that is not lower than the client's current level of physical conditioning. Choosing a movement that is too regressed may slow the client's progress.

Progression of Movement Sequences

As a Personal Training Specialist, you are responsible for choosing a progressive movement sequence that will further develop the client's motor skills needed for function or performance. Failure to do so may slow the process of reaching the intended goals of the program. After practicing and mastering the baseline movement sequence, the client is ready to be taught a progressed version of the sequence. This process may be required if the person wishes to return to function or performance after an injury. Progression is also necessary when a client wants the challenge of a more difficult exercise to develop greater strength, agility, or hypertrophy. Another example of progressing the squat exercise is the following:

1. Body-weight squat (baseline standard)
2. Barbell front or back squat (progression 1)
3. Barbell front squat with overhead press (progression 2)
4. Two-dumbbell squat with overhead press (progression 3)
5. Single-dumbbell squat with overhead press (progression 4)
6. Single-dumbbell squat with overhead press on an unstable surface (progression 5)

Any exercise may be progressed in a number of ways to simulate the client's specific environments of work, sport, or life activities. Figure 8.3 shows the variables that can be changed to progress or regress an exercise.

All the preceding variables for regressive and progressive foundational movement sequences may be modified by the Personal Training Specialist to reproduce a lifestyle, workplace, or sport-specific environment. Tempo may be increased or decreased to develop postural endurance or power output requirements of the movement sequence.

The goal is to create a program that physically prepares clients to function optimally and corrects movements that they do not perform efficiently. When designed correctly, a functional program creates a stable, mobile, resilient body that allows clients to do all the physical tasks they desire to perform.

To serve each client optimally, you must design a program that uses progressive sequences of movement to challenge stability within the scope of her or his specific goals. As clients acquire the skills necessary for each version of an exercise, they can then move on to the next version as appropriate. Although progression is usually desirable, you may have a client who achieves a level of skill and wishes to go no further. If the reason for this is sound, perhaps because the risk of performing the next version outweighs the benefit of the exercise, you may want to challenge the previous level in a different way, such as with additional resistance, less rest, or with other variables. In all cases, the safety of the client outweighs all other considerations.

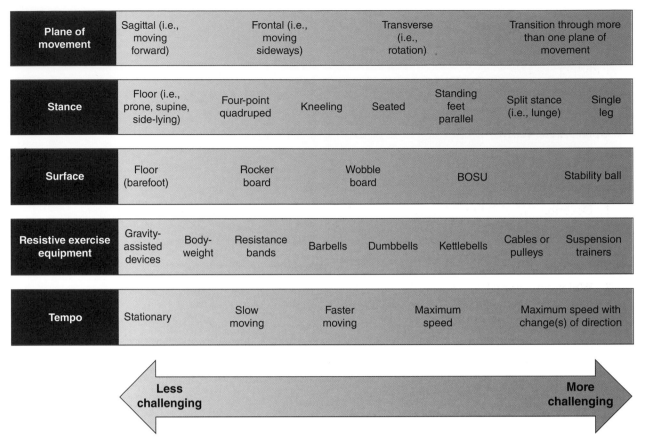

Plane of movement	Sagittal (i.e., moving forward)		Frontal (i.e., moving sideways)		Transverse (i.e., rotation)		Transition through more than one plane of movement	
Stance	Floor (i.e., prone, supine, side-lying)	Four-point quadruped	Kneeling	Seated	Standing feet parallel	Split stance (i.e., lunge)		Single leg
Surface	Floor (barefoot)		Rocker board		Wobble board	BOSU		Stability ball
Resistive exercise equipment	Gravity-assisted devices	Body-weight	Resistance bands	Barbells	Dumbbells	Kettlebells	Cables or pulleys	Suspension trainers
Tempo	Stationary		Slow moving	Faster moving		Maximum speed		Maximum speed with change(s) of direction

Less challenging ⟵   ⟶ **More challenging**

FIGURE 8.3   Continuum of exercise variations. Personal Training Specialists can progress an exercise by varying the plane of movement, stance, surface the exercise is performed on, equipment used, and tempo.

Summary of Main Points

1. Both static and dynamic postural stabilization require the recruitment of stabilizing muscles as well as major muscle groups.

2. Performing routine movements of daily life requires the nervous system to practice the process of stabilization continuously.

3. Applying the concepts of open and closed kinetic chain exercise is necessary when designing safe and effective programs.

4. In human movement terms, a skill may describe the learned ability to carry out a task with pre-determined results.

5. Biomotor abilities are a movement skill set that a person is born with, and the person needs little instruction to maintain or advance its efficiency.

6. Foundational movement sequences are an important element to include in each client's exercise program.

7. Choosing a movement that is too regressed may slow your client's progress.

8. Progression is necessary when a client wants the challenge of a more difficult exercise to develop greater strength, agility, or hypertrophy.

9. Any exercise may be progressed in a number of ways to simulate the environments of work, sport, or life activities.

Key Concepts for Study

Functional movement

Righting reflexes

Equilibrium reflexes

Performance training

Open kinetic chain

Closed kinetic chain

Biomotor abilities

Foundational movement sequences

Regression

Progression

Review Questions

1. Describe the difference between open and closed kinetic chain exercises.

2. Define functional training and explain its importance to clients.

3. Which type of reflex is primarily used when the body attempts to maintain its position on an unsteady surface?

   a. righting reflex

   b. myotatic reflex

   c. equilibrium reflex

   d. stretch reflex

4. Which of the following is not an example of an appropriate exercise progression?

   a. using kettlebells instead of dumbbells

   b. moving slowly instead of standing still

   c. moving in the transverse plane instead of the sagittal plane

   d. using a four-point quadruped instead of standing with feet parallel

5. Which of the following would be more appropriate for the beginner client?

   a. static stability exercises

   b. dynamic stability exercises

   c. complex stability exercises

   d. none of the above

6. The active movement sequences include all of the following except

   a. climbing

   b. twisting

   c. squatting

   d. pulling

7. When it comes to understanding posture, stability, and movement, people who are said to be natural-born athletes are likely to have a high level of

   a. biomotor skills

   b. biomotor abilities

   c. physical fitness

   d. active sequences

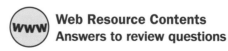

Web Resource Contents
Answers to review questions

PART II Case Study Questions

1. Using the information provided in the three case study profiles, what would your primary program focus be for Catherine, Lisa, and Thomas during each component of their workouts (i.e., cardiorespiratory training, resistance training, flexibility training)?

2. Catherine read online that flexibility training could help her maintain proper joint functioning and mobility as she gets older. Using the FITT principle and concepts discussed in chapter 7, describe the important characteristics of Catherine's flexibility training.

3. Given her previous experience and current fitness goals, Lisa believes that she would need to spend at least 90 minutes in the gym on most days of the week to get the results she desires. With your understanding of training guidelines and Lisa's physical activity profile, answer the following questions:

   a. What is Lisa's client type?

   b. How would you apply the FITT principle to her cardiorespiratory training?

   c. Lisa's resting heart rate is 71 BPM. What would her target training zone be in BPM?

   d. Given Lisa's busy schedule, how can you reduce her workout time from 90 minutes to 60? (Refer to table 4.6.)

4. Thomas comes to his first session with an article in his hand. He asks you to put him on an advanced Tabata interval-training program to save time and get results quickly. How do you explain to Thomas why this kind of workout may not be a good idea for his first training session?

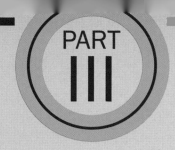

PART

III

Screening and Assessment

Combining both traditional and cutting-edge screening and assessment tools, this section of the manual teaches you how to understand your clients' starting point for the programs you will develop to complement their personal health and fitness goals.

In these chapters you will learn the importance of pre-exercise screening and assessments and why Personal Training Specialists need to perform both before designing and delivering training programs. After you master this section, you will be ready to work with your clients safely and effectively.

Passive Screening and Assessments

Gregory S. Anderson, PhD
Chad Benson, MSc
Mark Stone, BSc

LEARNING OUTCOMES

After completing this chapter, you will be able to

1. explain the reason for using health screening with all clients;

2. discuss the necessity for having all clients complete and sign a PAR-Q+ form;

3. understand how to implement a health-screening questionnaire;

4. identify a Personal Training Specialist's *Standards of Practice* with reference to medical conditions;

5. explain how to assess postural imbalances visually;

6. describe and recognize the postural stress results of upper and lower crossed syndrome; and

7. understand the process of conducting standard health assessments (e.g., HR, BP, and body composition) using various methods.

Before working with a client, you must gather as much information as possible to ensure that you, the Personal Training Specialist, are doing everything you can to support the client in succeeding with her or his goals, as well as preventing her or him from becoming injured in any way. In part 3 of this manual, we introduce you to both passive and dynamic screening and assessment protocols designed to give you a wealth of information that will allow you to create safe, effective, enjoyable, and time-efficient programs for your clients.

This chapter covers passive screening and assessments, which can be accomplished without risk to the client, and the following chapter covers dynamic assessments, which require movement and therefore carry some increased risk and need for care. Assessments should be performed by a Personal Training Specialist or qualified health professional to ensure that the information is valid, reliable, and reproducible.

Preparation must always precede the assessment. Before an assessment, clients should be told what to wear, when and where the assessment will take place, and not to exercise or consume caffeine or alcohol for 12 hours before the assessment. After clients arrive, they should fill out a PAR-Q+ (if they have not done so already), have the assessment session explained to them, and then sign an informed consent document. The Personal Training Specialist should have copies of the PAR-Q+ and the signed informed consent document kept on file.

The following is canfitpro's recommended order of steps for screening and assessment. The first three steps in assessment are covered in this chapter. The last two steps are covered in chapter 10, "Dynamic Assessments."

1. Pre-exercise screening (e.g., PAR-Q+, health history questionnaire)
2. Passive postural assessment (front, back, and side)
3. Standard health assessment (e.g., HR, BP, body composition)
4. Dynamic postural assessment
5. Fitness assessment:
   a. Cardiorespiratory fitness assessment, muscular capacity assessment
   b. Flexibility assessment

Always repeat the assessment sequence in the same order for consistent results.

Pre-Exercise Screening

Every Personal Training Specialist and facility has the legal and ethical obligation to ensure that clients entering the facility are reasonably safe. This obligation is part of your **duty of care** to your clients, and any breach may result in negligence. Negligence may leave Personal Training Specialists or the facility (or both) liable for damages should a client be injured because of inadequate screening and assessment, defective equipment, faulty supervision, incompetent instruction, or Personal Training Specialists' working outside their *Standards of Practice*. Therefore, to provide a safe and effective training environment, you must screen clients for health problems before allowing them to use your facility or before you develop a fitness program for them.

Pre-exercise screening is a crucial first step in the personal training process. You need to understand your clients' health before you counsel them, plan an exercise program for them, or even decide whether you are capable of becoming their Personal Training Specialist.

Your clients' personal health history is a serious and private matter, and all information must be kept confidential. If you encounter a client who has significant medical concerns or risks outside your expertise, you should encourage the client to search for a more qualified exercise professional or qualified health professional. A qualified exercise professional works with high-risk clients, including those with chronic medical conditions. A Personal Training Specialist may be considered a qualified exercise professional in the context of the referrals or recommendations given by the PAR-Q+ and ePARmed-X+. In the case of specific medical conditions or in working with certain population groups, the Personal Training Specialist's qualifications will depend on additional certifications, education, and training acquired.

Purposes of Pre-Exercise Screening

Pre-exercise screening is part of your *Standards of Practice* as a Personal Training Specialist and therefore part of your legal responsibility. This screening is designed to identify clients who have medical conditions that leave them at risk of injury or death when performing moderate to vigorous physical activity. Pre-exercise screenings allow you to do the following:

1. Be professional and fulfill legal responsibilities (*Standards of Practice*)
2. Identify a possible need to refer clients to qualified health professionals
3. Understand clients better and establish good communication
4. Identify areas of strength or weakness based on previous injury
5. Determine safe and effective exercises
6. Develop a precise, individualized exercise program

Pre-exercise screening must be able to identify clients who have any of the following:

- Diagnosed disease
- Signs or symptoms of a disease that is not yet diagnosed
- Increased cardiac risk
- Risks inherent in new activity because of age

Screening for each of these factors provides the minimal evaluation required before you can allow clients to train in a facility or take them on as personal training clients.

Diagnosed Disease

Clients with diagnosed disease or severe limitation who have not been given guidelines for exercise should seek further information before becoming more physically active or engaging in a fitness assessment. They should complete the specially designed online screening and exercise recommendations program (i.e., the ePARmed-X) and visit a qualified exercise professional to work through the results and gain additional guidance.

Signs and Symptoms

Signs and **symptoms** of a disease process may be well established before diagnosis by a medical practitioner and act as early warning signals. Signs and symptoms of cardiorespiratory, metabolic, or respiratory disease that should prompt medical referral include

- pain and discomfort in the chest, lower jaw, or left shoulder;
- ankle swelling;
- feelings of rapid, throbbing heart rate;
- severe pain in leg muscles when walking;
- unusual fatigue and general feelings of lethargy;
- difficulty breathing when standing or at night;
- shortness of breath at rest or during light activity; and
- feelings of dizziness or fainting.

Cardiac Risk Factors

Personal Training Specialists should be well aware of cardiorespiratory risk factors and be adept at screening clients for these risk factors:

- Men and women over the age of 45 years and unaccustomed to regular vigorous- to maximal-effort exercise
- Family history of heart disease (a father or grandfather having a heart attack or dying suddenly before the age of 55 years or a mother or grandmother having a heart attack or dying suddenly before the age of 65 years)
- Smoking
- High blood pressure or hypertension (systolic pressure greater than 140 or diastolic pressure greater than 90)
- High cholesterol levels (total cholesterol over 200 milligrams per decilitre of blood)
- Diabetes (type 1 or type 2)
- Insufficient physical activity (less than 150 minutes of moderate-intensity cardiorespiratory activity per week or less than 75 minutes of vigorous-intensity activity per week)

Age-Related Risk

Men and women over the age of 45 years who are not accustomed to regular vigorous- to maximal-effort exercise are encouraged to consult a qualified exercise professional before engaging in this intensity of exercise. Although medical exams may not be required of active people who have no other cardiac risks and want to participate in light to moderate exercise programs, they should be mandatory if the potential clients were previously sedentary, are initiating a new exercise regimen, or combine an age risk with any other risk factor.

Physical Activity Readiness Questionnaire

To begin the client screening process, have the client complete and sign a Physical Activity Readiness Questionnaire for Everyone (PAR-Q+). This form is used as an initial health-screening tool and is administered before clients begin a physical activity program. The PAR-Q+ includes seven general questions designed to identify clients who must proceed to complete a series of follow-up questions about their medical conditions before participating in a new exercise program. It also covers two pre-screening topics: **diagnosed disease** and signs and symptoms. Clients' responses to the PAR-Q+ give you an idea of their known health problems and medical conditions that might be affected by exercise. But the PAR-Q+ is only a general pre-screening tool.

If clients answer yes to one or more questions on the PAR-Q+, they must complete the follow-up questions about their medical conditions. If they answer no to all of the follow-up questions about their medical conditions, they are ready to become more physically active after they have signed the participant declaration. If they answer yes to one or more of the follow-up questions about their medical condition, they must provide further information before becoming more physically active or engaging in a fitness appraisal. They must complete the specially designed online screening and exercise recommendations program, the ePARmed-X+ (at www.canfitprointeractive.com), or visit a certified fitness professional for assistance to complete ePARmed-X+ and for further information. As a Personal Training Specialist, you should not work with clients who have existing health risks until you have gained adequate experience working with healthy adults and the clients have been cleared for unrestricted physical activity by their medical practitioner.

You have the legal responsibility to have a signed PAR-Q+ for all clients whom you train and to adhere to the physical activity guidelines presented therein. Because health is a dynamic process that can change in a short time, clients should complete the PAR-Q+ on an annual basis or any time they have been away from your care for more than a month. The PAR-Q+ is available in the web resource that accompanies this book and is provided at the end of this chapter for reference as form 9.1. A copy of the PAR-Q+ can also be downloaded free by professional members of canfitpro from canfitpro INTERACTIVE (www.canfitprointeractive.com).

 The PAR-Q+ for Everyone is included in the web resource at www.HumanKinetics.com/FoundationsOfProfessionalPersonalTraining.

Health History Questionnaire

To gather more information about a client's health, you may wish to develop a second health-screening questionnaire to supplement the PAR-Q+. This second tool might include the following items:

1. Client details (e.g., name, address, phone numbers, emergency contact)
2. Current medical conditions (e.g., diabetes, asthma, arthritis)
3. Medication use and allergies
4. Current or past injuries
5. Treatment from qualified health professionals
6. Cardiac risks (e.g., high BP, high cholesterol)
7. Family health history
8. Past and present exercise history
9. Past and present nutritional information
10. Past and present work history

Many Personal Training Specialists use a standardized form for all clients or develop their own version of a questionnaire that works best for their interests and needs. An example of a health history questionnaire can be found in the web resource and is provided at the end of this chapter for reference as form 9.2. If any information gathered on the questionnaire raises a red flag or is outside your level of expertise, consult with a certified health professional to get recommendations for programming prior to beginning any exercise program.

 See the web resource at www.HumanKinetics.com/FoundationsOfProfessionalPersonalTraining for a client health history form.

Other Resources

Several forms and questionnaires useful to Personal Training Specialists are available. These questionnaires monitor such items as physical activity, cardiorespiratory risk, and lifestyle. You may also want to use forms such as SMART goal-setting worksheets to counsel clients and set up activity programs. Many of these resources can be downloaded free by canfitpro professional members from canfitpro INTERACTIVE (www.canfitprointeractive.com).

Client Risk Stratification

From the combination of the answers on the PAR-Q+ and the health history questionnaire, you will have to determine the risk that clients will put themselves in when engaging in an exercise program and the precautions you should take. This process involves risk stratification, or placing your client into one of three categories—low risk, increased risk, or high risk—and basing your decisions on the risk profile outlined in figure 9.1.

Low Risk

A low-risk (apparently healthy) client is one who answered no to all questions on the PAR-Q+, exhib-

its no signs or symptoms of disease, and has no more than one major cardiac risk factor. These people are able to start a moderate-intensity exercise program and undergo fitness testing without a referral from a medical practitioner. Men and women over 45 years of age and unaccustomed to regular vigorous- to maximal-effort exercise should consult a certified fitness professional before engaging in exercise of this intensity.

Increased Risk

Clients at increased risk are those who have two or more coronary risk factors but exhibit no signs (e.g., high BP) or symptoms (e.g., chest pain on exertion)

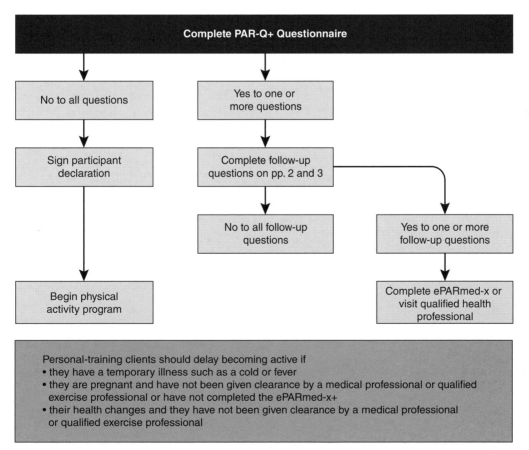

FIGURE 9.1 Pre-exercise screening guide. CHD = coronary heart disease.

Adapted, by permission, from T. Olds and K. Norton, 1999, *Pre-exercise health screening guide* (Champaign, IL: Human Kinetics), 29.

of cardiorespiratory or metabolic disorders. These clients may start a progressive moderate-intensity physical activity program under close supervision and should undergo clinically supervised maximal testing procedures before engaging in any vigorous physical activities.

High Risk

Clients should be referred to an appropriate qualified health professional for testing and exercise guidance if they have two or more coronary risk factors and exhibit positive signs (e.g., high BP) or symptoms (e.g., chest pain on exertion); have severe limitations; or have diagnosed cardiac, pulmonary, or metabolic disorders.

Referrals

After conducting the health-screening process, you will have a much better understanding of your clients' current health status and medical condition. Personal Training Specialists should not work with clients who have serious medical conditions. Any clients who answer yes to a question on the PAR-Q+ must complete the follow-up questions about their medical conditions. If they have two or more cardiorespiratory risk factors along with positive signs and symptoms, they should be directed to consult with a physician before engaging in a physical activity program. Any exercise guidance should be offered only after a doctor provides clearance for physical activity through the use of a form such as the ePARmed-X+ or other form that allows clients' doctors to provide specific guidelines for physical activity. Clients who are not cleared for unrestricted physical activity should be referred to the appropriate qualified health professional for exercise guidance.

Working with a client who is not cleared for unrestricted physical activity through either the screening process or medical referral puts the Personal Training Specialist at risk of being liable in the case of personal injury or health problems associated with the client being active. Although you may be well intentioned as a Personal Training Specialist, it is better to err on the side of caution when dealing with a potential or current client who is at high risk.

Passive Postural Assessment

After a client has been cleared for unrestricted physical activity, you should perform a passive postural assessment to determine whether you need to address any obvious postural concerns when designing a program. The benefit of a passive postural assessment is that you can passively observe the client (the client is at no risk since he or she is not exercising) to determine whether muscle imbalances are present because of tightness or weakness in one or more areas of the body.

Anatomical Reference— The Plumb Line

When observing posture, the plumb line can be used to bisect the body in the sagittal and frontal planes. If observing ideal posture and starting from the floor, the plumb line transects the anterior portion of the lateral side of the ankle and continues upward to pass through the centre of the knee joint and the superior portion of the femur. The line then passes through the centre of the rib cage, the glenohumeral joint, and the anterior one-third of the vertebrae in the cervical spine. It completes its path through the ear. From the front or the back, the plumb line bisects the distance between the heels, knees, the pelvic crests, the vertebral bodies of the spine, and the cranium. See figure 9.2.

Observing posture in the two planes is important in designing a fitness program. Careful observation increases awareness of faults in postural muscles of the body, as well as proprioceptive awareness of how the body is being carried or held in positions of work, sport, or play throughout the day.

All postural distortions restrict movement in the opposite direction. For example, when the right spiral line (see chapter 7) is facilitated, or tight, a right-sided chop or unilateral cable push is strong relative to the left-sided version of the same exercise. Similarly, and assuming equal coordination, a right diagonal lift (e.g., shoveling dirt or snow over the right shoulder) would be weak relative to the left. Because myofascial lines connect upper and lower segments, a series of changes to strength and weakness of movements in the lower body would be present.

If posture is out of balance, failure to make the appropriate changes can decrease the rate at which performance and aesthetic changes occur

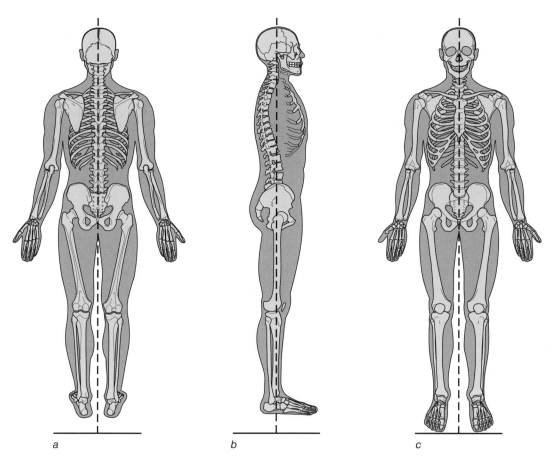

FIGURE 9.2 The position of the skeleton in ideal posture from *(a)* posterior, *(b)* lateral, and *(c)* anterior views.

in the body. In sport, fitness, or flexibility-related programs, improper posture may decrease optimal joint function, resulting in the potential for long-term injury and premature joint degeneration. When you conduct postural assessments with clients, the ones that show the greatest observable change from plumb line neutral will be an indication of the greater priority for preventive or corrective exercise.

 Postural imbalances usually develop over time because of daily movement patterns. Poorly designed exercise or fitness programs, ergonomically incorrect workstations, and repetitive movement-oriented occupations must be corrected biomechanically if the body is to reap the benefits of ideal posture and long-term musculoskeletal health and wellness.

Assessing Posture

During the screening process, the fitness professional must pay attention to imbalances that are present in a client's posture. As a trained Personal Training Specialist, you can observe imbalances that occur between muscle groups and joint systems. You will therefore be able to design programs that educate clients and help them achieve their goals.

Faulty alignment may indicate that the client is experiencing pain within a muscle or joint or experiencing a problem with **proprioception** (i.e., awareness of the body's movement and spatial orientation). You may need to refer the person out to an appropriate qualified health professional if a medical problem is apparent.

Common postural faults are usually the result of long, weak muscle groups on one side of the joint and short, tight muscle groups on the opposite side of the joint. These imbalances alter the function of the joint as well as passive and dynamic posture.

Assessing posture requires several skills including observation, land marking, critical evaluation, and program integration. The Personal Training Specialist needs to use all these tools to personalize program development for client progress. Successful movement evaluation, much like success in sport and life, depends on the ability to move through three-dimensional spaces. Therefore, the evaluation must examine posture from three angles: the front, side, and back.

Although a number of muscle function classification systems can be used for assessment, Vladamir Janda conceptualized muscle imbalances as a relationship of muscles that are prone to tightness and muscles that are prone to weakness. Muscles are known to work in partnership, as force couple pairs (Page, Frank, and Lardner, 2010) on opposite sides of the same attachment point. As discussed in detail in chapter 7, muscles are further interconnected by myofascial chains, or slings, that cross and connect muscles from several joints (Myers, 2009). These myofascial slings are proprioceptively rich and tend to respond best to rhythmic, low-level stretches. From this understanding of movement and muscle connections, Janda and Myers have identified several postural patterns that are common to sport, fitness, and life (Page, Frank, and Lardner, 2010). Here, we have chosen to examine two of the most common postural patterns.

Upper Crossed Syndrome

Upper crossed syndrome is a typical postural stress resulting primarily from imbalances displayed in the muscles that bridge and connect the head, neck, shoulder girdle, and thorax.

The facilitated muscles in upper crossed syndrome (i.e., those that present as short, tight, and inflexible) are shown in figure 9.3a. They include the pectorals (pectoralis minor), upper trapezius, levator scapulae, and the suboccipitals (muscles at the base of the skull). In addition, shortened internal rotators of the arm and upper segments of the rectus abdominis may be observed. Painful trigger points may be observed throughout the lateral and anterior muscles of the neck. Upper crossed syndrome may also produce short or tight gluteals and hamstrings.

In the case of facilitated muscle groups, short and tight classification does not indicate that the muscle is strong, even though hypertrophy may occur. Frequently, decreased sensory motor awareness and loss of coordination are present when a joint is affected by facilitated muscle groups.

Muscles that are prone to becoming lengthened and weakened in upper crossed syndrome are the long cervical spine extensors, deep cervical spine flexors, lower and middle trapezius, rhomboids, and serratus anterior (figure 9.3a). One of the greatest effects of upper crossed syndrome is the weakening of the diaphragm, which alters optimal breathing patterns.

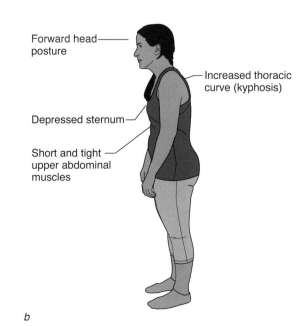

Weak:
Deep cervical spine flexors

Tight:
Suboccipitals
Upper trapezius
Levator scapulae

Tight:
Pectorals

Weak:
Long cervical spine extensors
Lower trapezius
Middle trapezius
Rhomboids
Serratus anterior

a

Forward head posture

Increased thoracic curve (kyphosis)

Depressed sternum

Short and tight upper abdominal muscles

b

FIGURE 9.3   (a) Muscle imbalances typical of upper crossed syndrome and (b) postural signs of upper crossed syndrome.

The physical presentations of a person with upper crossed syndrome are shown in figure 9.3*b*. In addition to increased curvature of the thoracic spine (**kyphosis**), upper crossed syndrome may be associated with decreased lumbar curvature, popularly known as a flat back. The typical seated workstation of a home or professional office may result in increased thoracic curve, decreased lumbar and cervical curve, and forward head posture. This presents itself by a C-shaped curve formed by the cervical, thoracic, and lumbar spine, and presents in the pelvis as reduced pelvic tilt. The C-curve posture encourages shearing forces throughout the cervical and lumbar spine, potentially resulting in painful disc protrusion or degenerative disk and degenerative joint disease. Suggested exercise progressions for a client with upper crossed syndrome can be found on canfitpro INTERACTIVE (www. canfitprointeractive.com).

Lower Crossed Syndrome

Lower crossed syndrome is a typical postural stress resulting primarily from imbalances in the muscles connecting the lumbar spine, pelvis, and femur. These muscles are known as the lumbo-pelvic-hip complex.

Facilitated muscles that present as short and tight in lower crossed syndrome are the iliopsoas, rectus femoris, and the lumbar portion of the erector spinae (figure 9.4*a*). In addition, shortened gastroc-nemius, soleus, distal hamstrings, adductors, tensor fasciae latae, and piriformis (a muscle in the gluteal region that laterally rotates the femur) may be observed. Significant weakness and inhibition will be demonstrated by the lower abdominals, gluteus maximus, gluteus medius, proximal hamstrings, posterior tibialis, quadrates plantae (in the plantar aspect of the foot), and, even though it is short and tight, decreased endurance of the lumbar erectors. Remember that in the case of long and weak muscle groups, decreased sensory motor awareness and a loss of coordination are associated with the function of the affected muscles and associated joints. Loss of both strength and endurance also occurs in the affected muscles.

Besides having postural changes in the lower body, people who demonstrate lower crossed syndrome typically present with forward head posture as well. Forward head posture can best be seen when looking at the client from the side (sagittal plane). The most prominent portion of the cheekbone protrudes past its alignment with the anterior portion of the clavicle. Other characteristics include rounded shoulders and depressed sternum (with the apex of the thorax at the level of T4), increased lumbar curve, and forward sway of the greater trochanter (superior femur) forward of the plumb line (figure 9.4*b*).

The lumbar curve test (figure 9.5) may be used as an estimate of the curve of the lumbar spine (**lordosis**).

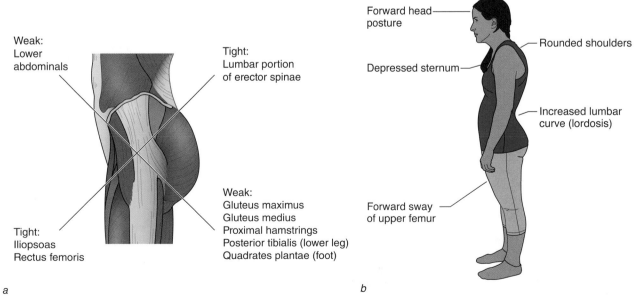

FIGURE 9.4 *(a)* Muscle imbalances typical of lower crossed syndrome and *(b)* postural signs of lower crossed syndrome.

This test can only be used to estimate whether a client or patient has too little, the correct amount, or too much curve to the lumbar spine.

To perform the test, have your client stand comfortably against the wall with heels, hips, and shoulders touching the wall. If she or he is able to slide the hand between the wall and the lower back to the point where the hand cannot slide past the spine, then the person may have just the right amount of lumbar lordosis. If the client cannot slide any part of the hand between the wall and the back at the level of the umbilicus, then she or he may have too little curve. If the client can slide the entire hand all the way through the space created by the curvature in the back and the adjacent wall, she or he most likely has too much lumbar lordosis.

The lumbar curve test as well as plumb line postural analysis should always be performed when the client is barefoot, because shoes with elevated heels increase inclination of the pelvis and curvature of the lumbar spine. The effect is caused by athletic shoes as well as fashion and dress shoes. You may also choose to perform the test again with the client wearing shoes, to demonstrate the way in which footwear may change their posture, compared to being barefoot.

The altered length–tension relationships of the affected muscles and joints in lower cross syndrome dramatically affect the ability of the lumbo-pelvic complex to stabilize and support weight load placed on the spine. When the spine is then subjected to extrinsic forces, such as carrying children, loading groceries, squatting, or deadlifting in the gym, it quickly tires and loses stability in the lower segments of the lumbar spine. These forces result in harmful compression, torsion, and shear on the lumbo-sacral region, often resulting in pain and spinal instability. Suggested exercise progressions for a client with lower crossed syndrome can be found at canfitpro INTERACTIVE (www.canfit-prointeractive.com).

www See the web resource at www.HumanKi-netics.com/FoundationsOfProfessional PersonalTraining for a form to record client performance on postural and fitness assessments.

Standard Health Assessment

After you have completed the postural assessment, you should document the results. If the client does not have any visible postural imbalances, or these imbalances do not pose any immediate danger to the client's health, you can proceed to the standard health assessment. This is the final stage of passive screening and assessment before beginning dynamic assessment.

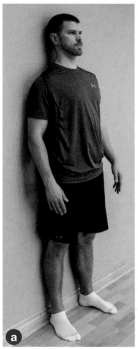
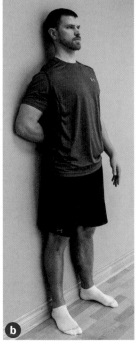

FIGURE 9.5 For the lumbar curve test, the client should stand against a wall without shoes *(a)*. The space between the wall and the naturally curved lower back is measured *(b)*.

If a client presents with postural imbalances that appear to be dangerous to his or her health or beyond your *Standards of Practice*, you should refer him or her to a qualified health professional for a more thorough assessment and exercise program design.

Resting Heart Rate

Resting heart rate (RHR) can be measured by placing the index and middle fingers on a pulse site (carotid artery, radial artery, or brachial artery; see figure 9.6) with light to moderate pressure. As a Personal Training Specialist, you can measure the client's resting HR during the standard health assessment. Alternatively, to get the most accurate reading, you can instruct the client to measure resting HR for at least 30 seconds in the morning before getting out of bed. Note that the first beat should be counted as zero. To determine beats per minute (BPM), simply multiply the 30-second value by two.

 When taking HR measurements, the first beat is counted as zero. An HR monitor can also be used to measure both resting and exercise HRs. To become more familiar with HR testing (and to compare resting HRs to exercise HRs) practice taking your own heart rate upon waking, during the day, and during exercise.

Whether HR is taken by you or the client, ensure that resting HR is always measured at a consistent time of day and that the client is uncaffeinated and unstressed (including recent exercise).

As clients increase their cardiorespiratory fitness, their resting HR gradually decreases, indicating that the heart is functioning more efficiently. Normal resting HR is approximately 70 BPM for men and 75 BPM for women. A resting HR of 100 BPM or higher is a warning sign to look more closely at the client's overall health and request a doctor's clearance before training the client. See appendix table C.1 for normative data on resting heart rate.

Resting Blood Pressure

In a clinical setting, resting blood pressure is measured using a stethoscope and a device called a sphygmomanometer (blood pressure cuff). Specialized courses are recommended should you wish to use this method with your clients. But within the exercise environment, a Personal Training Specialist can use a portable BP monitor, an automated testing station, or a documented reading from the client's medical professional. In most of these instances, the blood pressure is measured with the cuff on the client's upper left arm. The value recorded will have two numbers; the higher one is known as the systolic pressure, and the lower one is the diastolic pressure.

Systolic pressure is the amount of pressure on the walls of the arteries as the heart contracts, and it represents the work of the heart muscle. A normal resting systolic pressure is 120 mmHg.

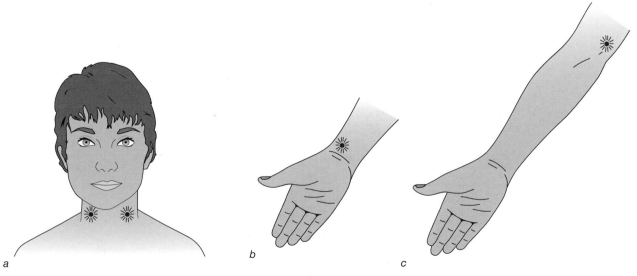

a　　　　　　　　*b*　　　　　　　　*c*

FIGURE 9.6 Locations of pulse sites in the *(a)* neck (carotid), *(b)* wrist (radial), and *(c)* arm (brachial).

Diastolic pressure is the pressure on the walls of the arteries as the heart relaxes and fills again, and it indicates resistance to peripheral blood flow. A normal resting diastolic pressure is 80 mmHg.

When assessing your clients, look for a normal resting BP of 120/80 mmHg or lower. If the resting systolic BP is 140 mmHg or higher or the resting diastolic BP is 100 mmHg or higher, you should refer the client to a doctor for clearance to exercise. Resting systolic BPs of 85 mmHg or lower are also problematic. Clients who have these lower BPs may be prone to dizziness and light-headedness, which must be considered when recommending exercises.

Alternative RHR and BP Considerations

If you do not test your clients' RHR and BP yourself, ensure that one of the following is completed:

- **Physician**—Ask your clients to provide their RHR and BP readings from their last medical examination (a form including the date and physician's name should be included).
- **Other**—Ask your clients to provide their RHR and BP readings from their last visit to their local clinic, drugstore, or gym where these were tested (a form including the date and location should be included, and BP should be measured and documented at least once every six months).

Body Composition

Many clients come to a Personal Training Specialist because they want to lose body fat and change their body composition by gaining muscle. Shedding extra body fat is a common goal for clients, and Personal Training Specialists face a constant challenge in helping their clients achieve this goal.

The purpose of assessing **body composition** is to divide the body into fat mass (all adipose tissue in the body) and fat-free mass (all other tissue including muscle, bone, and so on). Interest in body-fat content has grown over the past 50 years as it has become clear that obese people have a higher risk of heart disease, high cholesterol, high blood pressure and stroke, diabetes, several digestive and pulmonary disorders, degenerative joint diseases such as osteoarthritis, and even some cancers. Although these relationships exist, recent research indicates that the distribution of adipose tissue (i.e., where fat is located on the body) is most important in determining the health risk of obesity. Fat carried internally in the trunk area (visceral fat) carries the greatest risk, whereas peripheral fat under the skin (subcutaneous fat) carries a lower health risk. Hence, the lack of information on the distribution of adipose tissue in a measure such as percent body fat is a major limitation and links to health are not readily apparent.

Since the early 1940s, the field method of choice for assessing body composition has been anthropometric measurement of both skinfolds and girths. These tools help reduce the error of measurement, often fit the situation and client needs, and are useful in tracking changes in total amount and distribution of adipose tissue as well as changes in muscle mass. To track individual progress, plotting of basic anthropometric data is recommended. The median value of data taken in triplicate (the middle of three measures) reduces potential error in measurement. By comparing measures over time at regular intervals, you can track values associated with reduced health risk and those associated with increased health risk, and you may offer the client a better platform from which changes can be explained.

Skinfolds and Girths

Skinfolds measure the thickness of a double fold of skin and underlying adipose tissue (fat). Using a skinfold caliper, the thickness is measured by lifting the skinfold between the thumb and forefinger along the length of a fat pad at pre-determined locations. Skinfold measurements are an inexpensive way to examine site-specific body fat and to predict overall body composition. But these locations have to be precisely and consistently located for the measurement to be effective and accurate, so advanced knowledge or additional training in anatomy and anatomical landmarks is required. Once raised, the skinfold caliper is applied at 90° to the skin over the skinfold and then released so that it squeezes the skinfold gently. The measure is read from the skinfold caliper after two seconds.

Girths measure the total circumference of either a limb or the trunk at pre-determined levels. Girths include skin, fat, muscle, and bone. In combination with skinfolds, girth measurements are useful. If a skinfold measurement goes down but girth goes up, the muscle has grown in size, but if both the girth and skinfold measurements increase, girth has grown because of increased fat. Although girth measurement is a convenient and simple method of determining a baseline for your client, unless used in combination with skinfolds, it is difficult to evaluate the results or determine whether observed changes result from increases in lean body mass or decreases in body fat.

A chart containing height, weight, girths, skinfold measurements, sum of skinfold measurements, sum of trunk skinfold measurements, and sum of peripheral skinfold measurements may be an appraiser's most valuable tool. From these data, you can identify distribution patterns of adipose tissue and track absolute change in skinfold thickness over time. This information can then be used to reflect health risks, such as that associated with a low sum of trunk skinfolds but high waist girth (i.e., more **visceral fat**, which has a greater health risk). In this case, reduced waist girth would be the most appropriate indicator of a change in health risk. In someone with both high waist girth and a high sum of trunk skinfolds, a reduction in skinfold thickness and a corresponding reduction of waist girth should be the desired outcome of the training program.

Waist Girth Measurements

Waist girth is obtained to help identify fat distribution in the abdominal region, which is associated with increased health risk. Waist girth is taken with the subject standing with weight evenly distributed on both feet and the feet shoulder-width apart. A tape measure is placed so that it is level around the circumference of the waist at the level of greatest narrowing. Be sure not to indent the skin; use only enough tension to hold the tape horizontal and in the proper location. If noticeable narrowing is not apparent, take waist girth at the midpoint between the lowest floating rib and the top of the hip bone (iliac crest) or, in obese clients, two centimetres above the navel. See appendix table C.2 for normative data on waist girth.

Bioelectric Impedance Measurements

A popular method of measuring body composition is by **bioelectric impedance**. In this method, equipment sends a mild electrical current through the body from the wrist to the foot. The more lean tissue (muscle) the client has, the quicker the current travels because the water in the lean tissue provides little resistance; the fatter the client is, the slower the tissue conducts the current.

The benefits of bioelectric impedance are that it is quick, easy, and noninvasive; no technician is required; the analyzers are relatively inexpensive; and the analyzers may provide a computer printout that includes fat-free mass, fat mass, the ratio of fat to total body mass (i.e., percent body fat), and ideal weight. The drawbacks include the specificity of the equations (age, gender, obesity), the sensitivity of measured resistance to the placement of electrodes and hydration status of the client, and the variability among analyzers (even when made by the same company). Further, this method provides no indication of fat distribution, so the health-related concerns of increased or decreased body fat cannot be addressed.

When reporting data from bioelectric impedance, report absolute weights of fat-free tissue (lean tissue) and fat mass. Changes in these values, not the ratio of these values (i.e., percent body fat), should be encouraged based on clients' goals.

Predicting Health Risk

By using several measures related to fat distribution and the proportionality of the body (how heavy it is for its height), you can estimate the client's health risk. For example, a large waist girth indicates that fat is carried in the trunk, which carries a higher health risk than fat that is carried on the limbs. Hence, a waist girth of 0.88 metres or greater is considered a health risk for a female, and a girth greater than 1.02 metres is considered a health risk for a male.

Using clients' height and weight, you can determine their body mass index (BMI), which indicates whether they are carrying an acceptable amount of weight for their height. BMI is calculated by dividing the weight in kilograms by the height squared in metres (BMI = kg/m²). A BMI of less than 19 or greater than 25 puts clients at risk; a BMI greater than 30 often indicates obesity, although athletes with a great deal of muscle will also fall above 30, so you must be careful in your interpretation. Using the sum of skinfold measurements will help you make this decision. A large sum of skinfold measurements, a large waist girth, and a BMI over 30 suggest that the client is overweight because of increased body fat and thus is at a health risk, so weight loss (reduction of fat mass) would be an important goal for health reasons.

To determine disease risk from centralized fat deposition, the U.S. National Institutes of Health (NIH) and the National Heart, Lung, and Blood Institute (NHLBI) endorsed a simple clinical guideline for the identification and evaluation of overweight and obesity in 1998. By using the classical BMI categories for overweight and obesity and superimposing waist girth to determine the distribution of excess weight, they developed a prediction of health risk. Table 9.1 identifies those who are at increased health risk for diabetes, hypertension, and coronary heart disease.

Regardless of the measurement used to estimate body composition, you must understand that each assessment has room for error. In other words, they are only estimates. Use assessment results to track client progress rather than compare one client with another. Ratios should be avoided in body composition measurement. Because predicting percent body fat through any method is imprecise and does not provide information concerning regional fat and fat distribution, body fat is not recommended as a standalone measure. To date, the most highly recommended practice is to take several girths and skinfolds and graph the data to track changes in body composition. This approach will allow you to monitor changes in the distribution of body fat, which is more related to health risk and prevention.

 Percent body fat is often an overrated measure that is overemphasized by both Personal Training Specialists and clients. If performing assessments for health purposes, you must monitor where the fat is on the body, so percent body fat is of limited use. Body fat measurement is also prone to error. Do not use percent body fat as a standalone measure of health risk, and use it only to measure progress for a single client, not to compare clients with each other.

TABLE 9.1 Criteria for Increased Health Risks

Category	BMI (kg/m²)	DISEASE RISK RELATIVE TO NORMAL WEIGHT AND WAIST CIRCUMFERENCE	
		Men <102cm Women <88cm	Men >102cm Women >88cm
Underweight	<18.5	—	—
Normal	18.5–24.9	—	—
Overweight	25.0–29.9	Increased	High
Obese I	30.0–34.9	High	Very high
Obese II	35.0–39.9	Very high	Very high
Extreme obesity	>40.0	Extremely high	Extremely high

Adapted, by permission, from J.C. Griffin, 2006, *Client-centered exercise prescription,* 2nd ed. (Champaign, IL: Human Kinetics), 88-89.

Summary of Main Points

1. Performing health screenings of clients is an essential component of the initial stages of the personal training process.

2. Each client should complete and sign a PAR-Q+ form annually.

3. The use of a second health-screening form, such as a health history questionnaire, helps Personal Training Specialists collect additional information about a client's health history and current health status.

4. The information that clients share in health screening must be kept confidential.

5. The decision to perform a fitness assessment should be made by the client and the Personal Training Specialist.

6. Assessments should be performed by a Personal Training Specialist or qualified health professional to ensure that the information is valid, reliable, and reproducible.

7. Postural assessments should be conducted before proceeding to the standard health assessment.

8. A normal resting HR is 70 BPM for men and 75 BPM for women.

9. A normal resting BP is 120/80 mmHg.

10. Body composition assessments help identify whether the client has a health risk because of excess body fat. These assessments are most effective when the distribution of body fat is also evaluated.

11. Resting HR should be less than 100 BPM, and blood pressure should be lower than 140/100 to conduct any passive or dynamic assessments, or physical fitness testing.

Key Concepts for Study

Duty of care

Diagnosed disease

Signs and symptoms

Body fat percentage

Bioelectric impedance

Upper crossed syndrome

Lower crossed syndrome

Review Questions

1. Explain why it is important for a Personal Training Specialist to conduct pre-exercise screening for every client and list at least five types of information that should be gathered from the health history questionnaire.

2. Describe the ways in which postural faults can affect a client's training results.

3. Upper crossed syndrome presents

    a. long and weak pectorals, upper trapezius, and levator scapula

    b. short and tight pectorals, upper trapezius, and levator scapula

    c. short and tight middle trapezius and rhomboids

    d. strong diaphragm

4. Lower crossed syndrome presents

    a. short and tight iliopsoas, rectus femoris, and lumbar erectors

    b. long and weak iliopsoas, rectus femoris, and lumbar erectors

    c. strong gluteus maximus and hamstrings

    d. flat back or swayback posture

5. A BMI of 30 or higher may indicate that a client is

    a. overweight and at risk

    b. muscular and not at risk

    c. low risk

    d. a and b

6. The PAR-Q+ must be completed

   a. by every client, once per month

   b. by the client's physician

   c. only by clients with a family history of heart disease

   d. before the Personal Training Specialist begins working with any client

7. Bioelectrical impedance measurements allow the Personal Training Specialist to assess

   a. girth measurements and muscular strength

   b. body composition

   c. hip-to-waist measurement ratio

   d. relationship between height and weight

 Web Resource Contents

PAR-Q+

Client health history form

Fitness and postural assessment form

Answers to review questions

PAR-Q+

The Physical Activity Readiness Questionnaire for Everyone

The health benefits of regular physical activity are clear; more people should engage in physical activity every day of the week. Participating in physical activity is very safe for MOST people. This questionnaire will tell you whether it is necessary for you to seek further advice from your doctor OR a qualified exercise professional before becoming more physically active.

GENERAL HEALTH QUESTIONS

Please read the 7 questions below carefully and answer each one honestly: check YES or NO.	YES	NO
1) Has your doctor ever said that you have a heart condition ☐ OR high blood pressure ☐?	☐	☐
2) Do you feel pain in your chest at rest, during your daily activities of living, **OR** when you do physical activity?	☐	☐
3) Do you lose balance because of dizziness **OR** have you lost consciousness in the last 12 months? Please answer **NO** if your dizziness was associated with over-breathing (including during vigorous exercise).	☐	☐
4) Have you ever been diagnosed with another chronic medical condition (other than heart disease or high blood pressure)? **PLEASE LIST CONDITION(S) HERE:** _____	☐	☐
5) Are you currently taking prescribed medications for a chronic medical condition? **PLEASE LIST CONDITION(S) AND MEDICATIONS HERE:** _____	☐	☐
6) Do you currently have (or have had within the past 12 months) a bone, joint, or soft tissue (muscle, ligament, or tendon) problem that could be made worse by becoming more physically active? Please answer **NO** if you had a problem in the past, but it *does not limit your current ability* to be physically active. **PLEASE LIST CONDITION(S) HERE:** _____	☐	☐
7) Has your doctor ever said that you should only do medically supervised physical activity?	☐	☐

☑ **If you answered NO to all of the questions above, you are cleared for physical activity.**
Go to Page 4 to sign the PARTICIPANT DECLARATION. You do not need to complete Pages 2 and 3.

▶ Start becoming much more physically active – start slowly and build up gradually.

▶ Follow International Physical Activity Guidelines for your age (www.who.int/dietphysicalactivity/en/).

▶ You may take part in a health and fitness appraisal.

▶ If you are over the age of 45 yr and **NOT** accustomed to regular vigorous to maximal effort exercise, consult a qualified exercise professional before engaging in this intensity of exercise.

▶ If you have any further questions, contact a qualified exercise professional.

⬤ **If you answered YES to one or more of the questions above, COMPLETE PAGES 2 AND 3.**

⚠ **Delay becoming more active if:**

✓ You have a temporary illness such as a cold or fever; it is best to wait until you feel better.

✓ You are pregnant - talk to your health care practitioner, your physician, a qualified exercise professional, and/or complete the ePARmed-X+ at **www.eparmedx.com** before becoming more physically active.

✓ Your health changes - answer the questions on Pages 2 and 3 of this document and/or talk to your doctor or a qualified exercise professional before continuing with any physical activity program.

!"#$%&'()*+,-.*/01234*!"5567"%6)&"8 -9:
01-01-2016

FORM 9.1   PAR-Q+ pre-exercise screening form.

Reprinted with permission from the PAR-Q+ Collaboration and the authors of the PAR-Q (Dr. Darren Warburton, Dr. Norman Gledhill, Dr. Veronica Jamnik, and Dr. Shannon Bredin).

PAR-Q+

FOLLOW-UP QUESTIONS ABOUT YOUR MEDICAL CONDITION(S)

1.   **Do you have Arthritis, Osteoporosis, or Back Problems?**

If the above condition(s) is/are present, answer questions 1a-1c   If **NO** ☐ go to question 2

1a.	Do you have difficulty controlling your condition with medications or other physician-prescribed therapies? (Answer **NO** if you are not currently taking medications or other treatments)	YES☐ NO☐
1b.	Do you have joint problems causing pain, a recent fracture or fracture caused by osteoporosis or cancer, displaced vertebra (e.g., spondylolisthesis), and/or spondylolysis/pars defect (a crack in the bony ring on the back of the spinal column)?	YES☐ NO☐
1c.	Have you had steroid injections or taken steroid tablets regularly for more than 3 months?	YES☐ NO☐

2.   **Do you have Cancer of any kind?**

If the above condition(s) is/are present, answer questions 2a-2b   If **NO** ☐ go to question 3

2a.	Does your cancer diagnosis include any of the following types: lung/bronchogenic, multiple myeloma (cancer of plasma cells), head, and neck?	YES☐ NO☐
2b.	Are you currently receiving cancer therapy (such as chemotheraphy or radiotherapy)?	YES☐ NO☐

3.   **Do you have a Heart or Cardiovascular Condition?** *This includes Coronary Artery Disease, Heart Failure, Diagnosed Abnormality of Heart Rhythm*

If the above condition(s) is/are present, answer questions 3a-3d   If **NO** ☐ go to question 4

3a.	Do you have difficulty controlling your condition with medications or other physician-prescribed therapies? (Answer **NO** if you are not currently taking medications or other treatments)	YES☐ NO☐
3b.	Do you have an irregular heart beat that requires medical management? (e.g., atrial fibrillation, premature ventricular contraction)	YES☐ NO☐
3c.	Do you have chronic heart failure?	YES☐ NO☐
3d.	Do you have diagnosed coronary artery (cardiovascular) disease and have not participated in regular physical activity in the last 2 months?	YES☐ NO☐

4.   **Do you have High Blood Pressure?**

If the above condition(s) is/are present, answer questions 4a-4b   If **NO** ☐ go to question 5

4a.	Do you have difficulty controlling your condition with medications or other physician-prescribed therapies? (Answer **NO** if you are not currently taking medications or other treatments)	YES☐ NO☐
4b.	Do you have a resting blood pressure equal to or greater than 160/90 mmHg with or without medication? (Answer **YES** if you do not know your resting blood pressure)	YES☐ NO☐

5.   **Do you have any Metabolic Conditions?** *This includes Type 1 Diabetes, Type 2 Diabetes, Pre-Diabetes*

If the above condition(s) is/are present, answer questions 5a-5e   If **NO** ☐ go to question 6

5a.	Do you often have difficulty controlling your blood sugar levels with foods, medications, or other physician-prescribed therapies?	YES☐ NO☐
5b.	Do you often suffer from signs and symptoms of low blood sugar (hypoglycemia) following exercise and/or during activities of daily living? Signs of hypoglycemia may include shakiness, nervousness, unusual irritability, abnormal sweating, dizziness or light-headedness, mental confusion, difficulty speaking, weakness, or sleepiness.	YES☐ NO☐
5c.	Do you have any signs or symptoms of diabetes complications such as heart or vascular disease and/or complications affecting your eyes, kidneys, **OR** the sensation in your toes and feet?	YES☐ NO☐
5d.	Do you have other metabolic conditions (such as current pregnancy-related diabetes, chronic kidney disease, or liver problems)?	YES☐ NO☐
5e.	Are you planning to engage in what for you is unusually high (or vigorous) intensity exercise in the near future?	YES☐ NO☐

FORM 9.1   *> continued*

PAR-Q+

6.   **Do you have any Mental Health Problems or Learning Difficulties?** *This includes Alzheimer's, Dementia, Depression, Anxiety Disorder, Eating Disorder, Psychotic Disorder, Intellectual Disability, Down Syndrome*

       If the above condition(s) is/are present, answer questions 6a-6b   If **NO** ☐ go to question 7

6a.	Do you have difficulty controlling your condition with medications or other physician-prescribed therapies? (Answer **NO** if you are not currently taking medications or other treatments)	YES☐ NO☐
6b.	Do you have Down Synrome and back problems affecting nerves or muscles?	YES☐ NO☐

7.   **Do you have a Respiratory Disease?** *This includes Chronic Obstructive Pulmonary Disease, Asthma, Pulmonary High Blood Pressure*

       If the above condition(s) is/are present, answer questions 7a-7d   If **NO** ☐ go to question 8

7a.	Do you have difficulty controlling your condition with medications or other physician-prescribed therapies? (Answer **NO** if you are not currently taking medications or other treatments)	YES☐ NO☐
7b.	Has your doctor ever said your blood oxygen level is low at rest or during exercise and/or that you require supplemental oxygen therapy?	YES☐ NO☐
7c.	If asthmatic, do you currently have symptoms of chest tightness, wheezing, laboured breathing, consistent cough (more than 2 days/week), or have you used your rescue medication more than twice in the last week?	YES☐ NO☐
7d.	Has your doctor ever said you have high blood pressure in the blood vessels of your lungs?	YES☐ NO☐

8.   **Do you have a Spinal Cord Injury?** *This includes Tetraplegia and Paraplegia*

       If the above condition(s) is/are present, answer questions 8a-8c   If **NO** ☐ go to question 9

8a.	Do you have difficulty controlling your condition with medications or other physician-prescribed therapies? (Answer **NO** if you are not currently taking medications or other treatments)	YES☐ NO☐
8b.	Do you commonly exhibit low resting blood pressure significant enough to cause dizziness, light-headedness, and/or fainting?	YES☐ NO☐
8c.	Has your physician indicated that you exhibit sudden bouts of high blood pressure (known as Autonomic Dysreflexia)?	YES☐ NO☐

9.   **Have you had a Stroke?** *This includes Transient Ischemic Attack (TIA) or Cerebrovascular Event*

       If the above condition(s) is/are present, answer questions 9a-9c   If **NO** ☐ go to question 10

9a.	Do you have difficulty controlling your condition with medications or other physician-prescribed therapies? (Answer **NO** if you are not currently taking medications or other treatments)	YES☐ NO☐
9b.	Do you have any impairment in walking or mobility?	YES☐ NO☐
9c.	Have you experienced a stroke or impairment in nerves or muscles in the past 6 months?	YES☐ NO☐

10.   **Do you have any other medical condition not listed above or do you have two or more medical conditions?**

       If you have other medical conditions, answer questions 10a-10c   If **NO** ☐ read the Page 4 recommendations

10a.	Have you experienced a blackout, fainted, or lost consciousness as a result of a head injury within the last 12 months **OR** have you had a diagnosed concussion within the last 12 months?	YES☐ NO☐
10b.	Do you have a medical condition that is not listed (such as epilepsy, neurological conditions, kidney problems)?	YES☐ NO☐
10c.	Do you currently live with two or more medical conditions?	YES☐ NO☐

PLEASE LIST YOUR MEDICAL CONDITION(S) AND ANY RELATED MEDICATIONS HERE: _____

_____

GO to Page 4 for recommendations about your current medical condition(s) and sign the PARTICIPANT DECLARATION.

 OSHF
Ontario Society for Health and Fitness

Copyright 2016 PAR-Q+ Collaboration   3/4
01-01-2016

FORM 9.1   *> continued*

PAR-Q+

☑ **If you answered NO to all of the follow-up questions about your medical condition, you are ready to become more physically active - sign the PARTICIPANT DECLARATION below:**

▶ It is advised that you consult a qualified exercise professional to help you develop a safe and effective physical activity plan to meet your health needs.

▶ You are encouraged to start slowly and build up gradually - 20 to 60 minutes of low to moderate intensity exercise, 3-5 days per week including aerobic and muscle strengthening exercises.

▶ As you progress, you should aim to accumulate 150 minutes or more of moderate intensity physical activity per week.

▶ If you are over the age of 45 yr and **NOT** accustomed to regular vigorous to maximal effort exercise, consult a qualified exercise professional before engaging in this intensity of exercise.

⬢ **If you answered YES to one or more of the follow-up questions** about your medical condition:
You should seek further information before becoming more physically active or engaging in a fitness appraisal. You should complete the specially designed online screening and exercise recommendations program - the **ePARmed-X+ at www.eparmedx.com** and/or visit a qualified exercise professional to work through the ePARmed-X+ and for further information.

⚠ **Delay becoming more active if:**

✓ You have a temporary illness such as a cold or fever; it is best to wait until you feel better.

✓ You are pregnant - talk to your health care practitioner, your physician, a qualified exercise professional, and/or complete the ePARmed-X+ **at www.eparmedx.com** before becoming more physically active.

✓ Your health changes - talk to your doctor or qualified exercise professional before continuing with any physical activity program.

● You are encouraged to photocopy the PAR-Q+. You must use the entire questionnaire and NO changes are permitted.
● The authors, the PAR-Q+ Collaboration, partner organizations, and their agents assume no liability for persons who undertake physical activity and/or make use of the PAR-Q+ or ePARmed-X+. If in doubt after completing the questionnaire, consult your doctor prior to physical activity.

PARTICIPANT DECLARATION

● All persons who have completed the PAR-Q+ please read and sign the declaration below.

● If you are less than the legal age required for consent or require the assent of a care provider, your parent, guardian or care provider must also sign this form.

I, the undersigned, have read, understood to my full satisfaction and completed this questionnaire. I acknowledge that this physical activity clearance is valid for a maximum of 12 months from the date it is completed and becomes invalid if my condition changes. I also acknowledge that a Trustee (such as my employer, community/fitness centre, health care provider, or other designate) may retain a copy of this form for their records. In these instances, the Trustee will be required to adhere to local, national, and international guidelines regarding the storage of personal health information ensuring that the Trustee maintains the privacy of the information and does not misuse or wrongfully disclose such information.

NAME _____   DATE _____

SIGNATURE _____   WITNESS _____

SIGNATURE OF PARENT/GUARDIAN/CARE PROVIDER _____

──── **For more information, please contact** ────
www.eparmedx.com
Email: eparmedx@gmail.com

Citation for PAR-Q+
Warburton DER, Jamnik VK, Bredin SSD, and Gledhill N on behalf of the PAR-Q+ Collaboration. The Physical Activity Readiness Questionnaire for Everyone (PAR-Q+) and Electronic Physical Activity Readiness Medical Examination (ePARmed-X+). Health & Fitness Journal of Canada 4(2):3-23, 2011.
Key References
1. Jamnik VK, Warburton DER, Makarski J, McKenzie DC, Shephard RJ, Stone J, and Gledhill N. Enhancing the effectiveness of clearance for physical activity participation; background and overall process. APNM 36(S1):S3-S13, 2011.
2. Warburton DER, Gledhill N, Jamnik VK, Bredin SSD, McKenzie DC, Stone J, Charlesworth S, and Shephard RJ. Evidence-based risk assessment and recommendations for physical activity clearance; Consensus Document. APNM 36(S1):S266-s298, 2011.

The PAR-Q+ was created using the evidence-based AGREE process (1) by the PAR-Q+ Collaboration chaired by Dr. Darren E. R. Warburton with Dr. Norman Gledhill, Dr. Veronica Jamnik, and Dr. Donald C. McKenzie (2). Production of this document has been made possible through financial contributions from the Public Health Agency of Canada and the BC Ministry of Health Services. The views expressed herein do not necessarily represent the views of the Public Health Agency of Canada or the BC Ministry of Health Services.

OSHF
Ontario Society for Health and Fitness

This document has been adapted (with permission) for inclusion in *canfitpro* documents.

Copyright 2016 PAR-Q+ Collaboration   4/4
01-01-2016

Health History Form

Name: _____

Address: _____

Home phone: _____ Work phone: _____

Date of birth: _____ Occupation: _____

Height (cm): _____ Weight (kg): _____ BMI: _____ [BMI = wt (kg)/ht (m)^2]

Fat mass (kg): _____ Fat-free mass (kg): _____

Blood pressure: Systolic _____mmHg Diastolic _____mmHg Pulse: _____BPM

Cardiovascular Risk

Please mark each statement that is true.

_____ You are a man over the age of 45 years.

_____ You are a woman over the age of 55 years.

_____ You are physically inactive (active less than 30 minutes three times a week).

_____ You are overweight (9 kg [20 lb] or more, or BMI over 30).

_____ You presently smoke or have quit within the past six months.

_____ You have high blood pressure or take blood pressure medication.

_____ You have been told you have high cholesterol.

_____ Your father or brother had a heart attack or heart surgery before the age of 55.

_____ Your mother or sister had a heart attack or heart surgery before the age of 65.

Existing Medical Conditions

Please check the appropriate conditions.

_____ Anemia   _____ Epilepsy   _____ Thyroid problems

_____ Arthritis   _____ Heart condition   _____ Ulcer

_____ Asthma   _____ Hernia   _____ Other: _____

_____ Cholesterol   _____ Obesity   _____

_____ Diabetes   _____ Pregnancy   _____

Medications

Are you currently taking any medications? _____ Yes _____ No

If yes, please list the condition and what medication is required.

Condition: _____ Medication: _____

Condition: _____ Medication: _____

Condition: _____ Medication: _____

Condition: _____ Medication: _____

> continued

FORM 9.2 Sample client health history form.

Allergies

Do you have any allergies? _____ Yes _____ No

If yes, please list and indicate whether medication is required.

Allergy: _____ Medication required: _____

Allergy: _____ Medication required: _____

Injuries

Do you have pain, or have you injured any of the following areas?

_____ Neck   _____ Shoulder: R, L   _____ Hip: R, L

_____ Upper back   _____ Elbow: R, L   _____ Knee: R, L

_____ Lower back   _____ Wrist: R, L   _____ Ankle R, L

Please explain: _____

Exercise Habits

_____ Intensive occupational and recreational exertion

_____ Moderate occupational and recreational exertion

_____ Sedentary work and intense recreational exertion

_____ Sedentary work and moderate recreational exertion

_____ Sedentary work and light recreational exertion

_____ Complete lack of occupational or recreational exertion

Is there any reason why you can't exercise regularly? _____ Yes _____ No

Explain: _____

Lifestyle

	Always	Sometimes	Rarely
I get seven to eight hours of sleep per night.	_____	_____	_____
I am physically active three times a week.	_____	_____	_____
I have regular medical checkups.	_____	_____	_____
I eat three to five servings of vegetables daily.	_____	_____	_____
I eat two to four servings of fruit daily.	_____	_____	_____
I eat six to ten servings of grains and cereals daily.	_____	_____	_____
I eat two to three servings of meats and nuts daily.	_____	_____	_____
I make a conscious effort to eat healthy.	_____	_____	_____
I follow a strict diet.	_____	_____	_____
I have no stress in my life.	_____	_____	_____
I am a very happy person.	_____	_____	_____
I am highly motivated.	_____	_____	_____

FORM 9.2   > *continued*

Goals

	Goal	Time frame	Commitment
1.	_____	_____	_____
2.	_____	_____	_____
3.	_____	_____	_____

Family Physician

Name: _____

City: _____

Phone number: _____

Contact in Case of Emergency

Name: _____

Phone number: _____

Relation: _____

Personal Training Specialist

By signing this form, I certify that I have asked for and understand the pertinent information required for me to make an informed decision.

Signature: _____ Date: _____

Client

By signing this form, I certify that I have fully disclosed all pertinent information in an honest and truthful manner.

Signature: _____ Date: _____

FORM 9.2 > *continued*

From canfitpro, 2016, *Foundations of Professional Personal Training,* 2nd ed. (Champaign, IL: Human Kinetics).

191

Dynamic Assessments

Gregory S. Anderson, PhD
Brian Justin, M.Kin
Chad Benson, MSc

LEARNING OUTCOMES

After completing this chapter, you will be able to

1. discuss the value and purpose of postural, foundational movement and fitness assessments;

2. understand the criterion used for dynamic postural assessment;

3. explain how cardiorespiratory fitness is assessed;

4. discuss how muscular strength and endurance are evaluated; and

5. explain how to assess flexibility for most clients.

Many Personal Training Specialists use a dynamic assessment to complement their clients' fitness training. Performing a dynamic assessment gives you a clear indication of your clients' current health status and fitness level. This information is invaluable in fine-tuning program design. To follow best practices and use programs that have the greatest potential to improve clients' health and fitness, all Personal Training Specialists should complement the information gathered from passive screening and assessments with dynamic assessment tests.

Dynamic assessments are useful for

- identifying where your client's posture is weak or strong during specific movement patterns;

- identifying your client's actual fitness level for cardiorespiratory endurance, muscular resistance, and flexibility;

- determining your client's strengths and weaknesses for the purpose of goal setting and counseling;

- isolating significant injuries or risk factors that might affect your client's ability to exercise with a Personal Training Specialist;

- developing an individualized and accurate exercise training program for each client that takes into consideration her or his unique needs, desires, and lifestyle factors;

- establishing a baseline and setting a standard for your client to measure future progress; and

- motivating your client, thus increasing exercise adherence and compliance.

The question you must address during the assessment is how much information you will need to design a safe, effective, enjoyable, and time-efficient exercise-training program, compared with your client's desire to understand his or her current fitness level. For example, asking an unfit client who is moderately overweight to perform difficult fitness tests may undermine that client's self-esteem. On the other hand, a regular exerciser might desire a full battery of fitness tests to evaluate his or her personal progress and success. You must determine what the client's priorities are and then decide what postural and physical fitness tests are necessary and appropriate for the assessment.

 As a Personal Training Specialist, you can obtain useful information through the screening and assessment process, but your clients must be interested in and motivated by the assessments and results. You can decide with your clients to perform a full assessment, using all of the tests, or to do a partial assessment with only select tests. However, if you and a client choose not to perform all the assessments, be especially conservative with your initial program design, as you may not have the same depth of detailed information to assist in designing the program as you would gather from a full assessment.

Before designing programs for your clients, you have to evaluate the results of the complete screening and assessment process you have chosen to implement. This detailed evaluation will help you determine the appropriate exercise-training program to help your clients safely achieve their overall health and fitness goals. You need to become skilled in each aspect of the screening and assessment process to implement it properly with clients.

As introduced in chapter 9, the following is canfitpro's recommended order for assessments. The dynamic assessments in steps 4 and 5 will be covered in this chapter.

1. Pre-exercise screening (e.g., PAR-Q+, health history questionnaire)
2. Passive postural assessment (front, back, and side)
3. Standard health assessment (e.g. HR, BP, skinfolds, girth)
4. Dynamic postural assessment
5. Physical fitness assessment:
   a. Cardiorespiratory fitness assessment
   b. Muscular strength and endurance assessment
   c. Flexibility assessment

A light warm-up should precede the dynamic postural and physical fitness assessments. Always repeat the assessment sequence in the same order for consistent results.

Although this dynamic assessment sequence was chosen to help you foresee and therefore minimize risks and serious injury in exercise, a certain measure of risk is involved in having your client complete these assessments. Because some of these movements may be unfamiliar to your clients, delayed onset muscle soreness or injury may occur, so you should advise them of such possibilities before starting the dynamic assessment process.

Dynamic Postural Assessment

Building on the passive postural assessment described in the previous chapter, a dynamic postural assessment will allow you to evaluate a client's ability to move into and out of a neutral position. This will affect the potential for each exercise in the training program to have its intended effect. As mentioned in the discussion about the myofascial pathways (chapter 7), good posture has been shown to reduce the likelihood and degree of injury. The relationship is reciprocal: good posture helps create good movement patterns, and good movement helps improve posture.

In your assessment of dynamic posture, you will likely identify areas where clients lack the strength to stabilize themselves during movements. This kind of joint instability and weakness can create a loss of power and coordination and is therefore a hindrance to efficient movement as well as functional and athletic performance.

A dynamic postural assessment will allow you to assess your clients' ability to

1. passively achieve neutral posture in preparation for movement,

2. create reproducible three-dimensional movement in and out of a neutral spinal position, and

3. allow muscles to move (lengthen and shorten) while maintaining joint and postural stability.

These assessments measure the client's ability to complete one repetition correctly for a series of tests. Although typical fitness programs rarely, if ever, train clients using one repetition of a small number of movements, each dynamic assessment test specifically requires such an approach to ensure that posture is evaluated and to give you the information required to design appropriate programs for each client. To train your clients effectively, you must also gather information about their capacity to tolerate fatigue. For this reason the assessment tests also contain aspects designed to examine the ability of your client to withstand both volume and intensity. Thus, these tests are also referred to as tests of functional capacity.

Although you will gain an introductory understanding of how to conduct dynamic assessments and incorporate some of the results into your program design, you may also choose to deepen your knowledge and further develop your skill set through specific courses on postural assessment and corrective exercise programming.

Equipment Required for Dynamic Postural Assessment

When administering the dynamic postural assessments, ask your client to wear athletic shoes and comfortable but form-fitting clothes. Close-fitting clothing will help you see the client's body position better and evaluate the client's movement errors.

The following equipment is also recommended:

- A metric (100 cm) and imperial (36 in.) measuring stick
- Flexible plastic (not cloth) measuring tape
- Empty wall, approximately 2.5 to 3 metres in height
- Wooden dowel or broomstick 2.5 to 5 centimetres in diameter
- Half foam roller or 2.5-by-10-centimetre plank (or a second wooden dowel)
- Yoga mat or 2.5-centimetre-thick foam fitness mat

Scoring the Dynamic Postural Assessment

As mentioned in the chapter about flexibility, to create an accurate picture of three-dimensional posture, mobility, and stability, you should observe your clients in all three planes of movement. Thus, the dynamic postural assessment tests evaluate posture from the front, side, and back as well as movement in the sagittal, frontal, and transverse planes.

The dynamic postural assessments have certain criteria that must be accomplished to obtain a high score. The scoring is broken down into four basic categories:

- A score of 0 is given if the client does not pass the clearing tests or has pain during any part of the movement. If 0 is obtained on any test, you should refer your client to a rehabilitative professional or corrective exercise specialist before integrating exercises that require the same restricted movement pattern.

- A score of 1 (low function) is given if the client cannot achieve the established range-of-motion requirement and cannot perform the movement pattern without major compensations.

- A score of 2 (moderate function) is given if the client can perform the movement but must use poor mechanics and compensatory patterns to accomplish the movement or established range-of-motion requirement.

- A score of 3 (high function) is given if the client can perform the movement without any compensations, according to the established range-of-motion criteria.

If the test result is asymmetrical (different on each side), the lower of the two scores should be recorded as the client's score. Mobility and stability exercises should be included in your client's program, appropriate to the assessment-based level of function. Therefore, the training sessions you create should include activities that help the client strengthen weak areas and stretch those that are tight. You can also integrate your understanding of the myofascial pathways to address the adjacent muscles as described in the chapter about flexibility.

As a Personal Training Specialist, you can use the overall dynamic postural assessment score to create a client's program using appropriate movements, activities, and exercises. You can work on the client's movement issues by focusing on either the results of specific tests or the client's total dynamic postural assessment score. You should give individualized mobility and stability programs to your clients that are appropriate to their assessment-based level of function. Movement errors on any of the assessments can be used as a guideline for generating safe, effective, enjoyable, and time-efficient programs. These tests often reveal a client's movement imbalances; if one muscle is dominant or strong, its antagonist is commonly weak. Strong patterns typically benefit from mobility exercises, whereas weak patterns usually benefit from muscle strengthening.

As a general approach to selecting exercises to help clients improve their dynamic posture and stability, each stage of assessment scoring can be addressed as follows:

Score = 0
- Incorporate any exercises, stretches, or mobility techniques recommended by a rehabilitative or corrective exercise specialist.
- Have the client perform gentle static stretches for tight muscles.
- Include exercises that activate and strengthen the weak, or antagonist, muscles.
- Retest approximately four weeks later to evaluate improvement.

Score = 1
- Have clients perform static or slow dynamic stretches for noticeably tight muscles during their personal training sessions, as outlined in chapter 7.
- Incorporate exercises into training sessions that activate and strengthen the weak, or antagonist, muscles, as well as the core.
- Asymmetrical core activation and flexibility exercises are recommended to address imbalances.
- Retest approximately four weeks later to evaluate the client's improvement in the restricted movement patterns.

Score = 2
- Have clients perform static or slow dynamic stretches for any tight muscles, on their own or during the session, based on the guidelines outlined in chapter 7.
- Include exercises that activate and strengthen the weak, or antagonist, muscles, as well as the core.
- Asymmetrical core activation and flexibility exercises are recommended to address imbalances.
- Evaluate the client's improvement during the next fitness assessment.

Score = 3
- Incorporate core activation and flexibility exercises (for both sides of the body) related

to the activities and dominant muscle groups involved in the planned workout.

- In addition to doing their regular training program, clients can perform specific mobility, flexibility, and core activation exercises on their own as needed.

When assessing movement errors, you can evaluate clients without using the formal scoring system. In these situations, you should consistently select the same test variation for each client when reassessing.

The dynamic assessment tests and their scores can also act as a baseline measure from which functional progress can be determined. With this method, comparison to normative values is not essential, but the Personal Training Specialist must clear the client on each level of the test to determine the client's current functional level.

In cases when you can create a competitive environment and challenge groups of clients with similar fitness levels, these tests permit both client and group comparative scoring. With proper and

When to Refer

In addition to situations in which clients cannot perform the movement pattern without major compensations (i.e., functional score = 0), you should also refer them to a rehabilitative or corrective exercise specialist when they present chronic pain, show minimal improvement in pain-free range of motion, or continue to make movement errors or compensations. Such specialists include orthopedic specialists, physiotherapists, athletic therapists, massage therapists, chiropractors, and other appropriately qualified exercise professionals.

consistent implementation, you can compare and contrast results among populations or with values obtained by different Personal Training Specialists (for the same or different client groups).

ASSESSMENT TESTS

canfitpro's Dynamic Postural Assessment Sequence consists of the following tests:

1. Seated spinal rotation test
2. Straight leg raise (lumbopelvic stability test)
3. Overhead squat test

 ## 1. Seated Spinal Rotation Test

Myofascial Sling
Anterior functional line, posterior functional line, and upper portion of the spiral line

Functional Capability or Capacity
- Range of motion in spinal rotation and associated myofascia
- Neutral spine awareness during rotation

Functional Relevance
This test gives you information regarding a client's mobility and symmetry in the transverse plane. Proper rotation will affect the successful execution of functional movements including the chop and lift, sport-specific rotational movements, and all resistance training exercises requiring rotation. Asymmetrical results on the other dynamic assessments will relate to the results of this seated spinal rotation. A history of low back pain and the inability to balance and maintain an upright posture (sometimes at high intensity and speed) will also affect a person's success while performing rotational movements.

The seated spinal rotation test, straight leg raise test, and overhead squat test were created by Chad Benson for nashFIT (www.nashfit.ca) and have been adapted for this textbook.

Setup and Procedure

- The client sits upright in an arms-crossed, legs-crossed position, and the dorsum of the feet touch the base of a pole or doorjamb.
- Instruct the client to hold and maintain contact of a dowel against the collarbones at shoulder level. The elbows and upper arms should hang down in front of the torso (as pictured).
- Instruct the client to rotate the right or left shoulder in an attempt to move the dowel toward the pole or doorjamb.
- Note the angle achieved and use a metre stick to measure the distance in centimetres between the dowel and pole or doorjamb.
- Repeat on the opposite side.

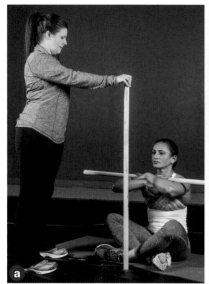 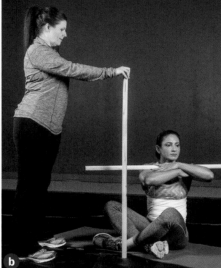 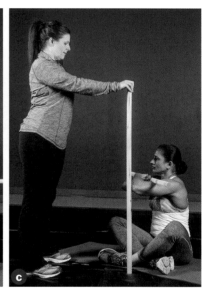

Start position   **End position left**   **End position right**

Movement Errors

- Setup: torso not upright
- Pain while trying to perform the movement
- Upper back rounded or flexed (i.e., thoracic kyphosis)
- Dowel not parallel to floor, torso side bend, or lateral flexion of spine
- Asymmetrical rotation (i.e., >25 cm difference in distance between right and left side)

Note: If two or more of these errors occur, the client has not passed that level.

Scoring

Score = 0: pain or greater than 35 cm from doorjamb (or 40 cm from pole)

Score = 1: more than 20 cm and less than 35 cm from doorjamb (or between 25 cm and 40 cm from pole)

Score = 2: more than 5 cm and less than 20 cm from doorjamb (or between 10 cm and 25 cm from pole)

Score = 3: less than 5 cm from doorjamb (or less than 10 cm from pole)

Note: The client's overall score for this test is based on symmetry. For example, if your client scores 1 on the right side and 2 on the left, the overall score for that test should be recorded as a 1.

2. Straight Leg Raise—Lumbopelvic Stability Test

Myofascial Sling

Posterior superficial line and deep longitudinal line

Functional Capability or Capacity

- Posterior sling mobility and range of motion
- Lumbopelvic neutral spine awareness and stability

Functional Relevance

This movement requires predominantly sagittal and transverse plane control (i.e., maintaining core neutral) and assesses the client's ability to maintain three-dimensional stability of the pelvis during movement. Bending over and walking are common daily life functions that benefit from hinging, unilateral leg raise, and movements based on forward leg swing. Thus, the hip hinge is incredibly important in everyday life, fitness, and sport.

Successful execution of many functional resistance movements is highly dependent on the client's ability to hip hinge while maintaining neutral lumbopelvic alignment at high intensities. Example of these movements include squatting, lunging, pulling movements, and common resistance training and yoga or Pilates exercises that involve bending, raising the legs, or single-leg balance while hinging (e.g., abdominal leg raise exercises, standing cable extensions, bent-over row, deadlifts, kettlebell swings, standing head to knee pose, and warrior III pose).

Setup and Procedure

Instruct your client to lie supine with the arms at the sides. The knees should be fully extended, and the feet should be 15 centimetres apart or closer.

Part 1

- Kneel behind the client's head and look toward the client's pelvis and feet.
- Direct the client to flex the right hip—while keeping the right knee fully extended—to briefly raise the right leg 10 to 15 centimetres off the floor. The left leg should remain motionless as the right leg is raised. Return the right leg to the floor and repeat the procedure with the left leg. (Be sure the client keeps the right leg on the floor as the left leg is raised.)
- After a brief pause, direct the client to repeat the movements, one leg at a time, but have the client contract the abdominal muscles as each leg is raised. Place your hand under the client's lower back and determine if that corrects any previously noted movement errors. (If so, then drawing in the core and using bracing techniques will greatly help this client.)

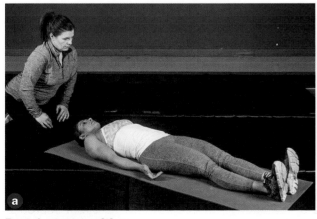

Part 1 start position

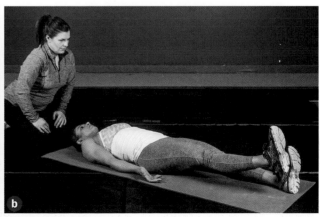

Part 1 end position

Part 2

- Stand on the left side of the client with your right foot placed on the floor and directly under the client's left knee. The back of the client's left knee should be resting on the top of your right foot.
- Direct the client to dorsiflex the right ankle so that the right foot is perpendicular to the floor and, while pressing down with the left leg on top of your right foot, direct the client to slowly flex the right hip to raise the leg up (with the right knee still fully extended) as far as possible under control.
- At the highest position, direct the client to pause momentarily so you can discern the position of the right heel and any errors in the movement.
- Direct the client to return the right leg to the floor.
- Change sides to stand on the right side of the client with your left foot placed on the floor and directly under the client's right knee.
- Direct the client to repeat the procedure with the left leg.

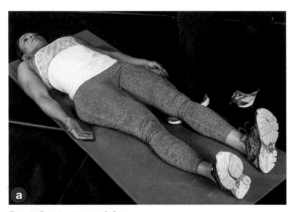

Part 2 start position

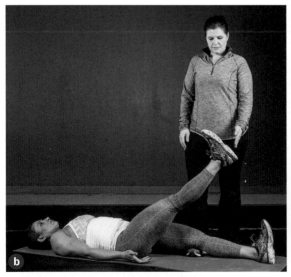

Part 2 end position, score of 1

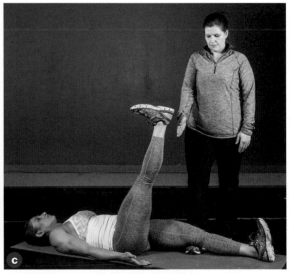

Part 2 end position, score of 3

Movement Errors

- Inability to keep the knees fully extended as a leg is raised.
- Leg externally rotates at the hip as the hip flexes.
- Breathing changes from belly breathing to rib cage breathing.
- Bulges appear in the abdomen as a leg is raised.
- Inability to keep the lower back in a neutral position as a leg is raised.
- Change occurs in the plane of the anterior superior iliac spine (ASIS).

Scoring

Score = 0: The client cannot perform the movement pain-free or achieve a neutral lower back position.

Score = 1: The client can lift a single leg off the floor with limited core neutral pressure change on your hand (part 1) and minimal knee flexion (part 1 or 2). In part 2, with your foot under the client's knee, the client is able to lift the opposite leg up to be vertically aligned with your ASIS that is the farthest from the client's head. If the client's pelvis significantly rotates bilaterally or asymmetrically in either part 1 or 2, a score of 1 is assigned.

Score = 2: The client can lift a single leg off the floor with no core neutral pressure change on your hand (part 1) with the knee fully extended (part 1 or 2). In part 2, with your foot under the client's knee, the client is able to lift the opposite leg up to be vertically aligned with your navel. If the client's pelvis has minimal and symmetrical rotation during any part of the test, a score of 2 is assigned.

Score = 3: The client can lift a single leg off the floor with no core neutral pressure change on your hand (part 1) with the knee fully extended (part 1 or 2). In part 2, with your foot under the client's knee, the client is able to lift the opposite leg up to be vertically aligned with your ASIS that is the closest to the client's head (or beyond). If the client's pelvis has minimal and symmetrical rotation during any part of the test, a score of 3 is assigned.

Note: The client's overall score for this test is also based on symmetry. For example, if your client scores 1 on the right side and 2 on the left, the overall score for that test should be recorded as 1.

3. Overhead Squat Test

Myofascial Sling

Includes components and influence from several myofascial lines.

Functional Capability and Capacity

- Mobility of extremities around stability of posture
- Neutral spine awareness and hip hinging

Functional Relevance

If you were to perform one catch-all dynamic postural test, the overhead squat would be the ideal choice. This test challenges upper- and lower-body mobility, postural control, lumbopelvic stability, head-to-toe sagittal plane biomechanics, and neuromuscular coordination. This movement relates to functional activities such as crawling, running, and jumping. Although it is a sagittal plane, symmetrical movement, this version of the overhead squat test allows asymmetrical analysis and influence from the other planes.

Although the overhead squat by itself isn't directly linked to all functional and sport-specific movements, it is relevant to activities that require mobility of the extremities and a stable posture. Success in this test directly correlates to a client's ability to use triple extension and flexion movement patterns such as the squat, deadlift, lunge, clean, snatch, press, and push press under load. Variants of the overhead squat can also be seen in yoga as chair, sitting, and warrior poses. The test has two parts: Success in part 1 of the test depends on movement range of motion, whereas part 2 of the test measures the muscular endurance of the pattern. Inability to perform a full-range-of-motion overhead squat is a clear indication that the client's joint alignment has compensated as result of lifestyle, sport, or fitness habits. Those who score higher are able to perform squat and overhead pressing exercises with greater range of motion and velocity with reduced risk of injury.

PART 1: RANGE OF MOTION

Setup and Procedure

- The client stands with feet shoulder-width apart and facing a pole or wall, 7.5 to 15 centimetres from the wall. The taller your client is, the farther her or his feet will be from the wall.
- Have the client grasp a dowel at arm's length with the hands one arm's width from each other.
- Instruct the client to raise the dowel over the head until the point at which the client's lower back begins to arch.
- Instruct the client to squat down while attempting to hold the dowel in the same overhead positon.

The levels of testing for the overhead squat assessments are considered progressive, and they should be performed in sequence to evaluate your client's ability to perform the movement. Each successful level (thigh below parallel) requires an increasingly more challenging combination of mobility, joint stability, and postural adjustments. Progress to the next level only if the client has successfully completed the previous level.

Level 1: Heels approximately 1 to 2.5 centimetres above the level of the floor with the femur below parallel to the floor

In level 1, the client performs the squat with the heels elevated approximately 2.5 centimetres off the floor. You can use a half foam roller, a plank 1 to 2.5 centimetres high by 10 centimetres long, or a second wooden dowel to achieve this elevation. Clients with limited ankle mobility (often because of tightness in the calf muscles) will find this level easier to perform than a conventional squat because less dorsiflexion is needed to execute the desired ROM.

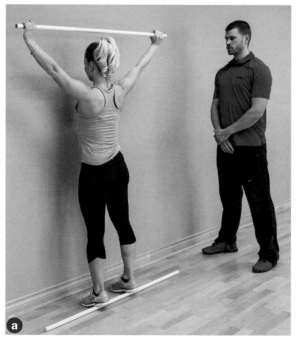

Start position

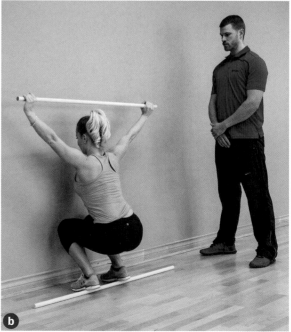

End position, level 1 pass

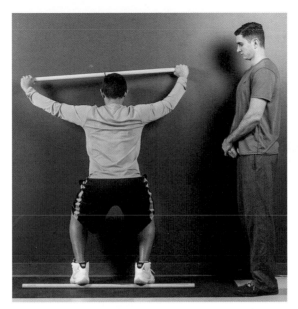

Level 1 with imbalance

Level 2: heels on floor, femur below parallel

In level 2, the client performs the squat without elevation of the heels. This level requires a greater level of mobility and joint control than the previous level.

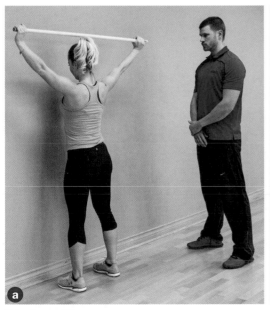

Start position

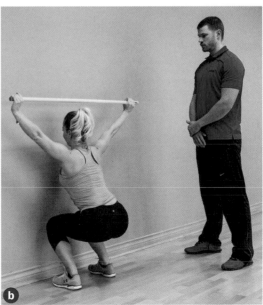

End position, level 2 pass

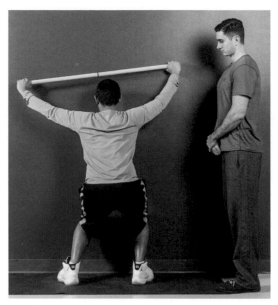

Level 2 with imbalance

Level 3: toes elevated (approximately 2.5 cm) and femur below parallel

In level 3, the client's toes are elevated approximately 2.5 centimetres on the half foam roller, 2.5-by-10-centimetre plank, or wooden dowel. This is the most challenging level, and only a select few clients will be able to achieve it on the first assessment.

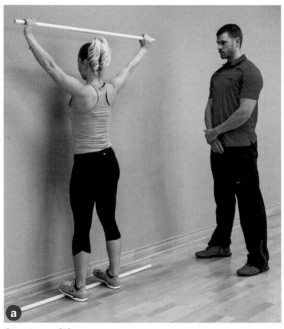

Start position

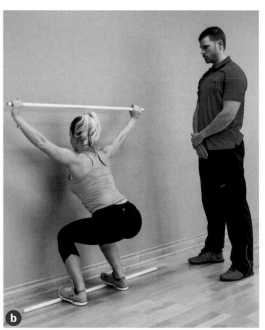

End position, level 3 unsuccessful

Movement Errors

- Forearms, rather than hands, are equidistant from the sides of the head.
- One or both elbows are not fully extended in the overhead position (record which elbow is the most flexed).
- Dowel is held in a position that is over or behind heels.
- Dowel is rotated backward or farther from the wall on one side compared with the other.
- Stable body position cannot be maintained.
- Thoracic spine is not held in a neutral position.
- Sacral spine is not held in a natural arch or iliac crest is in a forward, backward, or laterally tilted position.
- Hips shift away from the midsagittal plane.
- Loss of vertical alignment between the knee and the second toe (on the same side).
- Lower leg and thoracic spine are not held in a position parallel to each other.
- Pronation or supination occurs at either ankle.

The client qualifies as passing the level if no substantial errors are made or if not more than one detectable error is made.

Scoring

Score = 0: The client experiences pain at any position during the movement or cannot perform level 1 with the femur below parallel.

Score = 1: The client successfully performs the full range of motion (femur below parallel) with the heels elevated on a plank, half foam roller, or wooden dowel.

Score = 2: The client successfully performs the full range of motion (femur below parallel) with both heels flat on the floor.

Score = 3: The client successfully performs the full range of motion (femur below parallel) with both heels on the floor and the toes elevated on a plank, half foam roller, or wooden dowel.

*If the client achieves level 2 or 3, proceed to part 2 of this test.

PART 2: CAPACITY TESTING

Procedure

To assess muscular and postural endurance, have the client hold the level 2 position for as long as possible, without pain (up to 90 seconds). This part of the overhead squat assessment measures the client's resistance to fatigue and capacity to maintain optimal posture.

Scoring

Score = 0: The client is unable to keep the thighs parallel to floor and the arms in line with the ears.

Score = 1: The client holds the squat position for 0 to 30 seconds without losing balance or stopping.

Score = 2: The client holds the squat position for 31 to 60 seconds without losing balance or stopping.

Score = 3: The client holds the squat position for 61 to 90 seconds without losing balance or stopping.

*Reminder: If the client obtains level 0, refer him or her to a rehabilitative or corrective exercise specialist.

 See the web resource at www.HumanKinetics.com/FoundationsOfProfessionalPersonalTraining for a form to record client performance on postural and fitness assessments.

The best way to become proficient at performing each assessment is through practice. After reading through each of the dynamic assessment protocols, it is helpful to practice these new skills on yourself and a friend.

Cardiorespiratory Fitness Assessment

Cardiorespiratory fitness is defined as the efficiency of the cardiovascular, respiratory, and muscular systems at delivering and extracting oxygen for energy production and mechanical muscle work. A number of fitness tests measure cardiorespiratory fitness. The measurement of this fitness parameter is expressed as $\dot{V}O_2max$, also known as *maximal oxygen uptake* (see chapter 4).

The most accurate way to measure cardiorespiratory efficiency is through direct measurement of oxygen uptake during a maximal graded exercise assessment. This approach requires specialized laboratory equipment and can be quite expensive. A more common approach is the use of **submaximal tests** to estimate oxygen uptake, or $\dot{V}O_2max$.. This evaluation can be done using a timed distance (e.g., 2.5 km run or Rockport Fitness Walking Test), using distance per unit of time (e.g., 12-minute mile, or 7.5-minute kilometre), or evaluating the client's heart rate response to graded submaximal exercise. Many submaximal tests can be used to evaluate cardiorespiratory fitness, including steps, a treadmill (walk or run), or a stationary bike or cycle ergometer. A graded exercise assessment means that the intensity of the exercise is gradually increased (i.e., grade, resistance, speed).

In a submaximal graded exercise assessment, the client performs the exercise at increasing intensity without exceeding 85% of the age-predicted HRmax (see chapter 4). The Personal Training Specialist evaluates how the client responds to the increasing difficulty by measuring the HR in BPM. At the conclusion of the assessment, the Personal Training Specialist evaluates how hard the client was able to exercise before reaching the 85% barrier. The harder the client can exercise, the higher the calculated $\dot{V}O_2max$ is and the more fit the client is.

The Rockport Walking Institute has developed a walking test to assess cardiorespiratory fitness for men and women within the age range of 20 to 69 years. The test is safe to administer and is useful for assessing sedentary and older clients. To administer this test, instruct clients to walk 1.6 kilometres (four laps around a standard 400-metre track on the inside lane, or on a treadmill) as quickly as possible. Then take the client's HR immediately at the end of the test along with the time in minutes it took to do the walk. An HR monitor would be useful, but if you are manually taking the HR, a 15-second pulse count using the radial pulse will do. Clients should warm up and stretch actively for 5 to 10 minutes before the test, and they should wear good walking shoes and loose-fitting clothes. To estimate the client's maximal oxygen uptake based on the Rockport Fitness Walking Test, use the following generalized equation:

$$\text{For body weight (BW) in kilograms:}$$
$$\dot{V}O_2max = 132.853 - 0.0348\,(BW) - 0.3877\,(age) + 6.315\,(gender) - 3.2649\,(time) - 0.1565\,(HR)$$
$$\text{Gender = 1 for males and 0 for females;}$$
$$\text{time = minutes.}$$

You can compare your results to those in table 10.1.

TABLE 10.1   Average Values for Maximal Oxygen Uptake

Age	$\dot{V}O_2max$, males (ml/kg/min)	$\dot{V}O_2max$, females (ml/kg/min)
18–25	42–46	38–41
26–35	40–42	35–38
36–45	35–38	31–33
46–55	32–35	28–30
56–65	30–31	25–27

Adapted from the CPAFLA manual from CSEP.

 ## Learning to Judge Intensity

One important reason to have clients perform submaximal cardiorespiratory fitness assessments is to educate them about the relationship between HR and exercise intensity and compare HR to RPE. If you teach clients how exercise should feel at different intensities, they will have a better idea of how hard to exercise during cardiorespiratory training.

MUSCULAR CAPACITY ASSESSMENT

Many Personal Training Specialists assess muscular strength and endurance to help them develop an effective and accurate resistance training program. Attempting to measure a client's absolute strength is difficult and dangerous because it is the maximum amount of force that can be exerted one time, or in a one-repetition maximum (1RM), explained in chapter 6. The alternative tests that follow are easy and reasonably safe to perform. The results give you a good indication of your clients' muscular strength and endurance, which will help you develop an appropriate starting place for resistance training. You will also have a clear method of comparison so you can see whether your programs are increasing muscular strength and endurance in your clients.

Assessments for predicting muscular capacity can be categorized into normative and nonnormative tests.

NORMATIVE STRENGTH TESTS

Normative tests have values that rate the level of performance (i.e., poor to excellent) of the item being evaluated. These values are based on specific age populations. A large number of subjects have been examined to establish the values, so you can compare your clients' results with the rating to quantify their fitness level for the item you are assessing. For the results to be accurate when assessing individual clients, you must use the same testing **protocol** that was used to establish the norms.

Grip Strength Test

You can predict upper-body strength using a hand-grip dynamometer, which requires the client to squeeze the handle with maximal effort using both the right and left hands. The results of this test show a good correlation with actual upper-body strength because grip strength is needed to complete lifts for the upper body and even to perform some lower-body exercises (e.g., deadlift).

Setup and Procedure

1. Have the subject grasp a dynamometer. Be sure to adjust it so that the second joint of the fingers fits snugly under the handle. Lock the grip in place.
2. The client should hold the dynamometer in line with the forearm at the level of the thigh away from the body. The hand and dynamometer should not touch the body during the test.
3. Instruct the subject to squeeze the dynamometer forcefully while exhaling (to avoid buildup of intrathoracic pressure).
4. The client alternates hands, performing two trials per hand.
5. Combine the maximum scores for each hand and record them. Compare with age-adjusted norms.
6. See appendix table C.5 for normative data on grip strength.

10-Repetition Maximum Test

Instead of performing a 1RM test, which carries a high risk for injury, you can perform a 10RM test (resistance at which no more than 10 repetitions can be performed) of a specific movement pattern and use the results to estimate the client's 1RM. The 10RM test can be used with healthy adults who have lifting experience. Typically, the bench press, leg press, squat, lat pull-down, and shoulder press are used, but you can use any resistance exercise that you want to assess that your client is familiar with. To predict a 1RM from the 10RM, simply divide by 0.75.

Setup and Procedure

1. Have the client warm up for 5 to 10 minutes to increase core temperature.
2. Instruct the client to perform 5 to 10 repetitions at 50% of expected 10RM.
3. After a 1-minute rest and some light active stretching, the client performs 5 repetitions at 75% of expected 10RM.
4. Increase the load to the client's expected 10RM.

After using the 10RM test to estimate 1RM, you can also compare your clients' estimated 1RM to their body mass by simply dividing the 1RM load in kilograms by their body weight in kilograms. The result will give you a ratio of strength to body mass that you can monitor and compare with future tests or with normative data for applicable tests. Be sure to familiarize yourself with the exact protocols used during the development of the norms.

NONNORMATIVE STRENGTH TESTS

Nonnormative tests do not possess any data for comparison and therefore have no established ratings. In these tests, the data obtained by your individual clients are compared with their own future performance to monitor improvement. You can set the protocol for your test as long as your procedures for future tests remain consistent in subsequent assessments. These nonnormative tests are particularly useful when you are working with equipment that is specific to the environment or to the client's sport or activity (e.g., working with limited equipment in a home gym or testing an athlete on equipment that closely mimics movements required in her or his sport).

Percent-Improvement Tests

Many of the muscular resistance and endurance tests use traditional protocols that have little application to clients' daily movement and exercise patterns. As an alternative, you can use an approach to muscular resistance and endurance tests made popular by exercise physiologist Douglas Brooks: the percent-improvement approach. The following procedure can be used with whatever exercise you decide to assess:

Setup and Procedure

1. Pick a movement pattern that you would like to assess.
2. Find a resistance level at which your client can perform 10 repetitions (10RM) of that movement pattern as outlined in the 10RM assessment discussed previously.
3. After the appropriate load is found, record it on your data sheet.
4. Reassess in four to six weeks to evaluate whether any improvement has occurred as evidenced by an increase in repetitions of that load.
5. Calculate the client's percent improvement by dividing the difference between the previous and most recent tests by the initial test result and then multiplying the result by 100. For example, if your client improved by completing 15 repetitions of a load he or she could previously lift only 10 times, you would subtract 10 from 15, which is 5. Then you divide 5 by 10 (initial test result) to obtain 0.5. When you multiply 0.5 by 100, you get a 50% improvement.
6. If you want to track this movement pattern after the reassessment, complete another 10RM test to find the new strength level.

The drawback of this type of test is that you do not have any normative data for comparison. The advantages of this type of test are that you can create your own test parameters, assess specific movement patterns, and track changes in your clients' strength and endurance. If you want to assess them more on endurance, you can perform a 15RM test; if you want to assess more on strength, you can complete a 6RM test. This type of test allows you to gather meaningful data that you can use in your client's individualized program.

NORMATIVE MUSCULAR ENDURANCE TESTS

Three tests for muscular endurance are outlined in this text. The first one is a push-up test in which the client performs as many push-ups as possible until muscular failure occurs. This test can be done with the client in a push-up position on the knees or toes, and it indicates muscular endurance in a pushing movement pattern. The second test described is the horizontal pull-up, which allows you to evaluate your client's upper-body muscular endurance during a pulling movement pattern. The third test measures endurance of the abdominal muscles by having the client perform a maximal number of curl-ups in 60 seconds. The more curl-ups a client can perform, the better her or his muscular endurance is. Note that a sedentary client may not be able to complete these endurance tests successfully. Thus, the push-up, horizontal pull-up, and abdominal curl-up tests are most applicable to clients who already have a base level of fitness.

Push-Up Test

This test assesses the client's upper-body strength and endurance, mainly in the pectorals, deltoids, and triceps. Standardization of the push-up hand placement and lever length allows you to compare results from one test to the next. The following equipment is recommended for the most accurate and useful results:

- 120- to 150-centimetre wooden dowel
- Rolled-up towel or tennis, lacrosse, or hockey ball
- Adhesive tape

Setup and Procedure

- Tape or secure the ball to the floor.
- Have the client lie in a prone position and place the hands shoulder-width apart so that the ball touches the sternum at nipple level.
- Place the dowel along the client's spine so that it contacts the base of the skull, the spine between the scapula, and the sacrum between the gluteal muscles.
- The test can be performed from the knees (with feet off the floor) or from the toes with the hips and knees fully extended and the ankles in neutral position (dorsiflexed).
- If the client is performing the push-ups from the toes, have him or her place the thumbs at shoulder level and shoulder-width apart. If the client is performing the push-ups from the knees, have him or her place the thumbs at eye level and shoulder-width apart.

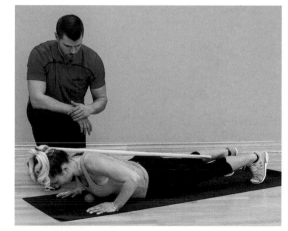

Start position

- Instruct the client to extend the hips and keep the thighs off the floor for the remainder of the test.
- Have the client perform as many repetitions as possible until technique breaks down over two consecutive repetitions or the client appear to strain forcibly. (Take note of total number of reps performed before fatigue sets in or significant movement errors occur.)

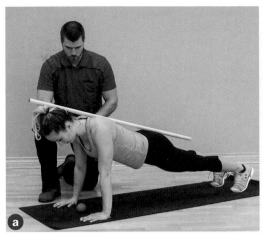 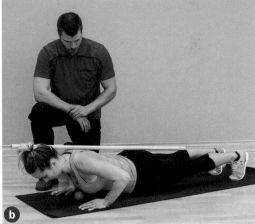

Successful rep position *(a)* **up and** *(b)* **down**

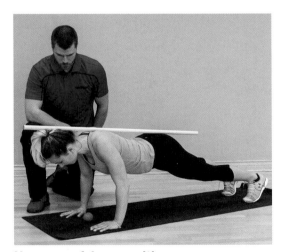

Unsuccessful rep position

Movement Errors

- The shoulder elevates during the push-up (note which side).
- The torso does not lift as a unit (i.e., does not maintain contact with the dowel).
- The knees do not remain fully extended (if the client is doing the push-up from the toes).
- If the client is performing the push-up from the toes, the thighs touch the floor; if the client is performing the push-up from knees, the hips touch the floor.

Scoring

From toes:

Score = 0: The client experiences pain or is able to complete no more than 10 repetitions.

Score = 1: The client successfully completes 11 to 22 repetitions.

Score = 2: The client successfully completes 23 to 40 repetitions.

Score = 3: The client successfully completes 41 or more repetitions.

From knees:

Score = 0: The client experiences pain or is able to complete no more than 8 repetitions.

Score = 1: The client successfully completes 9 to 20 repetitions.

Score = 2: The client successfully completes 21 to 35 repetitions.

Score = 3: The client successfully completes 36 or more repetitions.

Record the functional score obtained, whether the test was completed on the toes or on the knees, and the number of push-ups completed before failure.

Horizontal Pull-Up Test

This test assesses the client's upper-body strength and endurance, mainly in the latissimus dorsi, rhomboids, deltoids, and biceps. The pull-ups are performed from an adjustable-height squat rack or similar device and use a flat or adjustable bench.

Throughout the test, the client must maintain a straight body and pull the chest to the level of the barbell on each repetition. Standardization of the horizontal pull-up hand placement and lever length allows you to compare results from one test with the next.

Setup and Procedure

- Place the barbell on the squat rack slightly higher than the height of the bench (approximately 1 m from the ground).
- Secure a tennis ball to the barbell with tape, facing the floor.
- Have the client sit on the ground under and behind the bar, facing the bench with the feet toward the bench.
- With palms facing the bench and feet, the client grasps the bar using a shoulder-width grip, places the heels on the edge of the bench one at a time, and straightens the legs. The client lifts the hips until they are in a neutral position, the back is flat, and the arms are fully extended
- Adjust the position of the bench if necessary to ensure that the bar is directly above the nipple line.
- From the straight-arm neutral spine position (hang), the client performs pull-ups by pulling the chest to touch the tennis ball, reversing to full extension, and repeating.
- Low-functioning clients can perform from a 45° angle. To ensure consistency, note the distance of the feet to directly below the bar.
- Record the total number of reps performed before the client misses the ball on two successive reps.
- Failure is the inability to hold the torso neutral or complete a full ROM repetition.

Movement Errors

- Shoulders elevate on initiation of the pull (note which side).
- Torso and hips do not lift as a unit (i.e., lag in the hips).
- Excessive arching of the lower back occurs.
- Knees do not remain fully extended.

Scoring

If performing from flat position:

Score = 0: The client experiences pain or is able to complete no more than 5 repetitions.

Score = 1: The client successfully completes 6 to 10 repetitions.

Score = 2: The client successfully completes 11 to 19 repetitions.

Score = 3: The client successfully completes 20 or more repetitions.

If performing from 45° angle position:

Score = 0: The client experiences pain or is able to complete no more than 2 repetitions.

Score = 1: The client successfully completes 3 to 6 repetitions.

Score = 2: The client successfully completes 7 to 12 repetitions.

Score = 3: The client successfully completes 13 or more repetitions.

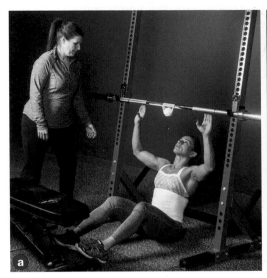
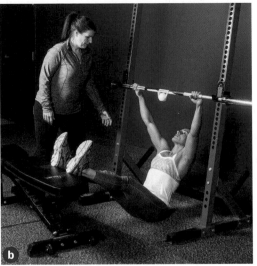

Setup

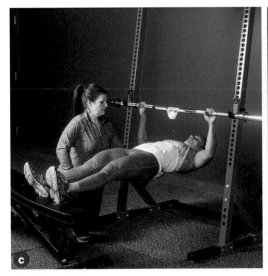
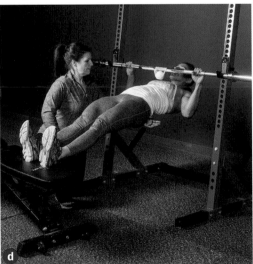

Start position

Successful rep position

Abdominal Curl-Up Test

Probably one of the most used tests of abdominal muscular endurance, the abdominal curl-up test gives reliable information regarding the strength and length relationship for the muscle groups that form the front and back of the torso. It also targets muscular resistance endurance of the abdominals and hip flexors. The core region acts as a stabilizer and mobilizer of the spine and is part of several myofascial lines. Clients who possess a lower crossed syndrome or weak abdominals often score poorly on this test.

Keep in mind that in this protocol you are primarily testing the muscle endurance of the rectus abdominis and external obliques in a trunk flexion pattern. This test does not give the whole picture of abdominal endurance, which requires more specific and comprehensive tests that are beyond the scope of this manual. Although the abdominal curl-up test is one of the most used assessments, it can be challenging to set up and standardize. You should practice with peers, watching for errors in repetitions so that you can improve the **standardization** of the test.

Setup and Procedure

1. Place two pieces of masking tape on a mat 10 centimetres apart.
2. Have the client lie supine with the head lying on the mat and the knees bent to 90°.
3. The client's arms should be fully extended with the fingertips at the zero mark. Instruct the client to keep the heels in contact with the mat throughout the test.
4. Set a metronome to 50 beats per minute.
5. Have the client curl up far enough that the fingertips touch the 10-centimetre mark while the client exhales. During the curl-up, the palms and heels must remain in contact with the mat. On the return, the head and shoulder blades must touch the mat with the fingertips touching the zero mark.
6. Instruct the client to perform as many curl-ups as possible, using the rhythm of the metronome as a guideline for pace (to a maximum of 25 in the 1-minute time limit).
7. Terminate the test if the client experiences undue discomfort, is unable to maintain cadence, or is unable to maintain the proper curl-up technique over two consecutive repetitions.
8. Compare the results with the data provided in appendix table C.7.

For nonnormative muscular endurance testing using this protocol, you can use the percent-improvement approach outlined previously.

FLEXIBILITY ASSESSMENT

Assessing flexibility is useful to Personal Training Specialists because detecting muscle imbalance and joint instability helps you develop exercise programs that can correct those weaknesses and reduce the client's risk of injury. Besides describing the assessments of dynamic posture and mobility, this section outlines two general tests that can be used to evaluate your client's flexibility.

 ## Sit-and-Reach Test

The sit-and-reach test is commonly used to measure forward trunk flexion. Sitting with legs extended and the upper body upright, the client reaches toward the toes using a sit-and-reach box. The distance that the client can reach forward determines relative flexibility in the hamstrings and low back muscles. The results can indicate areas of inflexibility that might put the client at risk for low back pain.

 Although the sit-and-reach test is a traditional test of posterior line flexibility, it cannot unilaterally assess the function of the line. This point emphasizes the importance of including the straight-leg raise dynamic assessment described earlier to gain more information on your client's mobility as it relates to rotational and gait patterns (i.e., functional and spiral lines).

Procedure

1. Have the client warm up for 5 to 10 minutes and perform two modified hurdler's stretches for 20 seconds on each leg (see appendix B).
2. Instruct the client to remove her or his shoes and sit with the soles of the feet against a sit-and-reach box at the 26-centimetre mark. The inner edges of the soles are placed within 2 centimetres of the measuring scale.
3. The client should reach forward with both hands as far as possible and hold that position for approximately two seconds. Be sure that the hands are parallel and that the client does not lead with one hand. The fingertips can overlap and should be in contact with the measuring device of the sit-and-reach box. Ensure that the knees stay extended but are not pressed down.
4. To assist with the attempt, the client should exhale and drop the head between the arms when reaching. Clients should not hold their breath at any time during the test.
5. Record your client's score (i.e., the most distant point reached with the fingertips) using the better of two trials.
6. Normative data is provided in appendix table C.8.

If a sit-and-reach box is not available, a metre stick or measuring tape may be used. At this point, the normative data for the sit-and-reach test would no longer be valid, but you could still get an accurate measurement of how a client was progressing from test to test.

Shoulder Flexibility Test

People use the shoulder joints in many sport movements, work activities, and activities of daily living. The shoulder flexibility test measures internal and external rotation of the shoulders. This assessment will help you determine whether your client has restrictions in rotation of the shoulder, which may lead to pain or injury.

Procedure

1. Have the client raise one arm, bend the elbow, and reach down across the back as far as possible.
2. At the same time, instruct the client to extend the other arm down, bend at the elbow, and reach up behind the back, trying to cross the fingers over those of the other hand. Watch for the client trying to arch the back to improve the score; correct this and have the client start the test again.
3. Measure the distance of finger overlap to the nearest half centimetre. If the fingers overlap, score a plus; if they fail to meet, score a minus.
4. Repeat with the arms crossed in the opposite direction. Average the two scores and compare the value with those found in appendix table C.10.

Scoring

Norms for the shoulder flexibility test are listed in appendix table C.10.

Based on your comfort level with the various fitness test protocols and the relevance to your client's needs, you must decide what fitness tests to use with each client on a regular basis. The assessments included here were chosen because they are relatively easy to implement, are low in cost, require little time to evaluate, and produce findings that you can use to create a safe, effective, and individualized program for each client.

 See the web resource at www.HumanKinetics.com/FoundationsOfProfessionalPersonalTraining for a form you can use to record client performance on postural and fitness assessments.

Sources of Error in Dynamic Assessments

When conducting any form of assessment, the Personal Training Specialist must avoid any errors that could affect the accuracy (i.e., validity and reliability) of results obtained. Test validity describes the degree to which the assessment measures the intended variable, and reliability describes the degree to which the results are consistent and could be reproduced if the test was conducted again using the same standard protocol. Both validity and reliability can be affected by client factors, testing equipment, the skill of the Personal Training Specialist, and the environment in which the assessments are conducted.

Client Factors

Before measuring your clients' physical fitness, familiarize them with equipment and assessment procedures. Some clients may have little experience with exercise and may need time to practice the movements involved (especially in tests that involve weightlifting). Sometimes you need to have the client try the movement while you give technique corrections before beginning the actual test. Additionally, you should always motivate your clients during the assessment and encourage them to do their best by giving positive feedback after each trial.

Equipment Used

The equipment used to conduct your assessments may affect your client's test scores. Therefore, be sure that all testing equipment is in proper working condition, and calibrated if necessary, before performing your assessments. This preparation will ensure client safety and accurate measurement of intensity, speed, distance, strength, and so on. You should also make certain that the equipment fits your client's body dimensions to avoid inaccuracies, potential injury, or client embarrassment.

Personal Training Specialist Skill

As a Personal Training Specialist, you need to use your observation skills, technique mastery, and familiarity with testing protocols to produce accurate test results. Be aware of the correct form and technique for each movement and be sure to standardize starting and ending positions in accordance with a standardized or personal-trainer-designed protocol.

Environmental Factors

Factors like room temperature, humidity, and the presence of other people may affect your client's test scores. Ideally, the room temperature should be 21° to 23° Celsius to maximize client comfort. You should aim for a clean facility that is not overcrowded so that you can limit potential discomfort or distractions for your client during the assessments.

Summary of Main Points

1. The decision to perform a dynamic fitness assessment should be made by the client and the Personal Training Specialist based on the client's individual needs, fitness level, and goals for the personal training program.

2. All fitness assessments should be performed by a Personal Training Specialist or qualified health professional to ensure that the information is valid, reliable, and reproducible.

3. A dynamic postural assessment is an evaluation of mobility and stability.

4. Cardiorespiratory fitness can be measured by assessing heart rate response as the client performs an exercise that gradually becomes more difficult.

5. Using muscular endurance and resistance assessment, a Personal Training Specialist can develop an effective resistance training program.

6. An assessment of flexibility for all joints helps the Personal Training Specialist identify areas of weakness for each client.

Key Concepts for Study

Protocols

Submaximal test

Standardization

Nonnormative strength test

Review Questions

1. Why is the overhead squat test one key dynamic assessment that the Personal Training Specialist should have a client perform?

2. What is canfitpro's recommended order of assessments?

3. To create an accurate picture of three-dimensional mobility and stability, the Personal Training Specialist observes
   a. strength, endurance, and mobility
   b. mobility, posture, and stability in all planes of movement
   c. head-to-toe sagittal plane biomechanics
   d. none of the above

4. Postural assessments are useful for
   a. isolating significant injuries
   b. motivating the client
   c. establishing a baseline
   d. all of the above

5. In a submaximal graded exercise assessment, the client performs the exercise at increasing intensity without exceeding _____ percent of age-predicted HRmax.
   a. 65
   b. 75
   c. 85
   d. 95

6. To reduce the likelihood of client factor errors during assessment testing, the Personal Training Specialist should
   a. have the client perform the movement one time without any practice
   b. give positive feedback after each trial
   c. ensure that the room temperature is between 24 °C and 25 °C to maximize client comfort
   d. allow the client to practice the movement before doing the test but refrain from giving any technique cues

7. The seated spinal rotation test gives the Personal Training Specialist information regarding a client's
   a. mobility of extremities around stability of posture
   b. forward trunk flexion
   c. mobility and symmetry in the transverse plane
   d. extension and rotation in the sagittal plane

Web Resource Contents

Video clips showing the seated spinal rotation test, straight leg raise test, overhead squat test, push-up test, and sit-and-reach test

Fitness and postural assessment form

Answers to review questions

PART III Case Study Questions

Refer to the following assessment results (as well as previous information about each client) when responding to questions 1 through 4.

	Catherine	Lisa	Thomas
Resting heart rate (RHR)	81 BPM	71 BPM	80 BPM
Resting blood pressure	134/87 mmHg	115/78 mmHg	122/80 mmHg
Height	175 cm (5 ft 8 in.)	167.5 cm (5 ft 6 in.)	155 cm (5 ft 1 in.)
Weight	89 kg (196 lb)	79.5kg (175 lb)	55.5 kg (122 lb)
$\dot{V}O_2$max	28 ml/kg/min	39 ml/kg/min	38 ml/kg/min
Body fat %	33.7%	26.2%	21.6%
Push-ups	9	13	15
Curl-ups	10	16	13
Grip strength	R: 26 kg, L: 25 kg	R: 27 kg, L: 26 kg	R: 37 kg, L: 39 kg
Trunk forward flexion (sit-and-reach test)	17 cm	23 cm	32 cm
Straight-leg raise	Score = 1	Score = 2	Score = 3
Seated spinal rotation	Score = 2	Score = 1	Score = 2
Overhead squat	Score = 0	Score = 1	Score = 2

1. Using the information provided, which of the primary components of fitness are of greatest concern for
   a. Catherine?
   b. Lisa?
   c. Thomas?
2. Thomas views himself as a reasonably active person with a fairly high fitness level. Given his assessment results, how would you explain his actual current fitness level?
3. Catherine finds it difficult to maintain proper form while completing level 1 of the overhead squat assessment. What could this result indicate regarding Catherine's mobility and stability?
4. During Lisa's dynamic postural assessment, you notice that she has to bend her knees slightly to complete the straight-leg raise. Considering this observation, answer these questions:
   a. Which myofascial chains seem to be showing restrictions?
   b. How could you address these restrictions within Lisa's flexibility-training program?

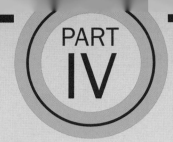

Program Design and Delivery

When designing a personal training program, you integrate all the knowledge and experience you have acquired to create the roadmap necessary for your client to succeed. From the concepts of program design to actual delivery of these programs, this part of the manual provides you with the framework used by canfitpro Personal Training Specialists to create safe, efficient, effective, and enjoyable programming that helps clients achieve their fitness goals.

Program Design Concepts

Rod Macdonald, BEd
Brad Schoenfeld, PhD

LEARNING OUTCOMES

After completing this chapter, you will be able to

1. identify the four elements of good program design;

2. understand the common principles of training;

3. determine best practices for exercise training and environmental considerations;

4. understand periodization and its application to program design; and

5. discuss program design terms and components.

All clients have a vision for what they want to achieve, and your responsibility as their Personal Training Specialist is to create a plan to get them there. Although the answer to the question "What is a program?" might seem obvious, many uneducated, unprofessional Personal Training Specialists do not grasp what a program actually is. Imagine trying to build a home without a blueprint. A program is the must-have blueprint that you will create to build your client's dream home (their goal). That imagery may help you begin to understand the importance of having a well-planned program for your client's goal. Program design, like home building, includes foundational elements. Without these foundational elements, the program you create may be weak and prone to discouraging or injuring the client.

Principles of Program Design

Based on what you have learned in previous chapters, you can see how the topics of cardiorespiratory training, resistance training, flexibility training, and foundational movement sequences, along with the information about health and fitness screening and assessments, provide what you will need to create a sound program. In addition to these topics, the concepts in this chapter are essential for you to understand in designing a program.

The programs you design for your clients are critical to their success. In every program, you will combine a diverse array of elements that utilize your theoretical knowledge, your experiences with other clients, and a little experimentation based on sound research and proven principles of training.

The best personal training programs have four elements in common: They are safe, effective, efficient, and enjoyable. Creating a quality program is both an art and a science, and all four elements are required before optimal results can be obtained. As with the legs of a table, if one element is missing or not strong enough, the client may become disillusioned or injured, and the personal trainer–client relationship can collapse (see figure 11.1).

Besides being safe, enjoyable, and efficient, your programs must be effective in delivering results. But success depends on numerous factors that occur before, during, and even after you design the program. A Personal Training Specialist may spend hours creating a program tailored to the needs of a specific client. A well-designed program will not only help your client achieve his or her goals safely but also be a resource that you can refer back to, assessing what exercises and approaches to training worked and are likely to produce results for the same and subsequent clients.

The following are common program design terms that you will see in this chapter and that will help

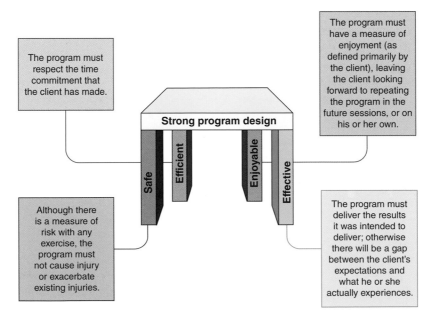

FIGURE 11.1   A strong program design should resemble a sturdy table.

you describe program components when working with your clients.

- **Repetitions (reps)**—A repetition is a single complete movement or exercise. For example, one rep of a pull-up consists of the concentric (muscle-shortening) motion during the upward pull phase and the eccentric (muscle-lengthening) motion during the lowering phase.

- **Sets**—A set is a combination of reps without rest. For example, 12 pull-ups performed consecutively would be one set of 12.

- **Load**—Load is the amount of resistance used for a given exercise. Keep in mind that the resistance provided by a dumbbell versus a machine versus tubing may vary significantly even if they are supposed to be the same. Always have the client attempt a new exercise variation with a lower load and then progress to the targeted load.

- **Tempo**—Tempo is the speed at which the exercise is performed. Tempo is usually described by two to four numbers, counted in seconds, for each rep. For example, a 4:0:2:0 tempo for the biceps curl would mean a four-second eccentric movement (i.e., extension of the elbow) followed by no pause before a two-second concentric movement (i.e., flexion of the elbow) followed by no pause before proceeding to the next rep. Pauses are sometimes used to hold a position either to eliminate momentum or to increase voluntary contraction of the targeted muscle group. If the tempo is indicated with only two numbers (e.g., 4:2), then the pauses are not indicated and the numbers shown are for the eccentric and concentric components of the rep, respectively.

- **Rest**—Rest is the time between sets or exercises. The amount of rest dictates how much recovery the energy systems receive, potentially changing the focus of the exercises and the ability to perform them with proper technique. For resistance training, a beginner needs a minimum of 30 to 60 seconds between sets of the same exercise to continue, but a period of one to two minutes is more likely to allow complete recovery for subsequent sets. To be more efficient, you may choose to use the rest time either to perform an exercise for a different muscle group or to stretch an area that is particularly in need of mobilization (as long as it is not the same muscle group that will be worked in any resistance exercises to follow).

Client Safety

As a result of the abundance of information available, a sometimes-dangerous shift has occurred in how some Personal Training Specialists work with their clients. Without some kind of philosophical approach to designing programs, Personal Training Specialists are prone to creating workouts on the fly, occasionally without much consideration of the volume, intensity, or difficulty involved. They may have been exposed to an interesting exercise or technique and want to use it with a client, or they may have become lazy and complacent over time. This casual approach is strongly discouraged because it is unprofessional and may be dangerous. A better approach is to train your clients to adopt a mastery approach.

Mastery

Regardless of how much planning goes into any program, some areas will inevitably need adjustment as the program is delivered for the first time, not to mention the longer-term adjustments needed as the client progresses. To support consistent and ongoing improvement, the best Personal Training Specialists embrace the concept of mastery.

Mastery is a learning methodology conceived by Benjamin Bloom in the late 1960s. His theory was that anyone could learn and subsequently master a task or subject if given the opportunity to do so at an appropriate pace. The great advantage of one-on-one personal training is that you have the ability to encourage mastery in your clients. Comparatively, small-group training or traditional group fitness classes offer limited opportunity for a person to go at her or his own pace if the group is proceeding to the next, possibly more complex element. If the participant does keep to a less complex movement pattern, she or he is likely to feel left out or discouraged. Encouraging mastery during personal training has two results; it will get your clients to their goals safely, and they will feel great about the process and your expert guidance.

The complexity of having to choose from countless combinations of exercises (along with the execution of those exercises) can be simplified if your program design is focused on developing mastery. Consider if you will, what a client really wants. Your client is not waking up in the morning thinking, "I really hope Joe makes a program for me that is extremely complicated and discouraging." What your client probably wakes up in the morning thinking (consciously or subconsciously) is, "I really hope Joe makes a program for me that gets me the results I want and helps me feel great." Unfortunately, some Personal Training Specialists inadvertently revert to programming excessively complex exercise sequences and miss the value and results of a simple program design that ensures success through mastery. As a Personal Training Specialist, you can use programs that are individualized and focused on mastery to help your clients achieve their desired results in a safe and enjoyable way.

Overprogramming may occur when a Personal Training Specialist plans a program that has too much volume (a large number of exercises), too much intensity (excessive heart rate or speed or too little rest), or too much technical complexity (exercises that are more complex than the client can perform safely or effectively). What you really need to achieve in any given program is progressive overload of the systems you are targeting. For example, having the client work toward mastering 3 exercises in one workout is more likely to be successful than having the client try to master 15 exercises in the same workout. Keep in mind that all clients will learn at a unique pace as they master the exercises given.

Focusing a client's workout on mastering foundational movements, breathing, posture, and body control gives the person a foundation on which to master more complex exercises. For example, the client should master shoulder shrugs, shoulder presses, stiff-legged deadlifts, and squats over several workouts before attempting a clean and press exercise. Unfortunately, many Personal Training Specialists go directly to the more complex exercise before having the client master the comparatively simpler components. In contrast, incorporating the concept of mastery provides a foundation on which Personal Training Specialists can design a successful program that either breaks all the elements down or brings them all together, which is the concept of segmentation and integration.

Segmentation and Integration

When creating programs for your clients, you will have to consider whether they would be better served by a segmented or integrated training approach. **Segmentation** refers to keeping the components of cardio, resistance, and flexibility separated from each other for the most part. This approach has been conventionally taught to Personal Training Specialists and is still the most popular way to structure a training program. An approach that blends the cardio, resistance, and flexibility of a program together, without a clear distinction between components is known as **integration**. Although a segmented approach makes up the majority of canfitpro's Personal Training Specialist certification, integrated training is often used with small or large groups of clients and in many group fitness classes.

In some ways, the ideal program for your client will be a progressive blend of both approaches to program design. Segmented programs are likely to be safer initially, and eventually providing increased integration will improve functional transfer and benefit most clients. In any case, you need to remember the importance of individualization and be sure that you are designing and modifying the program for one specific client.

After you understand and implement the concept of segmentation and integration, you have to plan your program in the context of a longer time frame, be it a month, year, or even longer. This concept is known as periodization.

Environmental Considerations

When designing the program, you need to be mindful of the environment in which the program will be performed. These considerations include physical obstacles or challenges that you may need to inform your client of (e.g., slippery floors, confined spaces, and so on) as well as climate-based challenges such as heat, humidity, or cold. For example, if the program will be performed in a hot, humid environment, you may need to schedule more breaks, lower the intensity, and encourage the client to hydrate. Conversely, if the program will be performed in a colder environment, the warm-up may need to be extended and the workout may need fewer breaks to prevent the client's body from becoming chilled. If it is not readily apparent, ask the client where he or she will be working out so that you can make any necessary modifications to avoid putting your client at greater risk of injury or discomfort.

Advantages and Disadvantages of Segmented Versus Integrated Programs

	Segmented programs	Integrated programs
Example	Warm-up followed by resistance training exercises followed by cardio exercise followed by flexibility exercises	Boot-camp-style instruction in which the client does complex movements like burpees, crawling, sprints, and so on
Advantages	May be easier to design the program May be easier to explain and demonstrate the program May be safer in general May be easier to track progress May be better for previously sedentary clients	May save time May be better for advanced clients May provide functional benefits
Disadvantages	May not provide as much functional transfer of fitness May take more time to complete all components	May be less safe because movements are more complex May sacrifice technique in favour of speed or repetitions May be more difficult to track progress May be difficult to know which part of which movements contribute most to which component of fitness

Periodization

Periodization is the systematic organization of training periods (typically measured in time) to facilitate the most efficient path from goal setting to goal attainment. Periodization allows the Personal Training Specialist to create a safe, easy-to-understand program that achieves short-term goals in the context of the client's longer-term goals. The ability to demonstrate to clients that you have a long-term plan for them will increase their confidence in you as well as ensure an enduring personal trainer–client relationship.

The genesis of periodization can be traced to the general adaptation syndrome theory of stress, which was first described by Hungarian scientist Hans Selye (1950). Selye proposed that the body undergoes a triphasic response when subjected to stress. He called the first phase the alarm stage. In this phase, the body perceives stress and reacts by initiating the fight-or-flight response carried out by the sympathetic nervous system. The second phase is called the resistance stage. In this phase the body ideally adapts by **supercompensation** so that the stressor can be dealt with more easily in the future.

The last phase, called the exhaustion stage, occurs when the stressor becomes too great for the body to handle. If this occurs, the body's resources become depleted, resulting in inability to maintain normal physiological function.

Your client's body may go through three stages in response to the demands of training exercises. In the alarm stage, the body primarily responds with the sympathetic system and experiences a short increase in energy to help meet the immediate demands. The resistance stage occurs when the body undergoes appropriate adaptations that will help the client better handle the demands of subsequent workouts. If your client is overtraining or challenged to the point of reaching the third stage (exhaustion), the body may lose optimal physiological function, causing a delay in the client's progress.

Physical activity is a stressor. When a client stimulates the body through exercise performance, the body will undergo a reaction of some kind. If the stimulus is not sufficient, no noticeable change will occur. If the stimulus is sufficient in intensity and duration, the body will not only compensate but supercompensate (Bompa, 2009), even from a single training session (see figure 11.2). In a single bout of exercise the client will have a lower level of performance at the end of the session than at the beginning, because of fatigue. But with supercompensation the body will not only return to the previous level of performance but experience an increase in performance when given the opportunity to recover.

In the case of multiple, successive training sessions, several scenarios may unfold. If the training stimulus is insufficient or too much recovery occurs between training sessions, little if any improvement may result (figure 11.3). If the stimulus is excessive or insufficient recovery occurs between training sessions, the client is likely to see a decrease in performance because of overtraining (figure 11.4). If the stimulus is just right, the client will see successive improvements in performance in response to appropriate use of progressive overload (figure 11.5). The goal of a periodized routine, therefore, should be to push the client toward the outer boundaries of the resistance stage without entering the exhaustion stage. As a client progresses from having rarely exercised to exercising on a regular basis, the potential to improve diminishes slightly. Consider, for example, Olympic athletes. Because they have taken their performance to a high level,

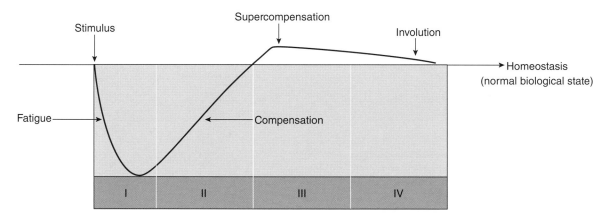

FIGURE 11.2 Supercompensation cycle of a training session.

Reprinted, by permission, from T.O. Bompa, 2009, *Periodization*, 5th ed. (Champaign, IL: Human Kinetics), 16. Adapted from N. Yakovlev, 1967, *Sports biochemistry* (Leipzig: Deutche Hochschule fur Korpekultur).

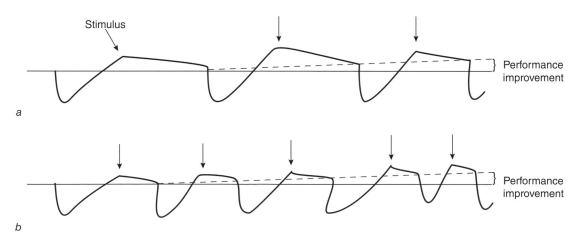

FIGURE 11.3 The sum of training effect. When *(a)* too much recovery occurs between bouts of exercise or *(b)* insufficient stimulus is used during training, the client will see minimal improvement.

Reprinted, by permission, from T.O. Bompa, 2009, *Periodization,* 5th ed. (Champaign, IL: Human Kinetics), 19. Adapted from D. Harre (ed.), 1982, *Trainingslehre* (Berlin: Sportverlag).

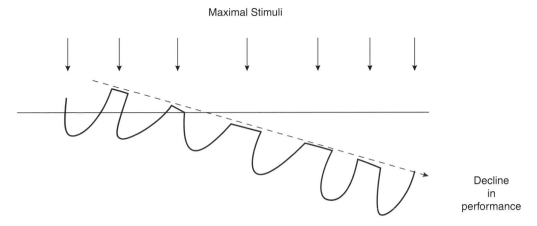

FIGURE 11.4 Decline in performance from prolonged maximal-intensity stimuli.

Reprinted, by permission, from T.O. Bompa, 2009, *Periodization*, 5th ed. (Champaign, IL: Human Kinetics), 19.

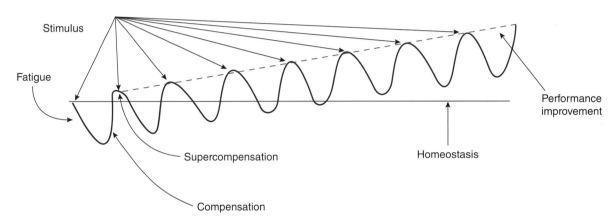

FIGURE 11.5 Successive improvements in performance.

they struggle to see even small improvements. In contrast, new exercisers may see staggering levels of improvement, sometimes increasing their strength or endurance 10 times or more compared with their capability when they began training. Although no one can maintain that pace of improvement indefinitely, a well-designed program can maximize the opportunity to improve.

The **sum of training effect** allows us to evaluate the overall outcome of a training program, based on the choice of stimulus, quality of recovery, and the subsequent gains or losses in fitness and performance. A real-life example of the *sum of training effects* can be seen in postal carriers. They are accustomed to walking many kilometres per week, up and down stairs and in sometimes challenging conditions. We might think that postal carriers

are extremely fit, but because the stimulus never changes significantly, they do not experience the effect of progressive overload over time. Initially, the sum effect of their training likely causes an increase in fitness because of the additional physical stimulus of their work. But after their bodies become accustomed to their routes, their fitness level quickly plateaus without further adaptation. An example of a possible decline in performance (i.e., a negative sum) would occur if you were to take a deconditioned person along a postal carrier's route. You would find that within one to two days, the deconditioned person would reach the exhaustion stage and be tired, sore, and possibly even injured because the stimulus was too great, in part because recovery between bouts of exercise was insufficient.

canfitpro Model of Periodization

Although multiple models of periodization are in use, canfitpro uses one that is adapted from the work of Tudor Bompa and is streamlined to apply specifically to fitness training. Like most methods of periodization, the canfitpro model is built from the following components:

- **Macrocycle**—This is the largest component of a periodized program, usually consisting of several months to several years (e.g., an Olympic athlete's four-year program).
- **Mesocycle**—This is the intermediate component of a periodized program, usually consisting of one to several months.
- **Microcycle**—This is the smallest component of a periodized program, usually consisting of one to several weeks. A microcycle is not usually shorter than one to two weeks because reliably measuring progress in such a short period is difficult.

The purpose of using periodization rather than a more instinctive or haphazard organization of training is that periodization both ensures confidence in the expected outcome and provides a record to look back at after a certain length of time (to examine what worked and what did not). Moreover, a properly designed periodized routine will help ensure that the client continues to make progress without becoming overtrained, thereby keeping the client safe and consistent in training. Periodization does not imply the creation of a rigid program that cannot be altered. On the contrary, a Personal Training Specialist using a periodized program is always able to substitute alternative exercises or methods of training based on the client's progress. Like a GPS navigation system used on a road trip, periodization provides a starting point and an expected route to the goal, but it can be altered to provide detours should unforeseen conditions arise.

Traditional periodization is based on preparing for sport using multiple modes of training to improve technical skill, psychological stamina, and tactical training, as well as fitness. The canfitpro model focuses almost exclusively on fitness as developed through cardiorespiratory, resistance, and flexibility training. Training for fitness is the domain of Personal Training Specialists, whereas teaching the skills and abilities related to specific sports are best left to qualified coaches of those sports. In other words, because most personal training clients are either training for fitness or using fitness to achieve other goals (e.g., weight management, health improvement, and so on), fitness is the focus of Personal Training Specialist's use of periodization. Although the fitness gained through personal training would undoubtedly improve the client's athletic capacity in a variety of sports, the sport itself is deemphasized and the technique of the fitness training is emphasized. When working with a client who also participates in competitive sport, the Personal Training Specialist is advised to collaborate with the client's coach, if she or he has one, to identify blocks of time when the client will be focusing more on the sport. If working with the coach is not an option, then you can work with the client to block off time when she or he may be competing or recovering from the sport. This approach allows you to balance the client's overall training and avoid overtraining. Figure 11.6 demonstrates an overview of an annual periodized program showing both intensity and volume of training.

Figure 11.6 demonstrates how a client's program might be spread out over 12 months (macrocycle) with progressive increases of training (combined intensity and volume). Each four-month period (mesocycles A, B, and C) in the client's program would focus on specific goals that build toward the larger goal. Within the mesocycles are month-long microcycles (microcycles 1 through 12) that include challenges that are more specific. The fifth and ninth microcycles are slightly lower in training load to permit recovery from the previously higher levels. These restorative periods, called unloading cycles, are essential components of a periodized routine. One of the biggest mistakes a Personal Training Specialist can make is continually pushing clients to the limits of their abilities without providing necessary recovery. Such an approach will ultimately result in an overtrained state, in which a client may experience impaired performance, delayed progress, or potential injury. Continued progress can be achieved only by including structured unloading cycles at strategic points throughout the mesocycle.

Application of Periodization to Program Design

To apply periodization to program design, stress must be balanced with recovery. This balance is based on the client's fitness, nutrition, and commit-

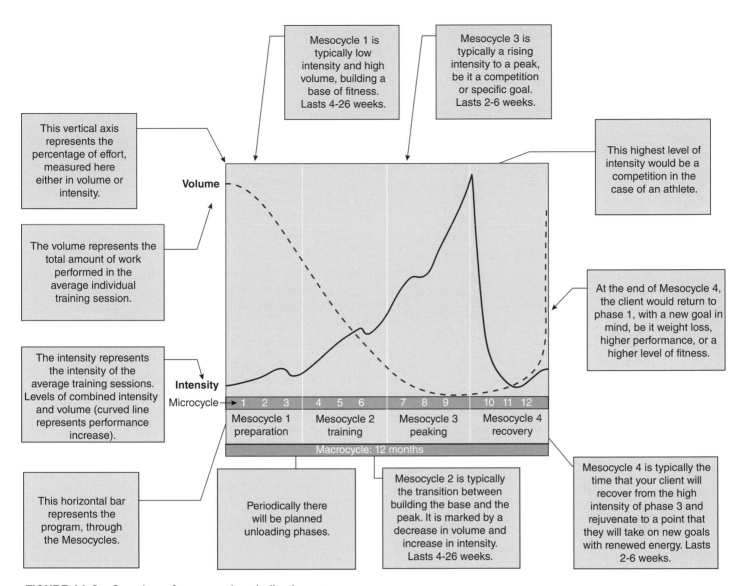

FIGURE 11.6 Overview of an annual periodized program.

ment to recovery (e.g., going downhill skiing after a substantial leg workout is not a commitment to recovery). In addition, erring on the side of allowing too much recovery is better than allowing too little. Balancing stress and recovery becomes more challenging when the client is working out more often than every other day. For example, if the client works with you on Mondays, Wednesdays, and Fridays but also runs on Tuesdays, Thursdays, Saturdays, and Sundays (which should have been revealed in the client's exercise history or in your ongoing communication), the heavy workload could have dramatic implications for how you structure the program.

Always ask about your client's physical activity outside your scheduled training sessions so that you can properly adjust the training program and prevent overtraining. For example, if your client plays soccer twice per week, you may adjust your cardiorespiratory programming to take into account this current activity.

Although not an absolute necessity, at least one full day should be set aside each week for either passive recovery (no exercise) or active recovery (low-impact, low-intensity exercise of relatively short duration). In addition, clients generally should be cautious of performing two maximally hard workouts on back-to-back days, especially for the same exercise, activity, or muscle group. If the time between exercise sessions is less than 24 hours, you should have your client perform a hard workout followed by a less intense workout the next time to allow adequate recovery. Note, however, that training experience, abilities, and other factors will ultimately influence how the client recovers from intense training sessions. Thus, program design must be tailored to the client's individual response.

Periodization of exercise variables can permit the combination of multiple modes of training within a week while reducing the likelihood of reaching an overtrained state. Without periodization, the combination of stresses might be too much and result in a chronic injury. Clearly, the program overall must be balanced, taking into account aspects of the client's training both within and outside the gym environment.

Figure 11.7 shows a detailed example of the use of periodization, designed for a client who has set a goal to increase endurance for a specific event or competition. Because the client's goal event occurs in the month of October, intensity increases as that time approaches. The client does not train only at high intensity, but the focus of the training is primarily high intensity. The client also performs an appropriate amount of low-intensity sessions as active recovery and as maintenance of the aerobic energy system. Each month has been broken into two- to three-week microcycles until September, when the next 8 to 10 weeks are broken into one-week microcycles. These shorter microcycles permit small adjustments to the program to accommodate adaptations required for the specific event or competition.

canfitpro's Principles of Training

When designing a client's program, canfitpro's training principles should be considered the foundational elements of periodization. Whether applied to resistance, cardiorespiratory, or flexibility training, both the Personal Training Specialist and the client must understand these principles (for complete descriptions of the principles, refer to chapter 2).

canfitpro's Training Principles (Revisited)

- **FITT**—When designing a personal training program, the frequency, intensity, time, and type of exercise must be considered.

- **Individualization**—Programs and modifications to programs must be made to accommodate every person's individual needs.
- **Specificity**—If clients want to improve an aspect of their performance, they have to train that aspect.
- **Progressive overload**—To improve, clients must continually challenge their fitness.
- **Recovery**—Recovery should not be seen as optional, but as a mandatory principle of training for every program. This principle becomes increasingly important as the clients' workouts become more stressful.
- **Structural tolerance**—The strengthening of tissues in and around joints (tendons, ligaments, and so on) will result in the ability to sustain subsequently greater stresses in training and to be more resistant to injury.
- **All-around development**—People who are well developed through all components of fitness are less likely to sustain injury and more likely to perform better in sport and in life.
- **Reversibility**—When training ceases, the body gradually returns to a pre-training state (i.e., "Use it or lose it").
- **Maintenance**—When a level of fitness has been achieved, it can be maintained with less work than was needed to attain it.

Selecting the Right Exercises

You can draw from an infinite number of possibilities in selecting the right exercises for your client to perform. As a new Personal Training Specialist, you may find this task intimidating, but you can take a few simple steps to find the most appropriate exercises for your client. For each exercise you might consider including in a client's program, ask the following questions:

- What muscle group are you targeting?
- What exercises can be performed where the client will be working out?
- Is the level of risk acceptable for each exercise?
- What potential challenges may I face in teaching this exercise?

Periodization for endurance training

Month	December	January	February	March	April	May	June	July	August	September	October	November
Competition												
Phase	Mesocycle A preparation		Mesocycle B training (transition from phase 1)			Mesocycle C training (transition into peaking phase)				Mesocycle D peaking		Mesocycle E recovery
Emphasis	General development		Specific development		Transition	Technical/Specific development		Transition		Performance/ Competitive development and maintenance		Maintenance/ Recovery
Cardio-respiratory system	Endurance		Endurance/ Power	Power				Power/ Endurance		Technical endurance		Maintenance/ Recovery
Muscular system	General strength		General endurance			Specific endurance				Maintenance		Maintenance/ Recovery
Flexibility and mobility	General development					Specific development				Maintenance		Maintenance/ Recovery
Technique			Simulation			General development				Specific development		Maintenance/ Recovery

a

☐ Indicates competition

Graph of intensity and volume of training by month

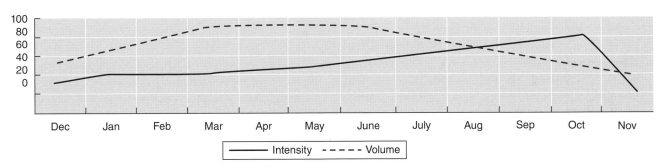

b

FIGURE 11.7   Detailed example of the use of periodization for a client training toward a specific endurance goal: *(a)* sample periodization program outline and *(b)* intensity versus volume.

Table 11.1 applies these four questions and provides strategies for exercise selection, using an exercise for the chest as an example. As you gain experience, exercise selection will become more instinctive and less formulaic.

Open Versus Closed Kinetic Chain Exercises

As discussed in chapter 8, "Foundational Movement Sequences," an ongoing debate exists as to whether the focus of a resistance training program should be on open kinetic chain exercises (OKCE) or closed kinetic chain exercises (CKCE). In an OKCE the foot or hand is free to move in space, such as in performing a seated leg extension or a lat pull-down or kicking a ball. In a CKCE, the foot or hand is typically fixed and cannot move throughout the exercise, such as in performing a barbell squat or a chin-up or getting out of a chair. Research has shown that CKCEs produce less stress on the joints because they typically use more muscle and are therefore more stabilizing to the joints. Real life, however, is a combination of open and closed kinetic chain movements. canfitpro's position is that including a combination of OKCEs and CKCEs is the best approach for most programs.

TABLE 11.1   Filtering Process for a New Personal Training Specialist (Chest Exercises)

Filtering question	Potential challenge	Possible solution
What muscle group are you targeting?	In this case you know that the client needs to strengthen the chest muscles, but you have to choose from thousands of chest exercises.	Select three to five exercises that you are confident teaching and that are effective.
What exercises can be performed where the client will be working out (equipment choice)?	If the client will be working out in a home gym, a program that includes a weight-machine chest press is not likely to be feasible.	Select three to five exercises, including both equipment-dependent and non-equipment-dependent exercises.
Is the level of risk acceptable for each exercise?	Some have higher risk (i.e., dumbbell chest press), and some have lower risk (i.e., machine chest press).	Rank the exercises by risk and required skill and match the exercise to the client's skill level.
What potential challenges may I face in teaching this exercise?	The client may ask a question about the exercise or muscle group worked.	Prepare for potential questions and instruct only those exercises that you can demonstrate with perfect technique.

Choosing the Right Equipment

When deciding what type of equipment to use within a program, you have many factors to consider, such as where the exercises are performed (e.g., at home or in a gym), whether anyone else will be using the equipment (it might be unavailable at times), and above all how feasible it is for the client, given his or her skill and confidence, to perform the exercise correctly.

 Always prioritize the safety or your client when selecting any exercise or equipment for the program.

Tables 11.2 through 11.4 demonstrate equipment options for resistance, cardiorespiratory, and flexibility training and their advantages and disadvantages.

Structuring a Workout

As a Personal Training Specialist, you will combine the program design elements discussed in this chapter to create a well-structured program for each client. In putting together these programs, you must ensure that each workout component (from warm-up to cool-down) is carefully planned and performed in the optimal sequence for client safety and success.

Warm-Up

All programs must include a warm-up to make sure the body and mind are ready for the workout. Without a warm-up, clients may have a less effective workout because of lack of diverted blood flow and lack of attention to the tasks at hand. A proper warm-up includes both general and specific components. A general warm-up serves to elevate core temperature and increase blood flow to target tissues. The focus of a general warm-up should be to perform light cardiorespiratory exercise that will result in breaking a light sweat. This goal can usually be accomplished with five or more minutes of aerobic activity at approximately 40 to 60% of maximal heart rate (3 to 4 on the 0 to 10 RPE scale). The warm-up should not result in undue fatigue because it will have a negative effect on subsequent exercise performance.

Virtually any modality involving large-muscle groups is acceptable, such as walking, running, cycling, and elliptical training. If clients will perform upper-body exercise in the session, doing exercise involving the arms such as jumping jacks, rowing, or active arms while jogging or on an elliptical machine can be beneficial. An additional benefit of a general warm-up is to allow clients to shift from their nontraining time into their training time. This transition will allow them to reduce stress, increase their focus on the workout ahead, and provide time

TABLE 11.2 Resistance Training Options

Resistance training options	Advantages	Disadvantages	Client skill level required
Body weight	• No cost • Can be performed anywhere; very functional	• Can be difficult for deconditioned or overweight clients	Moderate to high
Free weights (dumbbells, barbells, kettlebells)	• Simulate real-world resistance • Relatively low cost • Versatile application	• Sometimes hard to control • Require specific training for correct technique	Moderate to high
Weight or pulley machines	• Guide the client through a pattern of movement • Often include photos or images to help the client remember technique • Deconditioned or weak clients do not have to change heavy free weights because changes are usually made with a pin	• Standard machine size may not be optimal for shorter or taller clients • Can be complicated to set up and use • Each machine is usually practical for only one or two exercises • Require more space	Low to moderate
Cable-based machines	• Provide the client with some freedom of movement • Cables, unlike free weights, allow the resistance to stay constant throughout the range of motion • Some cable equipment is adjustable for the height of the client • One cable station can be used for multiple exercises	• Can be expensive and may require multiple attachments for additional diversity of movements	Moderate to high
Plate-loaded, leverage-based machines	• Less expensive than typical machines (uses manually loaded Olympic plates for resistance)	• Require more space than conventional machines because of swinging motion • Personal Training Specialist or client must lift and load each individual plate	Low to moderate
Pneumatic machines	• Allow the user to change the resistance with switches or foot pedals at any time • Permit explosive movement without momentum	• Do not accurately imitate real-world resistance • Very expensive • Require pneumatic compressor	Low to moderate
Elastic resistance	• Portable • Inexpensive • Can be used for virtually any exercise • Range of tubing resistance options permits use with all fitness levels	• Resistance increases through the range of motion • Can encourage eccentric part of the movement to be too fast	Low to high
Water resistance	• Creates resistance in all directions • Resistance accommodates force applied	• Requires pool • Not appropriate for everyone • More time consuming	Low to high
Air resistance (air compression)	• Resistance accommodates force applied • Buttons allow change in resistance, independent of speed	• Limited amount of equipment currently available • Costly	Low to moderate

TABLE 11.3 Cardiorespiratory Training Options

Cardiorespiratory training options	Advantages	Disadvantages	Client skill level required
Stationary bicycle (upright)	• Usually easy to learn • Can be a less expensive option for home equipment • Allows a variety of body positions, simulating the movements used in road cycling • Low impact	• Clients may find it boring • Minimal movement of upper body	Low
Stationary bicycle (recumbent)	• Usually easy to learn • Can be a less expensive option for home equipment • Recumbent bikes offer support to the lower back • Low impact	• Many clients find it boring • No movement of upper body	Low
Stair climber	• Minimal impact • Moderately expensive	• May not be appropriate for those with knee, hip, or ankle injuries	Low to moderate
Treadmill	• Usually easy to learn • Moderate impact	• Can be very expensive	Low to moderate
Rowing ergometer	• Provides nearly full-body workout • Less expensive than most cardiorespiratory equipment • Low impact	• Proper technique can be difficult to learn • Provides less feedback compared with other equipment • May not be appropriate for those with shoulder injuries	Moderate to high
Elliptical machine	• Low impact • Easy to learn	• Stride length is normally fixed and may not be correct for some tall or short clients • Not all units have upper-body option	Low to moderate
Cross-country ski machine	• Provides almost full-body workout • Low impact	• Can be difficult to learn technique • May not be appropriate for those with shoulder injuries	Moderate to high
Upper and lower climber	• Provides almost full-body workout • Low impact	• Many clients find it difficult and boring • May not be appropriate for those with shoulder injuries	Moderate
Upper-body ergometer	• Works the often-underused upper body • Offers an alternative to those without the use of their legs • Low impact	• Most clients do not have the upper-body endurance to get a good workout • May be difficult to learn proper technique • May not be appropriate for those with shoulder injuries	Moderate
Nonequipment cardio (walking; running; calisthenic movements such as burpees, jumping jacks, and so on)	• No cost • Can be performed anywhere; highly functional	• Advanced movements can be difficult, discouraging, and dangerous for deconditioned or overweight clients	Low to high

TABLE 11.4   Flexibility Training Options

Flexibility training options	Example	Advantages	Disadvantages	Client skill level required
Use of minimal equipment	Mat or floor exercises	• Portable • Inexpensive • Can be used for virtually any position	• Requires clients to get on the ground • Possible sanitation concerns	Low to high
Equipment based (machines designed for stretching)	Stretch trainer or stretch cage	• Does not necessitate getting on the ground • Gives diagrams for stretches to be performed	• Expensive • Does not work for all muscle groups	Moderate to high

for you as the Personal Training Specialist to check on their physical and mental readiness. The general warm-up should last five minutes or longer (approximately 10% of the total workout time).

The specific component of the warm-up is performed after the general warm-up. It is designed to enhance neuromuscular efficiency in performing a given exercise, especially if that exercise is resistance training in which adherence to technique and neuromuscular coordination is required for injury avoidance. By using exercises related to the activities in the workout, the neuromuscular system gets to rehearse the movement before it is performed at higher intensity. Exercise selection for the specific warm-up should therefore be as similar as possible to the chosen exercise. For example, performing a light set of the bench press would function as a specific warm-up before performance of heavy bench press sets. The push-up is also an acceptable exercise in this context, although its specificity falls short of the bench press movement itself. Specific warm-

Although you will design a program for the total time available, you can include optional exercises or ways to maximize time if the opportunity presents itself. For example, after clients are comfortable with a program, they could perform the warm-up and cool-down on their own. Going further, if you think that the resistance training component requires the most attention, you can have clients perform the cardiorespiratory training on their own (or vice versa) so that you can increase the time spent on that training component.

ups should be performed at approximately 50% of 1RM for about 10 to 15 repetitions. Again, fatigue should not be induced during warm-up activities; the goal is simply to enhance performance and safety in subsequent working sets. If the work performed after the warm-up uses body weight (e.g., calisthenic exercise) or is an intense cardio workout, the specific warm-up should include the same or modified movements performed at a progressive pace and range of motion. This approach allows you and the client to identify any concerns with mobility, technique, or injuries that the client forgot to mention. A dynamic mobility series can also be used to ease the client into the full ROM before beginning the more complex movements of the workout.

Resistance Versus Cardiorespiratory Training After the Warm-Up

The choice to include cardiorespiratory or resistance training after the warm-up depends on several things. From a time perspective, moving from the warm-up right into cardiorespiratory training is more efficient because the client is already likely to be on a piece of cardiorespiratory equipment. If you continue with resistance training after the warm-up, the client may have to do another warm-up before starting cardiorespiratory training later in the workout. But if the client's goals include an emphasis on muscular development, the resistance training should follow the warm-up so that the client has the most energy and enthusiasm for this component. Regardless of the workout order you select, any static flexibility training should be completed toward the end of the workout session to maximize its effects in a safe manner.

Flexibility

Flexibility training is usually incorporated into the cool-down (i.e., the point in the workout where the client gradually decreases exercise intensity to transition safely from activity back to rest). The advantage to performing flexibility-related exercises immediately after the cardiorespiratory component is that the client's soft tissues will be warmed up and more pliable; therefore, the muscles, tendons, fascia, and other connective tissue will be more receptive to flexibility training compared with stretching when they are not as warm. If flexibility training follows resistance training, the muscles will be pliable and receptive to flexibility training, although not to the same degree as they would be after cardiorespiratory training. Although static stretching should not be performed immediately before resistance exercises, some Personal Training Specialists choose to include dynamic stretching as part of the general or specific warm-up. This approach is most often used when training athletic people or when specific mobility issues need to be addressed before attempting other components of the workout.

Set Performance

When creating the resistance component of the program, you will have to decide how the client will perform each of the sets you have assigned. Most beginners start with straight sets (when they complete the sets on an even tempo, one at a time), whereas advanced clients may require more challenging ways to perform the sets. Table 11.5 lists a variety of approaches to set performance that can be introduced to clients as they develop their muscular strength and endurance and need greater challenge in various resistance exercises. The decision of

TABLE 11.5   Approaches to Set Performance

Type of set performance	Definition	Rationale	Example
Supersets and giant sets	Two or more sets are combined with little or no rest for the same or different muscle groups.	Supersets maximize efficiency and increase intensity.	Same muscle group: Cable chest crossovers are followed immediately by barbell bench press. Opposing muscle groups: Leg extensions are followed immediately by leg curls.
Drop sets (also known as rack running or strip sets)	The load used for a given exercise is reduced when exhaustion is reached to permit continued exercise.	By reducing the load, stress of muscle fibers can continue beyond the point that was possible at the starting load.	Biceps curls with 10 kg dumbbells, then 8 kg, then 6 kg, and so on.
Pyramid sets	Multiple sets are combined in an ascending or descending (or both) fashion.	By modifying the load and reps completed, both slow- and fast-twitch muscle fibers may be stimulated more completely.	Combination of sets of the following reps: 15, 10, 8, 6, 4, 6, 8, 10, 15.
21s	Superset that stimulates the upper half of the movement, the lower half of the movement, and the full range of the movement.	By splitting the movement, weak spots in the strength curve can be reduced.	Biceps curls using the lower half of the movement for 7 reps, the upper half of the movement for 7 reps, and the whole movement for 7 reps, for 21 reps total in the set.
Staggered sets	A set or exercise is performed between sets for a particular muscle group.	Using this downtime maximizes efficiency and allows more to be accomplished during the session.	Performing a set of abdominal crunches after each of three sets of shoulder presses.

Type of set performance	Definition	Rationale	Example
Circuit training	Sets of resistance, cardio-respiratory, and flexibility training are combined in a circuit with little or no time between sets.	Maximizing use of time allows more volume of training.	Completing one set of each exercise and repeating a full circuit three times: chest press, seated row, 2 min jump rope, biceps curl, triceps extension, crunches, 2 min jump rope, leg extension, leg curl, and 2 min jump rope.
Slow	By increasing time under tension, slow training dramatically increases either the concentric or eccentric (or both) parts of the rep.	Increased time under tension has been shown to be safe (momentum may be almost zero) and effective.	Tempo of 5:0:5:0 or other combination that reduces momentum.
Split training	Muscle groups are split up based on the goals of the client, the number of days she or he can work out, and personal preference.	Allows more total volume or intensity in a single session and increased focus on specific muscle groups.	See examples in table 11.6.

which set performance variations to use with a client should be based on individual training goals and the client's ability to perform the required movements with proper form and technique.

Advanced clients who want to perform resistance training four or more days per week may use split routines. In this approach, workouts focus on particular muscle groups on different days to avoid overtraining. See table 11.6 for examples of split-training schedules.

Adaptability

The final element to consider before you design a program is what kind of experience you want your client to have and what approach you will use to ensure success. Remembering the various aspects of the personal trainer–client relationship discussed in chapter 1, your approach should reflect your personality as well as the style your client will respond to best. For example, some clients enjoy

TABLE 11.6   Common Split-Training Combinations

Split	Sunday	Monday	Tuesday	Wednesday	Thursday	Friday	Saturday
3 days (full body—no split)	—	Whole body	—	Whole body	—	Whole body	—
4 days (split)	—	Chest Shoulders Triceps Core	Legs Back Biceps	—	Chest Shoulders Triceps Core	Legs Back Biceps	—
5 days (split)	—	Chest Shoulders Triceps Core	Legs Back Biceps	—	Chest Back Core	Shoulders Triceps	Legs Biceps Core
6 days (split)	—	Chest Triceps Core	Legs Shoulders	Back Biceps Core	Chest Triceps	Legs Shoulders Core	Back Biceps

being pushed to their maximum throughout the workout in a drill-sergeant style, whereas others prefer a gentler approach that guides them through their workout. Although you want to remain authentic to your personality, you should be adaptable enough to meet the needs of your clients. If you ever think that a Personal Training Specialist with a different approach would better serve a particular person, it may be in your best interest to help that client find a more suitable Personal Training Specialist.

Besides the theoretical knowledge you have acquired in the earlier chapters, the concepts in this chapter provide you with the foundation on which you can build a safe, effective, efficient, and enjoyable program for your clients. In the next chapter you will bring those concepts together as you learn how to design a customized program.

Summary of Main Points

1. Well-constructed personal training programs have four elements in common: They are safe, effective, efficient, and enjoyable.

2. Segmented programs are generally a safer approach to start with, eventually providing increased integration to improve functional transfer.

3. The goal of a periodized routine should be to push your client toward the outer boundaries of the resistance stage without entering the exhaustion stage

4. The general warm-up (40-60% of HRmax) helps prepare the body for the workout by elevating core temperature and increasing blood flow to target tissues.

5. The specific warm-up (10-15 repetitions at 50% of 1RM) is designed to enhance neuromuscular efficiency in performing a given exercise, especially if that exercise is resistance training.

6. You should create your own approach for programming to suit your style and your client's goals.

Key Concepts for Study

Periodization

Supercompensation

Sum of training effect

Progressive overload

Specificity

Review Questions

1. What are four elements of successful program design?

2. Describe the difference between the general and specific components of a client's warm-up.

3. Supercompensation refers to

   a. how the body responds after an effective warm-up

   b. the body's increase in fitness level after recovery

   c. the fatigue phase after a workout

   d. the building phase of the body as it is working out

4. The three components of periodization are

   a. beginner, intermediate, and advanced programming

   b. changes that occur in the workout program after month 1, month 2, and month 3

   c. microcycle, mesocycle, and macrocycle

   d. warm-up, cardiorespiratory training, and resistance training

5. When writing repetition speed as 3:0:2:0, what does the 3 represent according to can-fitpro's preferred tempo notation?

   a. the concentric phase of the exercise

b. the pause after the eccentric phase of the exercise

c. the pause after the concentric phase of the exercise

d. the eccentric phase of the exercise

6. The intensity for the warm-up should be _____ for the client?

   a. 3 to 4 on the 0 to 10 RPE scale and 40 to 60% of maximal heart rate

   b. 4 to 5 on the 0 to 10 RPE scale and 55 to 64% of maximal heart rate

   c. 3 to 4 on the 0 to 10 RPE scale and 45 to 55% of maximal heart rate

   d. 1 to 2 on the 0 to 10 RPE scale and 50 to 60% of maximal heart rate

7. If flexibility training follows immediately after resistance exercises, which of the following statements is true?

a. Muscles will be pliable and receptive to flexibility training but to the same degree as after cardio training.

b. Muscles will be pliable and receptive to flexibility training but to a higher degree than after cardio training.

c. Muscles will not be pliable and receptive to flexibility training.

d. Muscles will be pliable and receptive to flexibility training but not to the same degree as after cardio training.

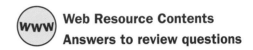

Web Resource Contents
Answers to review questions

Designing a Program

Rod Macdonald, BEd
Brad Schoenfeld, PhD

LEARNING OUTCOMES

After completing this chapter, you will be able to

1. design a customized personal training program;

2. know when to modify or change a program to the specifications of the client;

3. be comfortable with a typical personal training program; and

4. understand the difference between changing the exercise and modifying the performance of an exercise.

Although you can design a program in a variety of ways, until you develop a method that works optimally for you, using a standardized process provides both a path to follow and a way to ensure that you are not missing any information that may be critical to the success of the program. Figure 12.1 provides an overview of the program design steps discussed in this chapter.

How to Design a Program

If you use a systematic approach to designing programs and consider the following steps in your programming, your programs will be safer, more effective, more efficient, and more enjoyable.

Step 1: Information Gathering

Before any client programming begins, it is your responsibility as a Personal Training Specialist to gather information about the client, as discussed in chapters 9, 10, and 11 of this text. The details you should gather include the following:

- Health-screening results (PAR-Q+)
- Health history
- Exercise history
- Client preferences
- Client goals
- Predicted obstacles (time, client skill, and so on)
- Available equipment inventory
- Resources, if needed (exercise resources from books, articles, websites, and so on)
- Passive and dynamic assessment results

Without devoting proper attention to the information in this list, your ability to create an effective and safe program will be severely compromised. For example, if your client finds the stationary bicycle uncomfortable but you disregard that information

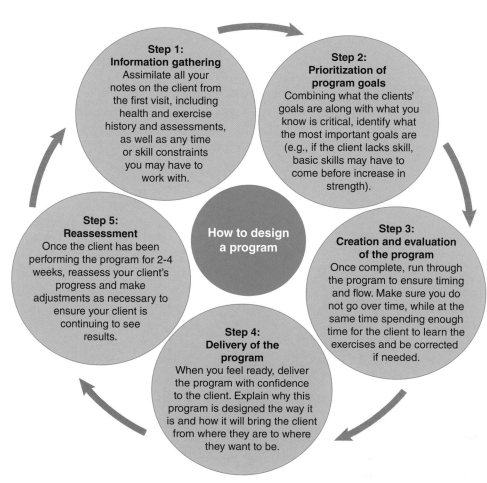

FIGURE 12.1   An overview of program design.

and instruct him or her to use that piece of equipment anyway, you will have a disgruntled and unmotivated client. If you have and respect that information, you can address it in an appropriate manner.

Step 2: Prioritization of Program Goals

Most clients have multiple goals, and you need to help them prioritize those goals. By working with your clients, you can help them better understand the process. In addition, you can recognize the obstacles that may prevent or delay them from achieving their goals. Many clients will have goals that are important to them, but they will be unable to achieve them without establishing certain skills and abilities. For example, if the client would like to lose 10 kg (22 lb) of adipose (fat) tissue but has never before worked out, resistance training with cardiorespiratory training should be combined as a program focus. But without a strong foundation of resistance training skills, the client will not achieve the goal of weight loss as quickly as she or he might otherwise. The program must therefore introduce resistance training and increase the client's skills so that she or he can maximize the results while still working out and doing activities that she or he is skilled at.

Step 3: Creation and Evaluation of the Program

Because the content of the program depends on its duration, you must start by considering how much time the client is willing to dedicate to a scheduled exercise program—how frequently and for how long he or she is able to train. Based on these constraints, you need to allow time for the client to perform the basic components of a program, including some, and potentially all, of the following:

- Warm-up
- Resistance training combined with, or separate from, cardiorespiratory training
- Flexibility training and cool-down
- Breaks between exercises or modes of training
- Unforeseen interruptions (unavailable equipment, client wanting to chat, and so on)

 By planning carefully, you will be able to combine or omit activities based on your client's goals as well as your focus for that portion of the periodized program. If the frequency of workouts is limited, you may choose to spend a longer time on certain activities during each session to enhance their effectiveness. Conversely, if the duration of each workout is limited, you can use a shorter time and higher intensity or change the way the sets are performed to maximize the time that your client has available for exercise.

Step 4: Delivery of the Program

After you have created the program, the next step is to deliver it to your client. Although the delivery of an exercise program is what many people consider a Personal Training Specialist's job, the fitness theory and program design concepts already discussed are crucial to delivering safe, effective, efficient, and enjoyable training sessions. The process of program delivery is addressed in detail throughout the next chapter.

Step 5: Reassessment

After you have followed all the previous steps of program design and delivery, you should periodically reassess your clients to determine what results they have obtained and what modifications are required. The frequency of reassessment may be different for each client, but it should typically occur every one to three months. You use the information you gather from reassessment to adjust priorities and program design, just as you used the information you gathered when you first began the program. In this way, program design is a circular, ongoing process.

Applying the Four Elements of Good Program Design

In chapter 11 we discussed the four elements of good program design. Specifically, it was noted that a properly designed program is safe, effective, efficient, and enjoyable. To achieve this objective, you must customize programs to the needs and abilities of your client. This approach is consistent with the principle of individualization, which states that because people are genetically unique and have different personalities and practical needs, they will necessarily respond to exercise in different ways. Therefore, the task of customizing exercise programs should be approached systematically.

First, programming should be aligned with your client's goals. One of the biggest mistakes you can make is to create the client's workouts based on your own fitness objectives. Such an approach is bound to cause frustration and disappointment for your client, ultimately straining the personal trainer–client relationship. For example, if the client's goal is to run a half-marathon, training your client to be a bodybuilder would be counterproductive. Similarly, a client who wants to lose weight would not be well served by your prescribing a power-lifting routine. Because each program delivers somewhat predictable results based on its design, you should create the program in a manner that is most consistent with the client's goals.

Second, you need to bear in mind the client's training status. Clients who are beginners should be approached differently from those who have substantial exercise experience. For novice exercisers, adaptations to resistance training during the first month or two are primarily related to developing neuromuscular coordination. The body is figuring out the best way to carry out movement sequences. Moreover, beginning clients are often deconditioned and prone to excessive muscular soreness. In these instances, your efforts in the early stages of training should be directed toward helping your client adjust to the demands of exercise rather than pushing to fatigue. Focus on instilling proper technique and movement sequencing. If a client is having trouble coordinating free-weight exercises, starting with machine-based movements may be best. This approach allows the development of resistance strength and reduces the risk of injury. Over time you can determine when to integrate exercises that are more complex.

Finally, you must account for any limitations specific to your client. This process begins with a review of your client's medical history. Risk factors, existing injuries, and other conditions must be considered here. For example, a client with a knee disorder may be unable to perform certain movements, and a client with hypertension should probably not lift heavy loads. You will also need to incorporate the results of any passive or dynamic assessments that you've conducted, as discussed in chapters 9 and 10. When in doubt about how to program for a client with an existing injury, postural concern, or mobility restriction, you should consult with the client's physician or a qualified exercise professional. Moreover, time-related limitations also need to be considered when constructing your client's program. A multiset, total-body routine might be in the client's best interests, but it will not be practical if the client is limited to training for 30 minutes in a given session. Therefore, you should balance your client's goals, abilities, and limitations when designing the program. Successfully managing these factors is where the science of training meets art.

Balancing the Program

When designing a program, you should focus on balancing the program so that all aspects of fitness are addressed and all the major systems and muscle groups are worked over the course of a given microcycle. As a rule, routines should encompass exercises in all three cardinal planes of movement (i.e., sagittal, frontal, and transverse). Humans are three-dimensional beings who carry out multiplanar movements during the course of everyday life. As discussed in chapter 8, these foundational movement sequences include but are not limited to twisting, pushing, and pulling movements performed in numerous directions, as they relate to cardiorespiratory, resistance, and flexibility training. In accordance with the principle of specificity, optimal functional transfer can therefore be achieved only by working the body in each of the respective planes. A balance between planar movements will help ensure optimal movement sequences as well as enhance physical symmetry.

Although balancing components is critical, it is relevant only within the context of the individual client. Within the overall balance, the focus should reflect the goals of the program and the client's training status. One client may need to work more on the upper body, whereas another may need to work more on the lower body. When clients come to you, they bring with them a variety of needs and goals that are often out of balance because of lifestyle, injury, or habitual posture. You need to have the creativity to design a program that is actually unbalanced to bring the client back into balance.

For example, if a client comes in with slightly forward-leaning posture not related to an injury or skeletal deformity, you may be able to help improve her or his default posture through personal training. As long as the client is able to return consciously to a neutral posture, the exercises you program can be used to train the body to maintain optimal posture. But you will need to deemphasize (not eliminate) chest and anterior shoulder exercises and emphasize rhomboid, posterior deltoid, and trapezius exercises, as well as open the chest and shoulders with flexibility training until the client returns to neutral posture. This unbalanced training approach will actually result in balance overall.

Although this type of unbalanced approach lends itself well to resistance training, it is also directly applicable to flexibility, such as when a client is more flexible in the upper body than in the lower body, and to cardiorespiratory training, such as when a client is a lifelong runner and does not require much cardiorespiratory training during your sessions.

As a Personal Training Specialist, you will need to consider all the previously mentioned factors to create the ideal program for each client. By following the steps outlined in figure 12.2, you will be able to integrate the key components of program design

 Although overall balance is important, an unbalanced training approach can be used to help clients work on specific elements of their physical fitness when imbalances or weaknesses have been observed during the assessments conducted by a Personal Training Specialist.

and create an individualized and effective personal training experience for each of your clients.

Modifying Programs

To ensure optimal success, successful Personal Training Specialists not only plan variety within their programs but also anticipate when their clients need variation. This section provides a toolbox of methods by which you can modify any exercise to make it progressively more interesting and challenging or, alternatively, easier and less challenging on days when clients may be feeling less energetic.

When to Change the Program

No strict rule dictates when to change your client's program, but the rule of thumb is to add some form of variation approximately every two weeks,

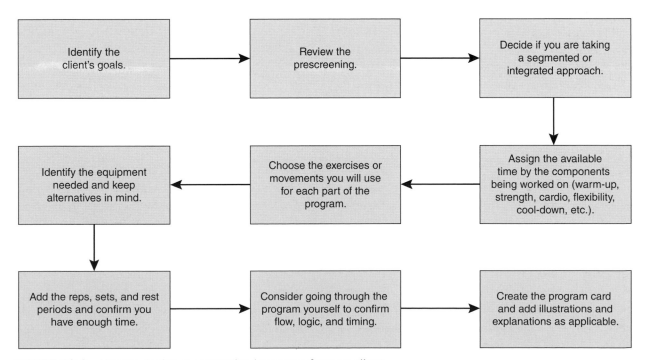

FIGURE 12.2 How to design a customized program for your client.

depending on how often the client is exercising and what his or her skill level is. Keep in mind that you need not change everything in the program, but you should change some aspects on a regular basis. For example, if your client is finding the squat challenging but the chest press easy, you might leave the squat as is and modify the chest press to make it more challenging. Carefully applying the principle of **progressive overload** will ensure that each client continues to improve his or her fitness in a safe and effective manner.

Tables 12.1, 12.2, and 12.3 show several training variables and examples of how you can safely incorporate them into a program.

When making changes to your client's program, follow these steps:

1. Tell clients when you first begin to train them that you will be making changes on a regular basis as necessary to ensure their progress toward their goals.
2. When clients are ready, inform them that you will be making a change to the program.
3. Based on their current level of ability and fitness, make changes slowly and incrementally (always underestimate rather than overestimate).
4. Anticipate areas of difficulty or risk given the changes.

TABLE 12.1   Resistance Training Progressions for Beginner to Advanced Clients

Variable	Progression	What this does	Example	Avoid
Speed of motion (tempo)	Go faster or slower.	Increases or decreases the effect of gravity or momentum, thereby increasing or decreasing the work that the muscle completes.	Use a 14 sec count instead of 6 or 7 sec count.	Going too fast or too slow (dangerous versus boring).
Range of motion (ROM)	Use partial ROM or full ROM.	Creates angle-specific adaptations.	Focus on the sticking point in the ROM.	Neglecting other points in the client's ROMs.
Set performance	Use supersets, drop sets, giant sets, and so on.	Modifies intensity, variety, and time.	Combine biceps curl and triceps extension.	Sacrificing proper technique on either exercise.
Stability	Gradually remove stability.	Involves additional synergistic muscle groups.	Perform seated biceps curl on a stability ball rather than on a bench.	Removing too much stability too soon.
Sensory perception	Gradually remove sensory feedback.	Increases the challenge by decreasing sensory feedback.	Close eyes during the set.	Putting the client at high risk for injury.
Recovery (rest interval)	Reduce recovery time.	Increases intensity by allowing less repletion of ATP stores.	Take 30 to 45 sec of rest instead of 60.	Exhausting the client.
Reps	Increase or decrease the number of reps.	Focuses results on either endurance or strength.	Drop the number of reps from 15 to 5 (and increase load).	Sacrificing technique for a higher load or more reps.
Sets	Increase the number of sets.	Increases volume and therefore the total amount of work.	Increase the number of sets from one to two.	Losing track of time (potentially doubling work).
Base of support	Narrow or widen the base of support.	Increases or decreases the need for balance.	Wider hands with push-ups or wider stance for squats.	Making the exercise so challenging that the risk is unacceptably high.
Lever length	Lengthen or shorten the lever used in the exercise.	By altering the lever length, you can change the effective resistance without changing the actual resistance.	DB side raises with arms extended vs. bent, or push-ups from the toes vs. knees	Sacrificing technique and form just to use a longer lever (for example, swayed back during full push-ups).

TABLE 12.2   Cardiorespiratory Program Progressions for Beginner to Advanced Clients

Component	Progression	What this does	Example	Avoid
Speed	Go faster or slower (with increased resistance).	Can modify the energy system being used.	Increase rpm, rate, or speed.	Going too fast or too slow (because this can cause incorrect technique).
Range of motion (rower, treadmill)	Focus on different aspects of the ROM.	Allows a focus on one aspect of the movement.	Take partial strokes on the rower in different phases of the stroke.	Spending too much time on a small part of the movement.
Resistance (incline on treadmill, level on bike and elliptical, wind damper on rower)	Increase resistance or tension.	Requires additional work and therefore additional calories.	Increase the incline on the treadmill instead of speed.	Making radical changes, potentially overloading the client.
Direction of movement (treadmill, elliptical)	Change direction.	Uses undertrained muscles and motor pathways, thus increasing caloric output.	Sideways shuffle on the treadmill or move backward on the elliptical.	Using awkward movement or excessive speed for the direction chosen.
Work-to-rest ratio (if using intervals)	Increase work time or decrease recovery time.	Can modify the energy system used.	Instead of working for 1 min and taking 1 min rest, try a 2:1 ratio.	Not allowing adequate recovery or overstressing the client with an excessive work interval.

TABLE 12.3   Flexibility Program Progressions for Beginner to Advanced Clients

Component	Progression	What this does	Example	Avoid
Speed	Go faster or slower.	Creates dynamic flexibility.	Move into a position dynamically.	Letting clients move too quickly or bounce.
Stability	Reduce stability.	Improves awareness of balance while using flexibility.	Do stretches on one foot.	Losing the effect of the stretch.
Transition	Move from one stretch to the next.	Creates a more fluid movement.	Move from a posterior deltoid stretch to a triceps stretch.	Focusing too much on transition and not enough on the desired stretch.
Duration	Hold the stretch longer.	Allows the muscle to relax more.	Try 45 sec instead of 15 sec.	Losing the point of tension or overstretching.
Breathing	Focus on breathing.	Integrates mind and body more completely.	Inhale and exhale according to length of stretch.	Letting clients hold their breath or lose focus on the muscle.

5. Assess results from the implemented changes.

6. Be flexible and make adjustments as necessary, possibly returning to the previous level of challenge until clients are more prepared.

7. Ask clients for feedback and make any necessary adjustments.

Changing the Exercise Versus Changing the Performance

Changing the exercise that your client is performing is not always necessary; you may be able to change simply how it is performed. For example, new clients who are performing a machine chest press may not need to progress to a barbell bench press if they are not ready to integrate free weights. Instead, they could perform the same machine exercise but increase the challenge by modifying the sets, reps, or tempo of the exercise or even how they position the body during performance, as described in table 12.1 (e.g., lift one or both feet off the ground to engage more core stabilizers in the chest press).

Be attentive to client feedback with respect to exercises. Understand that a number of factors influence exercise performance including body shape, limb length, and personal preference. If a client expresses a dislike toward an exercise, change it. Without exception, no exercise is essential to a routine. You can always come up with substitute movements that will effectively address the client's needs and abilities. Remember that adherence is paramount to the success of a program. If you are not sensitive to your client's desires, training and results will ultimately suffer.

Remain cognizant of the fact that environmental factors influence daily exercise performance. A client's capacity to train will vary somewhat from session to session. Many factors influence these daily variations, including stress, sleep, and hormonal changes, among others. Do not feel as if you have to push your client to the max on every workout. Gauge the client's motivation before the session. To ensure that your clients' training sessions will be safe, effective, efficient, and enjoyable, the programs you build must be flexible. This type of flexible programming has been shown to be effective in those who are internally motivated to exercise. Realize, however, that the success of this approach depends on the client's ability to make an honest assessment of his or her training state. Some clients always look to push themselves, whereas others consistently try to slack off. You need to get to know your client's mindset

and tendencies and employ flexible programming principles accordingly.

By applying a periodized approach to program design based on constant reassessment (and modifications for variety and injury prevention), you will increase the likelihood that your clients will achieve their goals and that you will have long-lasting, successful relationships with them.

There are many predesigned workouts and exercise ideas that your client may ask you to incorporate into their program based on recommendations in magazines, online, or from popular and successful Personal Training Specialists. It is important to review these programs with your client, explain any concerns you may have, and make individualized adjustments where necessary prior to implementing such workouts.

Sample Program Designs

Thousands of programs could be created for any client who has a specific goal. Table 12.4 and the sample periodized program that follows include just a few of the programs that you could use to achieve a variety of common goals. These examples are not the only ways to create programs of this sort; rather, they provide a reference as to what a safe and effective program might look like. Each program would require individualized modifications as the client progresses and would include a thorough warm-up and cool-down. When leading clients through a workout session, Personal Training Specialists typically have clients train larger muscle groups before smaller ones, and train the core muscles last.

TABLE 12.4 Sample Program Designs

Program component	Nonexerciser or occasional exerciser	Recreational exerciser	Recreational exerciser who has time constraints (limited number of workouts per week)	Committed exerciser or athlete	Committed exerciser or athlete with a goal to increase muscle hypertrophy	Dedicated exerciser or elite athlete
Frequency	1–3 days per week	3–5 days per week	1 day per week	4–6 days per week	5–6 days per week	5–6 days per week
Total volume	Low	Low	Low	Moderate	High	Moderate to high
Intensity	Low	Low to moderate	Moderate	Moderate	Moderate to high	High
Sessions per day	1	1	1	1–2	2	2
RESISTANCE TRAINING						
Sets	1–3	1–2	1	3–5	5–15	4–6
Reps	12–15	10–12	10–12	Varied	8–12	Varied
Recovery	30–60 sec	30–60 sec	30 sec	30–120 sec	60–120 sec	Varied
Set performance	Straight	Straight	Varied	Varied	Varied	Varied
Tempo	3:0:2:0	3:0:2:0	2:0:2:0	2:0:1:0 to 3:0:2:0	3:0:2:0	Varied
ROM	Full	Full	Full	Full	Varied	Varied
Stability	Full	Full	Full	Varied	Full	Varied
Sensory perception	Full	Full	Full	Varied	Full	Varied
Types of exercise	Mostly machines, stability ball, simple body-weight exercises	Machines, free weights, stability ball, body-weight exercises, basic cable or pulley	Machines, free weights, stability ball, body-weight exercises, basic cable or pulley	Machines, free weights, stability ball, body-weight exercises, cable or pulley, kettle bells, suspension straps, specialty equipment	Mostly free weights	Mostly free weights; can also use any equipment previously mentioned
Number of exercises	5–8	5–10	5	About 15	20–30	10–15
Sample exercises	Squat or leg press, leg curl, chest press, seated row, lateral raise, abdominal curl, back extension	Squat or leg press, leg curl, chest press, seated row, lateral raise, back extension, abdominal curl	Squat or leg press, chest press, seated row, abdominal curl, back extension	Leg press, leg curl, leg extension, chest press, chest fly, seated row, lat pull-down, lateral raise, posterior raise, biceps curl, triceps press, BOSU abdominal curl, reverse abdominal curl, plank, back extension	Squat, leg curl, leg extension, hip extension, calf raise, seated calf raise, flat bench press, incline bench press, decline bench press, shrugs, bent-over row, back extension, shoulder press, front raise, lateral raise, posterior raise, biceps curl, preacher curl, wrist curl, reverse wrist curl, triceps press, overhead triceps extension, lying triceps extension	Choice of exercises would be sport specific, adapted to increase functional transfer or to reduce imbalances (i.e., dumbbell chest press on stability ball versus machine chest press)

> continued

TABLE 12.4 > *continued*

Program component	Nonexerciser or occasional exerciser	Recreational exerciser	Recreational exerciser who has time constraints (limited number of workouts per week)	Committed exerciser or athlete	Committed exerciser or athlete with a goal to increase muscle hypertrophy	Dedicated exerciser or elite athlete
CARDIORESPIRATORY EXERCISE						
Duration	10–30 min	20–45 min	20–45 min	30–60 min	20–60 min	20–60 min or more
Intensity	50%–65% HRmax, RPE: 2–4	60%–75% HRmax, RPE: 3–6	60%–75% HRmax, RPE: 3–6	65%–85% HRmax, RPE: 4–7	65%–75% HRmax, RPE: 4–6	65%–90% HRmax, RPE: 5–9
Type	Walking, swimming, aqua fitness, stationary bicycle, basic group fitness	Walking, swimming, aqua fitness, stationary bicycle, treadmill, elliptical, stair climber, cycling or group fitness classes	Walking, swimming, aqua fitness, stationary bicycle, treadmill, elliptical, stair climber, cycling classes, intermediate group fitness classes, interval training	Walking, swimming, aqua fitness, stationary bicycle, treadmill, elliptical, stair climber, cycling classes, intermediate group fitness classes, interval training	Walking, swimming, aqua fitness, stationary bicycle, treadmill, elliptical, stair climber, cycling classes, intermediate or advanced group fitness classes, interval training, advanced circuits. Note: Most cardiorespiratory exercise for this group is maintained at low to moderate intensity to prevent hypotrophic adaptations	Walking, swimming, aqua fitness, stationary bicycle, treadmill, elliptical, stair climber, cycling classes, advanced group fitness classes, interval training, advanced circuits all previous types, sport-specific activities

Sample Periodized Program

Client: A 40-year-old female office worker who has a goal of increasing upper-body strength and losing five kilograms (11 lbs) of fat in three months

Month 1

Week 1

Exercise	Sets	Repetitions*	Rest interval
Seated row	1–2	12–15	2 min
Machine chest press	1–2	12–15	2 min
Leg press	1–2	12–15	2 min
Leg curl	1–2	12–15	2 min
Calf raise	1–2	12–15	2 min
Abdominal curl-up	1–2	12–15	2 min
Plank	1–2	Until it becomes difficult (up to 30 sec)	2 min

*For all tables in this program, this column represents a maximum repetition range. Select a load that allows the client to achieve this number of reps. If the client cannot complete the lower number, the load is too heavy and should be decreased. If the client can easily exceed the higher number of the range, the load is too light and should be increased.

Week 2

Exercise	Sets	Repetitions	Rest interval
Seated row	2–3	12–15	90 sec
Machine chest press	2–3	12–15	90 sec
Leg press	2–3	12–15	90 sec
Leg curl	2–3	12–15	90 sec
Calf raise	2–3	12–15	90 sec
Abdominal curl-up	2–3	12–15	90 sec
Plank	1–2	Until it becomes difficult (up to 45 sec)	90 sec

Week 3

Exercise	Sets	Repetitions	Rest interval
Seated row	3–4	12–15	60 sec
Machine chest press	3–4	12–15	60 sec
Leg press	3–4	12–15	60 sec
Leg curl	3–4	12–15	60 sec
Calf raise	3–4	12–15	60 sec
Abdominal curl-up	3–4	12–15	60 sec
Plank	2–3	Until it becomes difficult (up to 45 sec)	60 sec

Week 4

Exercise	Sets	Repetitions	Rest interval
Machine military press	3–4	8–12	60 sec
Lat pull-down (close grip)	3–4	8–12	60 sec
Machine chest press	3–4	8–12	60 sec
Leg press	3–4	8–12	60 sec
Leg curl	3–4	8–12	60 sec
Calf raise	3–4	8–12	60 sec
Abdominal curl-up (resisted if necessary)	3–4	Until fatigue	60 sec
Plank	1–2	Until fatigue	60 sec

Month 2

Week 1

Exercise	Sets	Repetitions	Rest interval
Machine military press	2–3	12–15	60 sec
Seated cable row	2–3	12–15	60 sec
Lat pull-down (wide grip)	2–3	12–15	60 sec
Machine chest press	2–3	12–15	60 sec
Squat	2–3	12–15	60 sec
Lunge	2–3	12–15	60 sec
Cable crunch	2–3	12–15	60 sec

Week 2

Exercise	Sets	Repetitions	Rest interval
Barbell chest press	3–4	10–12	90 sec
Seated cable row	3–4	10–12	90 sec
Lat pull-down (wide grip)	3–4	10–12	90 sec
Machine military press	3–4	10–12	90 sec
Squat	3–4	10–12	90 sec
Lunge	3–4	10–12	90 sec
Cable crunch	3–4	8–10	90 sec

Week 3

Exercise	Sets	Repetitions	Rest interval
Barbell chest press	3–4	6–8	2 min
Seated cable row	3–4	6–8	2 min
Lat pull-down (wide grip)	3–4	6–8	2 min
Machine military press	3–4	8–10	2 min
Squat	3–4	6–8	2 min
Lunge	3–4	6–8	2 min
Cable crunch	3–4	6–8	2 min

Week 4 (Unloading Cycle)

Exercise	Sets	Repetitions	Rest interval
Barbell shoulder press	1–2	12–15	90 sec
Seated row	1–2	12–15	90 sec
Lat pull-down (wide grip)	1–2	12–15	90 sec
Barbell chest press	1–2	12–15	90 sec
Barbell squat	1–2	12–15	90 sec
Lunge	1–2	12–15	90 sec
Cable crunch	1–2	12–15	90 sec

Month 3

Week 1

Exercise	Sets	Repetitions	Rest interval
Circuit:			
Dumbbell shoulder press	3	12–15	60 sec between circuits
One-arm dumbbell row	3	12–15	60 sec between circuits
Dumbbell chest press	3	12–15	60 sec between circuits
Cross-cable pull-down	3	12–15	60 sec between circuits
Bulgarian split squat	3	12–15	60 sec between circuits
Lateral lunge	3	12–15	60 sec between circuits
Romanian deadlift	3	12–15	60 sec between circuits
Farmer's walk	3	12–15	60 sec between circuits

Week 2

Exercise	Sets	Repetitions	Rest interval
Circuit:			
Dumbbell shoulder press	3	10–12	60 sec between circuits
One-arm dumbbell row	3	10–12	60 sec between circuits
Dumbbell chest press	3	10–12	60 sec between circuits
Cross-cable pull-down	3	10–12	60 sec between circuits
Bulgarian split squat	3	10–12	60 sec between circuits
Lateral lunge	3	10–12	60 sec between circuits
Romanian deadlift	3	10–12	60 sec between circuits
Farmer's walk	3	10–12	60 sec between circuits

Week 3

Exercise	Sets	Repetitions	Rest interval
Circuit:	3	6–8	60 sec between circuits
Dumbbell shoulder press	3	6–8	60 sec between circuits
One-arm dumbbell row	3	6–8	60 sec between circuits
Dumbbell chest press	3	6–8	60 sec between circuits
Cross-cable pull-down	3	6–8	60 sec between circuits
Bulgarian split squat	3	6–8	60 sec between circuits
Lateral lunge	3	6–8	60 sec between circuits
Single-leg Romanian deadlift	3	6–8	60 sec between circuits
Farmer's walk	3	6–8	60 sec between circuits

Week 4 (Unloading Cycle)

Exercise	Sets	Repetitions	Rest interval
Barbell shoulder press	1–2	12–15	90 sec
Seated row	1–2	12–15	90 sec
Lat pull-down (wide grip)	1–2	12–15	90 sec
Barbell chest press	1–2	12–15	90 sec
Barbell squat	1–2	12–15	90 sec
Lunge	1–2	12–15	90 sec
Romanian deadlift	1–2	12–15	90 sec
Cable crunch	1–2	12–15	90 sec

Summary of Main Points

1. The most important component of programming to perform before you begin to create a client's program is information gathering.

2. Personal training programming should be aligned with your client's goals.

3. When creating a workout program, always consider your client's exercise level, experience, mindset, and goals.

4. Although no strict rule dictates when to change your client's program, you should aim to incorporate progressive overload and add some element of variety about every two weeks.

Key Concepts for Study

Sum of training effect

Progressive overload

Specificity

Progression

Review Questions

1. List the five steps in program design.

2. List at least three variables that the Personal Training Specialist can change to make the client's cardiorespiratory training more challenging without changing the selection of exercise or equipment type.

3. A Personal Training Specialist should be performing client reassessments every

   a. workout

   b. week

   c. month

   d. one to three months

4. Which three factors must be successfully managed to accomplish a meeting of science and art in personal training?

   a. home programming, group-style training, and gym workouts

   b. cardio training, resistance training, and warm-up training

   c. client goals, abilities, and limitations

   d. Personal Training Specialist goals, abilities, and limitations

5. When training clients, the best approach is to

   a. train them to their maximum every workout

   b. overestimate their ability and change if needed

   c. underestimate their ability and change if needed

   d. be firm in programming, allowing only minimal changes

6. No strict rule governs when to change a client's program, but the general rule is to make a program adjustment at least once every _____, depending on _____ and the client's _____.

   a. two weeks; how often the client is exercising; skill level

   b. four weeks; the client's endurance level; timeline

   c. two weeks; the type of exercise that the client is performing; assessment score

   d. four weeks; the type of exercise that the client is performing; endurance level

7. If a client comes in with a slightly forward-leaning posture that is not related to an injury or deformity, which style of training would you use in his or her program?

   a. balanced approach

   b. unbalanced approach

   c. overcompensation

   d. supercompensation

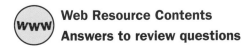

Web Resource Contents

Answers to review questions

Delivering a Program

Rod Macdonald, BEd
Brad Schoenfeld, PhD

LEARNING OUTCOMES

After completing this chapter, you will be able to

1. identify the five steps of program delivery;

2. understand the importance of charting every workout and identify best practices; and

3. understand how to prepare for the first personal training session and subsequent sessions.

The delivery of a program may be the most important aspect of programming. As a Personal Training Specialist, you are responsible for each client's understanding of the program you create for them. If your client understands the expectations of the exercises, the movement sequences, and the muscles that should be working, then your delivery is successful.

To prepare yourself to deliver a training program, you need to talk directly with the client to establish his or her expectations for the program. Before the first session with the client, you should schedule at least one conversation by phone, web cam, or, preferably, in person. This conversation may take place before or at the same time as a fitness assessment. It should include information about the upcoming sessions, business policies, and other important details you wish to discuss.

Many clients will not know what to expect from these first communications, let alone from a health and fitness screening and subsequent training sessions. You are responsible for communicating clearly what they should expect of the process, what your expectations are of them, and what expectations they should have of you. By setting the expectations ahead of time, you are creating an ideal setting for the first and subsequent training sessions.

Five Steps of Program Delivery

When delivering a program, you need to ensure that your client understands and properly executes each exercise. The five steps shown in figure 13.1 give you a template of how to deliver a program to your client and be successful every time.

Step One: Explain the Program

Before any physical personal training takes place, you should go over the program with your client. Begin by providing a brief overview of what you will be doing. Describe the types of exercises that will be included and the manner in which they will be carried out. Explain the rationale for the program and make sure your client understands how

it addresses her or his goals, needs, and abilities. Always ask the client whether she or he has any questions and clarify that your answers satisfy the client. This approach allows you to deal with any conflicts upfront, thus preventing minor issues from becoming larger problems down the road. Make it clear that the personal training program is a partnership between you and the client. Emphasize the importance of communication and encourage your client to voice any concerns that may arise. Establishing rapport early sets the stage for a mutually respectful relationship that will endure over time.

Step Two: Exercise Demonstration

When first taking your client through the routine, make sure to provide a thorough description of each exercise. In doing so, make an effort to appeal to different learning styles, including visual, auditory, and kinesthetic modes. Although people generally have a preferred learning style, most are multimodal and thus benefit from a variety of approaches. As such, employ a combination of all three modes in your descriptions. Demonstrating (i.e., demoing) the new exercises in a program is always a good idea. A good demo provides a visual image of the movement that your client can commit to memory. You should go through the exercise relatively slowly at first to emphasize movement sequencing and then demo it at the desired speed to provide proper context for performance.

As you initiate the demonstration, orally explain what you are doing. Make your description as simple as possible, avoiding the use of jargon. If possible, relate the exercise to that of everyday activities. For example, you can equate a one-arm dumbbell row with starting a lawnmower or describe the deadlift as akin to picking up heavy suitcases. These kinds of analogies make the image more vivid, enhancing retention for subsequent motor performance. Kinesthetic descriptions can include putting your finger on the target muscle of the client. For example, you could put your fingers on the client's triceps when doing an elbow extension to reinforce where the movement should be felt. Table 13.1 gives additional

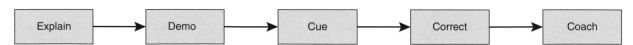

FIGURE 13.1   The five-step program delivery system.

TABLE 13.1   Sample Exercise Demonstration

What to do	What to say	Example
Take the client to the location of the exercise.	Introduce the exercise orally, mentioning the name, the muscle groups worked, and the purpose as it is relevant to the client.	"This is the leg press. It mainly works the hamstrings and quads (muscles in your thighs). It is a great exercise for improving jumping, picking up heavy objects, and overall fitness." (Relate the exercise to whatever is most relevant to the client.)
Demonstrate the adjustments of the exercise, if applicable.	Show the client where the adjustments are made and why.	"The adjustment on the leg press allows a person of almost any height to use it. It is located here. To adjust it, just pull on this lever and move up or down until your thighs are parallel to the platform."
Demonstrate the exercise.	Explain how to perform the exercise, including cues and things to avoid.	"Make sure that your back is stable and your eyes are facing forward. Start by pressing through the heels, making sure that your knees track over your toes. As you press, exhale throughout the movement and pause slightly at the end of the movement without locking your knees. Return to the start position by slowly lowering yourself and inhaling throughout the movement. Continue without pause until you get to 12 reps. If you cannot maintain technique or are otherwise uncomfortable during the set, return the weight to the platform."
Allow the client to try the exercise.	Talk the client through the movement, repeating the key instructions that you mentioned in your demo. Ask how and where the client feels the exercise.	"Where do you feel the most work being done? Are you pressing through the heels? That looks great. Continue breathing. I'll let you know when to stop."

 Be respectful of your client's personal space. Some clients may be modest or uncomfortable with physical contact by a Personal Training Specialist. Thus, make sure that you ask for permission before touching in any way.

examples of how to provide exercise demonstrations to your clients.

Step Three: Cue

Cueing is one of the most important aspects of proper program delivery. Simply stated, cueing refers to prompts that focus the learner's attention to a given aspect of the movement. **Cues** can be verbal or nonverbal, and they can be provided both during and after exercise performance. Verbal cues are most commonly used during training and can be provided both before and during exercise performance. For example, "Feet shoulder-width apart" and "Elbows in" are specific cues that direct your client's attention to key elements of the exercise. Following a few guidelines can help you offer effective verbal cueing. First, cues should be concise. As a rule, the cue should contain no more than three or four words. Second, limit the number of cues to no more than two or three at a time. Offering too many cues increases the chance that the client will forget one of them and can interfere with skill performance. Finally, use the same cues repeatedly so that the client forms a strong association between the cue and the exercise.

Nonverbal cueing generally involves kinesthetic prompts. For example, if a client tends to round his or her back during the squat, you can gently place your finger on the lumbar region as the client performs the exercise as a reminder to maintain a neutral spinal position. Nonverbal cues can be supplemented with verbal cues to enhance skill acquisition. In the case of a client who rounds his or her back while squatting, you can say, "Neutral back," as you touch the client's lumbar spine. Again, you need to gain permission from your client before making any physical contact.

Step Four: Correct and Spot

At times a client will not be able to grasp performance of an exercise despite repeated attempts at cueing. If that is the case, you should stop the exercise and attempt to assess the root cause. Ask your client whether something is difficult to understand. Have the client repeat back what is expected; often you will notice that the issue is a simple matter of miscommunication. If the client does in fact comprehend proper exercise execution, then consider other potential causes. Perhaps a flexibility issue limits movement, or maybe what the client thinks is happening is disconnected from the actual performance. If you are unable to address the issue, you may decide to move on to a different exercise temporarily while working to address the problem. Remember, continuing to have a client perform a movement improperly not only increases the potential for injury but also may have a demotivating effect that can negatively affect adherence if the client becomes frustrated, uncomfortable, or embarrassed.

Spotting is the act of closely following the movement of the client, sometimes with your hands on the client or the equipment to assist if she or he begins to fail in the movement. Make sure that you are in position to spot the client, particularly during the early stages of training. Depending on the exercise selected, the equipment being used, and the client's level of familiarity or skill with each movement, you can use various spotting techniques. Each of the exercise examples in appendix A provides a description of the most appropriate spotting techniques for that specific exercise. Clients sometimes perform poorly because they are afraid of injury, but knowing that you are there to assist if anything goes amiss can reduce their apprehension and thus enhance proper exercise performance.

When you are spotting a client, he or she must be aware of what you are doing and why, and you need to ask the client's permission if you are physically close to or touching him or her. In addition, your spotting technique and positioning must be strong enough to ensure that you are not injured should you be required to assist the client.

Step Five: Coach the Movement

Besides cueing and correcting the movement, you need to **coach** your clients toward success as they perform each exercise. The reinforcement and encouragement you provide will help clients push themselves toward improvement in their overall fitness and take them closer to their specific training goals. An important issue that Personal Training Specialists face is knowing when to push a client to the point of muscular failure. As a rule, the focus in the early stages of training should be on mastering exercise technique. This step involves developing the neuromuscular coordination needed to carry out the movement sequence with precision. When the client achieves mastery, you can proceed to push the client to muscle failure, thereby initiating a greater adaptation response.

The question then becomes how often you should push your client to the point of muscular fatigue. The principle of progressive overload dictates that gradually increasing the volume and or intensity of the program is essential to realizing ongoing adaptations. Thus, the more experience the client gains with resistance training, the greater the need is to go all out during performance. Although training to failure is important for maximizing results (particularly with strength and hypertrophy goals), doing so too often can lead to overtraining and thus negatively affect your client's training outcomes. Ultimately, the frequency of failure training depends on individual goals and abilities, and you should select the frequency according to the guidelines in table 6.12. Generally, the client should be pushed to her or his limits on at least some of the working sets, but not every set. As with all training variables, failure can and should be periodized into the workout scheme so that adaptations are optimized without bringing about overtraining.

Program Card

You should chart every client workout. The most common way to do this is to create a **program card** and carry it on a clipboard, or as a document on a tablet or smartphone. The most important elements to include in a program card are the following:

- Client name
- Workout date
- Exercises to be performed
- Number of sets and set performance
- Number of reps and tempo
- Amount of rest between sets

- Any relevant information about how the client felt during the session (i.e., tired, energetic, and so on)

Note that this list refers to recording repetitions rather than load in resistance training exercises. You should select a load that allows the client to achieve the desired number of reps based on the workout focus and the client's unique goals. When tracking your client's progress, write down the number of reps he or she was able to complete, because this component is more important to physical adaptation than the load used. Deemphasizing the load on the program card prevents the ego from getting involved. The load can be added to the comments section as a reminder of client progress and as an indicator of the appropriate starting load for the next workout.

When planning your client's program, emphasize the desired number of repetitions rather than the absolute amount of load. The desired number of repetitions is more closely related to the overall program focus and will dictate the load that your client will use for each exercise.

Charting client workouts offers several important benefits. First, charting provides a detailed record of performance that can be evaluated over time. Because you will be working with many clients, you are not likely to remember what you did with a particular client last week, not to mention last month. Having a written record of each session allows you to review your client's progress and compare it to expected results. In this way, you can determine the effectiveness of the program. You can make educated decisions about when and how to alter program variables. Moreover, if the program is not producing the desired outcome, you can make appropriate adjustments without wasting valuable time and effort. Keeping detailed records is also important from a risk-management perspective should your client incur an injury.

Charting workouts is also an excellent way to enhance client motivation. For example, showing a client that she or he lost two centimetres around the waist in two weeks or increased her or his bench press by 10 kilograms (22 lb) over the past month is highly motivational. This information can inspire the client to stick with the program and even intensify her or his efforts.

Finally, the program card used to chart workouts can be provided to clients if they will be working out on their own. In such cases you should tailor the card to the individual needs of the client. For instance, you might need to provide information on seat-height adjustment for various machines or sketch rough illustrations to remind the client of the exercise. Knowing your client's comprehension of fitness will help guide the selection of what additional information to include. Using an online workout builder that includes images and videos and provides space to input exercise parameters is useful and can be easier for your client to understand.

Visit canfitpro INTERACTIVE (www.canfitprointeractive.com) to check out canfitpro's preferred personal training tools to build workouts and programs. These tools include an online program builder, training logs, a video exercise library, and suggested fitness routines to help you create a safe, effective, efficient, and enjoyable program for each client.

We have included a completed sample program card, which is shown in figure 13.2. A blank program card is provided in the web resource as a template for your use. Keep in mind that many versions of program cards are available. If you work in an established facility, they may prefer you to use their card. If you work independently, you may wish to customize or create your own program card or use an online workout builder, such as the one provided on canfitpro INTERACTIVE (www.canfitprointeractive.com).

See the web resource at www.HumanKinetics.com/FoundationsOfProfessionalPersonalTraining for a blank version of the client program card.

Training Session

When you meet for the first training session, you must be prepared. Allow sufficient time to review your client's file and history to determine how you

Program Card

Client: _____   Phase: _____   Reassessment date: ___/___/___

Resistance Training Guidelines

Session date	W1/D1		W1/D2		W1/D3		W2/D1		W2/D2		W2/D3		W3/D1		W3/D2		W3/D3	
Tempo	3:0:3:0		3:0:3:0		3:0:3:0		3:1:2:0		3:1:3:0		3:1:3:0		4:1:2:0		4:1:2:0		4:1:2:0	
Rest	:30		:30		:30		:45		:45		:45		:60		:60		:60	
Set performance	Straight		Straight		Straight		Straight		Straight		Straight		Superset		Superset		Superset	
Exercises	**Reps**	**Sets**	**Reps**	**Sets**	**Reps**	**Sets**	**Reps**	**Sets**	**Reps**	**Sets**	**Reps**	**Sets**	**Reps**	**Sets**	**Reps**	**Sets**	**Reps**	**Sets**
Dumbbell squat	15	2					15	2					10	3				
Dumbbell deadlift	15	2					15	2					10	3				
Dumbbell stationary lunge	15	2					15	2					12	3				
Stability ball hamstring curl	15	2					15	2					12	3				
Plank	:15	2					:30	2					:45	2				
Seated medicine ball twist	15	2					15	2					15	2				
Seated row			15	2					15	2					10	3		
Lat pulldown			15	2					15	2					10	3		
Single-arm dumbbell row			15	2					15	2					12	3		
Cable reverse fly			15	2					15	2					12	3		
Dead bug			:15	2					:25	2					:40	2		
Superman			15	2					15	2					12	2		
Dumbbell chest press					15	2					15	2					10	3
Dumbbell shoulder press					15	2					15	2					10	3
Dumbbell lateral raise					15	2					15	2					12	3
Skull crusher					15	2					15	2					12	3
Side plank					:15	2					:15	2					:30	2
V-sit					:10	2					:15	2					:20	2
Notes																		

Client Goals

1. _____
2. _____
3. _____

Training Guidelines

Always warm up. Include a general warm-up (~8 minutes cardio at 40–60% HRmax) and a specific warm-up (50% 1RM for 10–15 reps).

Resistance training 3 times/week with cardiorespiratory training 3 times/week on off days.

Recovery day on Sunday.

Program Breakdown

	Sunday	Monday	Tuesday	Wednesday	Thursday	Friday	Saturday
Resistance training		Day 1		Day 2		Day 3	
Cardiorespiratory training			Day 1		Day 2		Day 3

Cardiorespiratory Training Guidelines

Day 1: Steady-state cardio for 30–45 minutes at 75–85% HRmax.

Day 2: Graded exercise for 15–20 minutes. Perform a light jog starting at a 1-degree incline, go up 1 degree every 2 minutes.

Day 3: High-intensity intervals for 10–15 minutes at a 1:1 work-to-rest ratio (1-min intervals at 90% HRmax).

Flexibility Guidelines

Stretch after each workout.

Complete standing pectoral stretch, cobra stretch, modified hurdler's stretch, overhead triceps stretch, cat stretch, standing calf stretch, cross-body posterior deltoid stretch, standing quad stretch, lat stretch.

FIGURE 13.2 Sample client program card.

Company information and logo here

are going to support the client, from the greeting all the way to the end of the session.

• When you meet a client for the first session, greet him or her and establish rapport. Start with small talk, perhaps about the weather, his or her kids, or simply how the day is going. Move into the exercise session in a way that suits the client's mood and personality. For example, if a client is lacking self-confidence, you might say how pleased you are to see him or her and acknowledge that the person should be proud of just being there. If, on the other hand, the client is always stressed and pressed for time, you can move more quickly into the session and facilitate stress reduction through slower movements and focused breathing. Refer back to chapter 1 for indications on how best to work with each client based on his or her personality characteristics.

• The goal of the first session is to orient the client to the program and lay the foundation for future sessions by teaching correct technique and increasing the client's self-confidence. If you have designed a program that should take 50 to 60 minutes to complete, you will need at least twice as long to go through the program the first time because you will have to demonstrate the exercises and make corrections throughout. To avoid feeling rushed as you guide your client through the first session, be prepared to reduce the number of exercises you introduce.

• To save time, have the client start the warm-up and use that time to preview what you will be doing during the session so that she or he knows what to expect. Ask the client whether any changes in health have occurred. Remind the client to tell you about any injuries sustained outside the training environment so that you can make the necessary adjustments.

• During the first session, you will have to orient clients to the program, show them where they can find the equipment, and demonstrate how to use the equipment (adjust seat height, remove and replace collars on a barbell, and so on). Your clients will likely be training without you from time to time, so they need to feel confident making those adjustments by themselves. If the program card does not have images, you should provide small illustrations or stick figures to help clients remember how to perform the exercise if the equipment does not

have such illustrations (weight machines typically do, whereas free weights do not). Include space on the program card where you can note adjustments in a logical way.

• After clients understand the equipment, you will have to demonstrate correct technique using cues that they will easily remember and relating the exercise to some benefit in their daily lives (e.g., "The barbell deadlift can help make picking up your children easier."). You can then allow clients to perform the exercise on their own. Clients must be able to perform the exercise correctly before you apply any additional challenges (i.e., increased resistance or intensity). Before proceeding to the next exercise, summarize the exercise and reinforce the effort the client has put forth.

After going through the entire program, ask clients whether they have any questions. Finish the session on a positive note by saying something like, "Great work! You really understand the need for good technique, especially on the squat. Do you have any questions before we wrap up?"

In subsequent training sessions, you need to continue to correct exercises and reinforce proper technique. Continually challenge clients by introducing new exercises or variations of existing exercises every few sessions. Demonstrations may not be necessary if the client already knows how to complete the exercise properly, but you should still give a demo for any significant changes or new exercises. Make sure that the client is ready for the challenge. If the change is significant, have the client try the exercise with little or no resistance first and then add resistance slowly.

When delivering training programs, something will inevitably occur that you are not expecting. As the saying goes, expect the unexpected. Even if you do not know exactly how to deal with the situation, you need to react in a calm and professional manner.

In general, when something unexpected comes up, remain calm, assess the situation, and (without reacting too quickly) respond with the most appropriate action. A helpful approach is to imagine what the most experienced and professional Personal Training Specialist would do in the same situation.

Summary of Main Points

1. As a Personal Training Specialist, you are responsible for your client's understanding of the program.

2. Explain the rationale for the program and make sure that your client understands how it addresses his or her goals, needs, and abilities.

3. Demonstrating (or demoing) new exercises or variations in a program is important for a client's learning.

4. You should chart the details of every client workout.

5. At the first training session, set aside time to review your client's file and history to determine how you are going to support her or his overall fitness journey.

Key Concepts for Study

Program card

Spotting

Cue

Coach

Progressive overload

Review Questions

1. List three important guidelines to follow when giving technique cues to clients.

2. What goal or goals should the Personal Training Specialist have for the first session with a client?

3. When demonstrating an exercise, what is the most important reason for going slowly at first?

   a. to make the exercise as challenging as possible for the client

   b. to make it is easier to cue

   c. to emphasize movement sequencing

   d. to allow the client to watch her- or himself in the mirror

4. Nonverbal cues can be supplemented with verbal cues to enhance

   a. coaching

   b. skill acquisition

   c. movement

   d. understanding

5. If the client cannot grasp the performance of a given exercise by the cues given, the Personal Training Specialist should

   a. keep going with the same cues and hope that the client gets it eventually

   b. stop the exercise and attempt to assess the root cause

   c. show the client again and instruct him or her to perform it just as you did

   d. stop the exercise immediately and move on to a different activity

6. To incorporate the principle of progressive overload, the Personal Training Specialist should

   a. always train a muscle to failure

   b. gradually decrease volume or intensity of exercise to limit negative adaptation

   c. gradually increase volume or intensity of exercise to realize ongoing adaptations

   d. give the client a higher amount of load than she or he can lift comfortably

7. What is the foremost reason for charting clients' workouts?

   a. A chart is a useful tool for clients who are visual learners.

b. The Personal Training Specialist can make appropriate adjustments if the program doesn't produce the desired outcome.

c. The Personal Training Specialist can track any injuries that clients might incur.

d. A chart provides a detailed record of performance that can be evaluated over time.

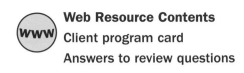

Web Resource Contents

Client program card

Answers to review questions

Injury Recognition and Prevention Strategies

Terry Kane, BPHE, BSc

LEARNING OUTCOMES

After completing this chapter, you will be able to

1. distinguish two types of pain that a client could experience;

2. define scope of practice and the implication for how you handle clients with undiagnosed pain;

3. define and describe the two types of musculoskeletal injuries that a client could experience;

4. describe and differentiate an acute musculoskeletal injury from an overuse musculoskeletal injury;

5. define and differentiate the signs of an injury and the symptoms of an injury;

6. define the goals and action steps you should take as a Personal Training Specialist in the management of acute and overuse injuries;

7. identify what to do if a client asks for your recommendations for undiagnosed pain or asks for your recommendations about treatment that she or he is receiving for an injury;

8. identify the importance and rationale behind securing written authorization from a qualified health professional before having an injured client resume exercising;

9. identify and differentiate the two categories of risk factors for common musculoskeletal injuries; and

10. identify what steps you can take to prevent both acute and overuse injuries.

At some point in your career as a Personal Training Specialist, one of your clients will complain to you of pain before, during, or following a training session. This chapter is intended to educate you on how to manage this situation in the most appropriate manner. The information contained in this chapter will not only empower you with strategies to advise your clients on what to do but also help you use this information to prevent injuries.

Not unlike a fire alarm, pain is a message that originates somewhere in the body to indicate a lack of normal tissue function or homeostasis. Essentially, pain is how the body tells us that something is wrong and needs investigation and possible treatment.

The two types of pain are categorized by their origin. Both can result in permanent disability or even death if ignored or mismanaged.

1. **Mechanical pain** is the result of damage to the musculoskeletal system in which pain is created by a mechanical action or motion (e.g., falling from a ladder to the floor).
2. **Systemic pain** is the result of a disease, infection, or medical condition (e.g., rheumatoid arthritis, heart disease).

Given the number of systemic conditions that can cause pain, and the specificity of treatment for each condition, the remainder of this chapter focuses specifically on mechanical musculoskeletal pain.

Understanding Scope of Practice

Scope of practice refers to the actions for which a person has been educated and is considered competent to perform, usually following successful completion of an examination by a recognized professional or academic organization. For a Personal Training Specialist, this is focused primarily on the development and delivery of safe and effective physical activity programs, and is referred to as the *Standards of Practice*, as outlined earlier in this text. Diagnosing the source of pain remains the domain of physicians and other qualified health professionals.

Despite your experience and knowledge, diagnosing a client's pain is beyond the scope of practice of a Personal Training Specialist. Given the potential for permanent disability and possibly death from either a delayed diagnosis or mistreatment, any client who reports undiagnosed pain to you should be referred to a physician. Further exercise should be postponed until medical clearance has been given by a physician or another qualified health professional (e.g., physical therapist) to resume it.

 Musculoskeletal injuries vary in their presentation, symptoms, severity, and treatment. Despite your personal experience, a client with persistent or undiagnosed pain should be referred to a physician or other qualified health professional.

Types of Musculoskeletal Injury

The two categories of musculoskeletal injury are defined by their mechanism of injury and onset of symptoms.

1. An **acute injury** results from the application of a single force or load, creating tissue damage and leading to immediate pain and dysfunction.
2. An **overuse injury** results from repetitive loading, leading to the gradual onset of pain and dysfunction over days or weeks.

Although both categories of injury are mechanical in origin, their symptoms and treatment differ depending on the injured tissue and severity of injury. To help you educate and direct your injured clients, the following sections describe a number of details specific to each category of musculoskeletal injury.

Acute Injuries

Acute injuries result from the application of a single force that exceeds the threshold of tensile strength of the loaded tissue, creating tissue damage and generating immediate pain. Table 14.1 gives examples of acute injuries that might affect various tissues. Determining the tensile strength of one tissue from another or from one person to another is impossible. Rather than assuming that all clients have the same capacity to exercise and giving them the same exercise program, the default in personal training is to err on the side of caution and individualize exercise programs to prevent injuries. A client's age, family medical history, personal medical history, and previous injuries can raise or lower the threshold of tissue strength and consequently change the risk of acute injury. As a result, Personal Training Specialists are required to have each client complete a PAR-Q+ form. You need to conduct an initial screening and assessment of each client before designing an exercise program.

Signs and Symptoms of Acute Injuries

Clients typically describe their injury based on how the injury feels (symptoms) and the resulting effect of the injury (signs). Symptoms of an acute injury can include one or more of the following: immediate pain, stiffness, muscle spasm, and tenderness to touch. Signs of an acute injury can include one or more of the following: immediate swelling at the injury site, bruising, redness and increased warmth at the injury site, loss of normal function at the injury site, loss of muscle strength, and loss of motion.

Immediate Management of Acute Injury

The two goals in the immediate management of an acute injury are minimizing the tissue damage and controlling the inflammatory response associated with the injury. The time required to recover from an acute injury depends largely on how well these goals are achieved in the 72-hour window of time following injury. Excessive inflammation that is allowed to establish itself at the site of injury can compound the effect of the injury, add additional treatment time to reduce it, and delay a return to full activity.

Based on these two goals and the importance of the initial 72-hour window, the following actions are encouraged in the event of an acute injury.

1. **Professional medical opinion**—Despite your personal experience and knowledge of injuries, any client with acute undiagnosed pain should be referred to a physician for a diagnosis as soon as possible. Musculoskeletal injuries vary in their presentation, symptoms, treatment, and severity and can result in a neurovascular injury (i.e., nerve, artery, or vein injury) that could lead to permanent disability and even death.

2. **Rest**—Discontinue any activity known to aggravate the condition and restrict motion through the injured tissue. This approach facilitates the formation of early repair tissue (primitive scar) at the site of injury, which is part of the body's healing process. Length of rest varies depending on the injured tissue and severity of injury.

3. **Ice**—Applying ice reduces the immediate inflammatory response, swelling, and pain. The frequency and duration of icing depend on how superficial the injured tissue is to the surface, how sensitive the patient is to cold temperatures, and whether the person has any medical condition for which icing would be considered contraindicated, such as lack of sensation to temperature or peripheral vascular disease. As a rule, ice should not be applied for longer than 20 minutes at a time and should not be reapplied until the tissue has regained full sensation (i.e., the area previously iced is no longer numb to the touch). When using a chemical ice pack instead of real ice, you should wrap it in a towel or cloth and visually inspect the skin periodically to prevent potential damage to the skin and nerves.

4. **Compression**—Compression of the injured tissues prevents swelling. Any time the injured tissue is below the level of the heart (e.g., leg injury), it should have some form of external compression

TABLE 14.1 Examples of Acute Injuries

Tissue	Injury	Possible mechanism of injury	Clinical diagnosis (made only by a medical professional)
Bone	Fracture	Tripping and falling on an outstretched arm	Fracture of distal radius
Ligament	Sprain	Rolling an ankle by falling off a piece of balance equipment	Sprained anterior talofibular ligament in ankle
Muscle	Strain	Rapid contraction during a plyometric exercise	Strained hamstring
Tendon	Rupture	Sudden lunge or plyometric exercise	Ruptured Achilles tendon

stocking or wrap on it. If a client changes posture, such as by lying down, and elevates the injured tissue above the heart, compression is no longer necessary. If the client lowers the injured tissue below the heart, then some form of compression would be helpful in minimizing the swelling.

5. **Elevation**—Elevating the injured tissue above the heart helps minimize swelling and is therefore encouraged if doing so is at all possible.

 Ice should not be applied for longer than 20 minutes at a time. If using a chemical ice pack, wrap it in a towel or cloth and take extra care to monitor the skin for potential damage.

Thus, the most effective strategy for managing an acute injury is (1) to see a physician as soon as possible; (2) unload and rest the injured tissue immediately; (3) lie down to elevate and ice the injured tissue; and (4) apply a compression bandage, wrap, or sleeve any time the injured tissue is below the level of the heart.

 The mnemonic **RICE** is a helpful way to remember the steps to managing acute injuries: rest, ice, compression, and elevation.

Responsibilities of the Personal Training Specialist

If your client experiences an acute injury, you should take the following steps to protect the client's health and prevent liability for further injury.

1. If your client has *not been examined by a physician*, getting that done should be your first recommendation.

2. If your client has seen a physician, you should know what the diagnosis is and whether the physician has endorsed continued exercise under your guidance. For your own liability protection and that of your facility, you should discontinue exercising with any injured client until you receive written endorsement from a qualified health professional.

3. If your client is currently undergoing treatment for an acute injury, you should ask the client to contact the treating qualified health professional to

determine whether exercising with you is indicated or contraindicated at that time. Because of privacy laws in Canada and the United States, other qualified health professionals cannot discuss a patient's injury with you without written permission to do so—an authorization form signed by the physician and the patient (your client). The most effective route to get feedback on your client's injury and exercise program is to give your client a copy of the exercise program and have him or her ask the other qualified health professional whether he or she is ready to resume training with you. To reduce the risk of complicating any injury, you should postpone any exercise program until you have written permission provided by your client's physician or another qualified health professional.

4. Unless otherwise instructed by the physician or other qualified health professional, you should recommend that your client continue intermittently icing the injury until the site of injury is no longer stiff and does not appear swollen, bruised, red, or warm to the touch. Although some clients may prefer to apply heat to an injury, heat increases blood flow to the injured tissue, can increase swelling, and may delay a return to full activity.

Overuse Injuries

Overuse injuries result from repetitive tissue loading over time in which no single load is sufficient to cause significant tissue damage and immediate pain. If the motion or exercise is repeated without adequate time to recover, tissue damage and inflammation will accumulate and ultimately cause discomfort and pain.

As with an acute injury, the presence of intrinsic risk factors such as muscle tightness, muscle weakness, history of injury, and altered biomechanics can increase the risk of an overuse injury (see table 14.2). Extrinsic risk factors such as running shoes that don't fit properly can also increase the risk of overuse injury. A common example of an overuse injury is **carpal tunnel syndrome**, which is the result of repetitive computer keyboard work day after day without sufficient recovery time.

Signs and Symptoms of Overuse Injuries

Symptoms of an overuse injury include one or more of the following: low-grade discomfort at the site of the injury, discomfort in activities of daily living other than exercise (such as descending stairs or sleeping), sensation of stiffness at the site of the injury, tenderness to touch, and progression in the intensity of pain with continued exercise or activity. Signs of an overuse injury include one or more of the following: alteration of normal biomechanics to avoid pain (e.g., limping downstairs to avoid patello-femoral pain), swelling, and loss of pain-free motion with normal activities.

Immediate Management of Overuse Injuries

The low level of pain and gradual onset associated with overuse injuries often mislead clients into believing that their pain

- is insignificant,
- will go away by itself, and
- does not require medical attention.

During the initial 72-hour window following the onset of pain or discomfort, clients are encouraged to rest and ice the injured tissues as outlined earlier in the section on acute injury.

The distinguishing feature of an overuse injury is the persistence of pain beyond 72 hours. Many common overuse injuries involve soft tissues located within 2.5 centimetres of a joint (e.g., pain at the elbow where the tendons of the forearm muscles attach). As a default, medical attention should be sought in the event of any undiagnosed slow-onset pain if it persists longer than three days and is noticeable in activities of daily living (e.g., walking, sitting, dressing, washing, sleeping). Under these circumstances, a physician should investigate the pain before the client returns to any exercise or sport known to trigger the pain. In the event that the client's pain occurs only with certain exercises, she or he should stop executing these exercises for 14 days and see a physician (or other qualified health professional) if the pain returns.

After clients have written permission from a qualified health professional to return to exercise, they need to be educated to the fact that despite the absence of pain, they may be vulnerable to reinjury for three to six months (depending on the injury). Although your clients can and should exercise during this period, they need to

- modify their training program,
- explore changes to their exercise technique or equipment, and
- monitor their symptoms with any progression in training volume.

Continuing to exercise or perform any activity that reproduces pain will make the injury worse and can result in permanent disability.

TABLE 14.2 Examples of Overuse Injuries

Tissue	Injury	Possible mechanism of injury	Clinical diagnosis (made only by a medical professional)
Bone	Fracture	Long-distance running	Tibial stress fracture
	Periostitis	Overuse of forearm Faulty mechanics in tennis	Epicondylitis (tennis elbow)
Tendon	Inflammation	Running on uneven terrain or in poor shoes	Achilles tendinitis
	Inflammation	Overuse in overhead movements	Shoulder impingement
Fascia	Inflammation	Repetitive trauma to foot with poor biomechanical support	Plantar fasciitis
	Inflammation	Friction of IT band at lateral femoral epicondyle	IT band friction
Cartilage	Inflammation	Repetitive weight-bearing or impact activity on degenerative joint	Osteoarthritis
	Inflammation	Repetitive load on a bent knee Biomechanical malalignment	Patellofemoral pain
Bursa	Inflammation	Repetitive load	Greater trochanteric bursitis
Skin	Inflammation	Friction between layers of skin	Blisters

Injury Prevention Strategies

As a Personal Training Specialist, you will have the trust of your clients in designing safe, appropriate, and progressive exercise programs that ensure their health and safety. Given that each client has a unique medical history, current health profile, and experience with exercise, you are responsible for identifying all risks of injury and preventing their occurrence.

Prevention of Acute Injuries

In terms of injury prevention, two categories of risk factors warrant consideration: intrinsic factors and extrinsic factors.

- **Intrinsic risk factors** are those that affect the tensile strength of a tissue during exercise and increase the risk of injury. These factors are personal to the client, such as muscle weakness, muscle inflexibility, muscle imbalances, joint laxity, discrepancy in leg length, psychological state of mind, and cognitive function. Other intrinsic risk factors that can increase the client's risk include a history of previous injury of the same body part or surrounding area, degenerative changes such as arthritis, history of surgery at the injury site, and the use of medications that can alter the perception of pain or reduce the client's ability to monitor the intensity of exercise accurately (e.g., beta blockers—a class of medication that slows the heart rate to treat abnormal heart rhythms and other conditions).

- **Extrinsic risk factors** are external to the client's physical and psychological status. They include environmental factors such as temperature and humidity, exercise equipment, and fitness apparel and footwear worn by the client.

As a Personal Training Specialist, you are responsible for preventing acute injuries by following these steps:

- Profile your client for the presence of any intrinsic risk factors.
- Use the client profile (PAR-Q+, interview, screening, and assessment findings) to select the safest and most appropriate exercises.
- Use the profile to determine safe and appropriate exercises for your client (use FITT principles: frequency, intensity, time, and type).

- Ensure that your client is instructed on proper technique in all exercises, including warming up and cooling down.
- Ensure that your client can independently demonstrate proper execution of all exercises, including safe operation of any associated exercise equipment (e.g., turning a treadmill on and off, setting up resistance training equipment, and so on).
- Ensure the safety of the exercise environment by maintaining all exercise equipment in proper working order (e.g., making sure that all safety features are fully operational).

Prevention of Overuse Injuries

Prevention strategies for overuse injuries focus on three concepts. In short, you should educate the client, choose the proper dose of exercise, and progress the exercise program wisely.

Client Education

In many cases, overuse injuries are preventable by communicating well with your clients and educating them. As mentioned earlier, a low-grade ache can turn into an overuse injury through continued participation in activity and aggravation of the original tissue damage. The concept of stopping exercise is particularly difficult for clients who believe in the old saying "No pain, no gain." Unfortunately, clients who believe in this saying commonly don't report

When noticing what seems to be an overuse injury in your client, you may feel frustrated, as the injury could affect your programming and your client's ability to achieve his or her goals. In these situations, remember to remain nonjudgmental and ask yourself these two questions:

1. Did you educate your clients about the importance of not exercising with pain?
2. Did you create an environment where your clients thought that they could acknowledge their pain to you?

Refer back to chapter 1 for descriptions of key qualities that a Personal Training Specialist should possess in order to build a trusting rapport with clients.

their pain. They continue to aggravate their injury until it's too late. The result is that they require medical treatment and time off to heal. One of the most important steps in preventing an overuse injury is to educate clients from the outset that there is *no gain with pain.* You also need to create an environment where clients feel comfortable telling you that they are sore without fear of ridicule or embarrassment.

Dose and Volume of Exercise

One of the most important physiological qualities we possess is the ability of the body to repair itself from damage and to adapt at any age. Whether your client is 20 years old or 80 years old, he or she has the capacity to undergo physiological adaptations to exercise. But age, family medical history, and personal medical history affect the capacity for change and the degree of potential change.

The primary cause of overuse injuries is an imbalance between the physiological tissue damage created by an exercise or motion and the degree of tissue repair that is achieved before repeating the exercise. Administering exercise is not unlike prescribing a medication. The key to preventing overuse injuries is ensuring that both the selected exercise and the volume of exercise are appropriate for the client, specifically in terms of frequency, intensity, and volume. Note that frequency refers to the number of times per week that a client can safely exercise without sustaining injury. This quantity depends largely on the intensity and volume of exercise in a given workout. The more intense and greater the volume of exercise is in a given workout, the more time is required for tissues to recover and repair before the workout is repeated. Volume refers not only to the duration or number of repetitions of a given exercise but also to the number of exercises for a given muscle group in the workout (e.g., squats, leg presses, and knee extensions all work the quadriceps and load the patella-femoral joint).

Before clients reattempt a given workout program or exercise, they should be entirely free of pain in the given muscle and surrounding joints. If clients are still experiencing pain or discomfort before a workout, they need more time to repair and recover before exercising the painful muscle group or joint.

Given the potential to create injury, encouraging clients to work through pain is negligent and unprofessional. Therefore, the key to preventing overuse injuries is recognizing the importance of selecting the most appropriate exercises for your client's profile and the safest dose of exercise.

Progressing a Training Program

When it comes to progressing an exercise program, you need to appreciate the physiological capacity of your clients to adapt to exercise. To avoid an imbalance, the rate of progression should not exceed the client's rate of adaptability for her or his age and health profile. For example, if a client has the capacity to adapt at 10% per week and you increase the exercise program by 20%, at some point in time the imbalance may result in tissue damage, inflammation, and pain. For most clients, 10% per week is a safe maximum increase in exercise. To reduce the risk of overuse injury in a new client with whom you are unfamiliar, err on the side of safety and limit any progression in a given exercise program to 10% per week in either intensity (load, resistance, speed) or volume (repetitions, sets, duration), but not both.

As a Personal Training Specialist, you have the responsibility of preventing an overuse injury by following these steps:

- Educate your clients about the consequences of exercising through pain.
- Educate your clients that exercising a painful muscle or joint will likely only make their pain worse and potentially force them to discontinue that exercise.
- Create an environment where clients are under no pressure to exercise with pain.
- Ask your clients before every training session whether they are pain free. If they are not, you must modify their program for that workout to avoid aggravating their injury and creating more pain.
- Profile your clients (PAR-Q+, interview, screening, and assessment findings) for the presence of any intrinsic risk factors, particularly excessive muscle tightness or any biomechanical abnormality that may arise through highly repetitive exercises or motions.
- Ensure that any equipment used by your clients fits well and is in good operational condition.
- Use the client profile to select the most appropriate exercises.

- Use the client profile to determine the dose (frequency, intensity, volume) of exercise.
- Using your profile, educate your clients about a safe and appropriate rate of exercise progression.
- Use appropriate forms to document injuries that your clients may have. A blank form is provided in the web resource and forms are also available through canfitpro INTERACTIVE (www.canfitprointeractive.com).

 See the web resource at www.HumanKinetics.com/FoundationsOfProfessionalPersonalTraining for a form to document a client's injury.

Summary of Main Points

1. Clients may at times complain of pain with exercise training.
2. As a Personal Training Specialist, you cannot ignore pain, nor can you diagnose or recommend treatment. You must stay within your scope of practice and act in the best interest of the client at all times.
3. If a client reports undiagnosed complaints of pain, you should refer the client to a physician.
4. If a client is undergoing treatment for an injury or has recently been discharged from treatment for an injury, you should secure written authorization from the treating qualified health professional before resuming training of the injured joint or muscle.
5. As a Personal Training Specialist, you can play a significant role in helping your clients manage their injuries by taking appropriate steps immediately, referring injured clients to a physician or other qualified health professional, and educating clients effectively.
6. Personal Training Specialists play a significant role in preventing musculoskeletal injuries by screening clients for potential risk factors, creating safe and appropriate exercise program designs, and ensuring a safe and effective training environment.

Key Concepts for Study

Scope of practice
Acute injury
Overuse injury
Sprain
Strain

Sign
Symptom
RICE (rest, ice, compression, and elevation)
Intrinsic risk factor
Extrinsic risk factor

Review Questions

1. Name four things that the Personal Training Specialist needs to know about the client to assess the risk of an acute injury.

2. Describe the two categories of risk factors that can lead to an overuse injury.

3. Which of the following is not indicated for a Personal Training Specialist to suggest in the event of an undiagnosed acute injury?

   a. securing a professional medical opinion

   b. resting the injured tissue

   c. heating the injured tissue

   d. compressing the injured tissue

4. Which type of pain occurs specifically because of disease, infection, or a medical condition?

   a. chronic pain

   b. acute pain

   c. mechanical pain

   d. systemic pain

5. Which of the following is *not* helpful in working with a client who has a history of a recent overuse injury?

   a. Secure a letter from an appropriate qualified health professional authorizing exercise for the affected injury.

   b. Explore changes to the exercise technique or equipment to reduce the chance of reinjury.

   c. Modify the training program to avoid that area.

   d. Recommend that the client take pain medication before exercising.

6. Which one of the following is an example of an acute injury?

   a. bursitis

   b. tendinitis

   c. stress fracture

   d. none of the above

7. A strain is damage to underlying _____, and a sprain is damage to underlying _____.

   a. bone; tendon

   b. muscle; ligament

   c. muscle; tendon

   d. tendon; ligament

Web Resource Contents

Form to document injury

Answers to review questions

15

Business of Personal Training

Mike Bates, MBA

LEARNING OUTCOMES

After completing this chapter, you will be able to

1. identify and explain the 4 Ps of marketing;

2. identify various pricing structures;

3. explain the pros and cons of various types of promotional efforts;

4. explain the steps you can take when selling your services;

5. identify how to build your clientele through referrals;

6. identify the key aspects of your professional image;

7. explain the best way to terminate a relationship;

8. identify the key aspects of risk management;

9. understand when you need to have insurance; and

10. explain policies and procedures.

As a Personal Training Specialist, you are running your own business. Whether you are working inside or outside a fitness club, it is ultimately your responsibility to market your services, make your sales pitch, keep your records and paperwork in order, develop and enforce policies and procedures, manage risk, and present yourself in a professional manner. It is true that some clubs will assist you in many of these areas, but your success will eventually come down to your ability to master them yourself. This chapter provides an overview of what you need to know in order to be successful in the business side of personal training.

Career Opportunities

Personal Training Specialists work in many capacities and are compensated in many ways. Each opportunity can be considered based on your preferences and expectations.

One of the most popular ways to get started in the fitness industry is to work as a Personal Training Specialist in a fitness centre. In this role, trainers either are paid by the hour or split their revenue with the club (e.g., club takes 50% and trainer takes 50% on any money collected from the trainer's clients). This is an ideal starting point for most entry-level trainers for the following reasons:

- It provides access to the established clientele of the club.
- Working at an hourly rate can often allow you to get paid before you have your own clientele.
- It provides access to a large amount and variety of equipment.
- There is minimal financial risk for you.
- The club will assist in marketing and selling your personal training services.
- Administrative support (e.g., scheduling, bookkeeping) is normally offered by the club.
- Insurance should be provided if the club is paying you.
- Training, continuing education, and support will likely be provided by the club.

Additional considerations when working for a fitness club include the following:

- Revenue is normally split with the club.
- You may have other duties at the club.
- Hours may not be as flexible as you would prefer.
- You are accountable to your supervisor and club.
- You are competing with other trainers for the same clientele.

A second potential job position has you working in a personal training or small-group training studio. In this situation the only people who use the studio are those who are paying for personal training. These locations are normally smaller than the average fitness club and cater only to people who are interested in personal or small-group training. Some of the advantages of this type of situation are as follows:

- The company helps you attract clients.
- The studio already has the equipment you will need.
- Insurance is provided if the studio is paying you.
- Training might be offered by the company.

Additional considerations when working in a personal training studio include the following:

- You have to split your profits with the company.
- Equipment is limited due to space limitations.
- You are accountable to your supervisor and studio.
- Hours may not be as flexible as you would like.

A third option for Personal Training Specialists is to work as a contract, or freelance, trainer. In these situations, you are running your own business. This might be in a private studio of your own, in clients' homes, as a mobile trainer, or in a fitness club to which you pay rent in order to use its facility. Some of the advantages of this approach include the following:

- You are self-employed.
- You can set your own hours.
- You may not have to share your revenue.

- You have more control and can decide how you want to run your business.

Additional considerations include the following:

- You must pay startup and ongoing expenses.
- You need to find your own clients and do your own marketing.
- You have to assume some financial risk.
- You need to have some entrepreneurial business skills.
- You need to purchase insurance.

As you can see, there are many options when it comes to working as a Personal Training Specialist in the fitness industry. You need to decide what is best for you and your particular situation. If you are unsure about where to start, you can always ask people who are working in the field for their thoughts and mentorship.

Marketing Your Services

When you get started in the fitness industry, clients will not be walking up to you offering to pay you for your services. To acquire clients, you will need to market your services so that potential clients are aware of you and what you can offer them. The traditional way to look at marketing is to break the process into four areas—product, price, promotions, and place. Also known as the *4 Ps of marketing,* these areas form the core of your marketing plan. The marketing plan is the comprehensive action plan that will generate clients for your business. In this chapter we take a closer look at the 4 Ps of marketing and how you can apply them to your personal training business.

Product

For our purposes, the product is actually you and your services. To be successful, you need to have a firm understanding of your product and how to set yourself apart from your competition. Based on the work of Mullin, Hardy, and Sutton (1999), we explore three factors to consider when looking at your product: differentiation, development, and positioning.

Differentiation is your ability to separate yourself from other personal trainers and make yourself unique. An example of this is a trainer who has some special educational experiences (e.g., university degree or specialized training), a unique workout, a focused client base (e.g., seniors, people looking to lose weight, people with no time), or special personal characteristics (e.g., being a great motivator). The more you can differentiate yourself, the more likely you are to be remembered. The concept of differentiation is a key starting point for all Personal Training Specialists as they consider what it will take for them to be successful.

In terms of *development,* it is critical that you constantly look for ways to offer new programming ideas or information that will keep clients motivated and working toward their goals. Here are just a few of the many ways to come up with ideas:

- Attend conferences and workshops.
- Ask your clients what they are looking for.
- Join industry groups and associations to keep up on trends and to network.
- Look at other industries to see what is working for them and then determine whether you can use similar ideas in your business.

The fitness industry is constantly changing, and we are continually finding new and better ways for people to improve their health and achieve their fitness goals. Generating new ideas for you and your clients is critical to your long-term success in the industry. Most successful trainers agree that one of the keys to their success is their ability to continually reeducate themselves and then incorporate this new information into how they work with their clients.

Positioning is the perception that people have about you and your business. This perception can be based on what they see in marketing, how you present yourself at your facility, or how others speak of you. Each of these factors leaves an image in a potential customer's mind. It is critical that you spend time thinking about the image you want people to have of you. Ask yourself what image you want to set and what message you want to communicate. It is crucial to ensure that you are consistent in your approach to positioning. People need to know what to expect and are looking for consistency. Every aspect of marketing that follows is done with this image in mind.

Price

There are many ways to price your services. Pricing for personal training will vary based on many factors, including geographic location, your experience and education, and the number of other personal trainers available. Generally speaking, you will be able to charge more for personal training in certain areas based on the cost of living and the economy in those areas. Trainers with more experience and education are also able to charge more for their services; the only stipulation is that you need to show people what they will get with this added experience and education.

The final factor to consider when setting a pricing structure for your services is the amount of competition you have, or the number of options potential clients have for personal training services. As with any other service or product, the fewer options customers have, the more they will have to pay. This is an example of demand outpacing supply. If there are more clients demanding personal training than there are personal trainers, the few trainers who are available will be able to charge a premium for their services. If you are competing against other trainers, you will need to take into consideration their rates and their services. As competition increases, clients will be able to consider all of the personal trainers available. A highly competitive market for personal training will normally force trainers to charge similar prices since clients often shop around for the best value. In these situations it is critical that you be able to sell yourself and differentiate yourself from other trainers.

Most Personal Training Specialists will sell their services as either individual sessions or packages of 10 or 20 sessions or sometimes more. Most of the time clients receive a discount based on the number of sessions that they purchase. Here is a potential pricing structure:

1 session	$50
10 sessions	$450 ($45 per session)
20 sessions	$800 ($40 per session)

Traditional sessions are about 55 minutes in duration to allow time to prepare and set up for the next client, but many trainers also offer 30-minute sessions that appeal to time-limited clients. Since 30-minute sessions are less expensive than 55-minute sessions, they may also help you address clients' concerns about the costs of higher-priced sessions. If the previous pricing structure were used, a 30-minute session could be priced in the following way:

1 session	$35
10 sessions	$300 ($30 per session)
20 sessions	$500 ($25 per session)

In theory, trainers should be able to make more money if they have clients training in 30-minute intervals because they are able to train more people and generate more income per hour.

Although these have traditionally been the most common ways to price sessions, they are not the only pricing structures. Small-group training is another approach to personal training that has increased in popularity in recent years. These types of sessions are normally conducted in small groups (2-4) but can be organized however the trainer wants. In small-group sessions there is normally a lower price per person, but overall the trainer will be generating more money than in a single-person session. Group training works best when

- the trainer has created a 4- to 10-week program based on a challenge or goal,
- clients have come together or have organized themselves, or
- the trainer has found clients with similar fitness goals.

One way to price group sessions is as follows:

Two people (20 sessions 45-55 minutes per session). Each person pays $300, for a total of $600 ($30 per session).

Four people (20 sessions at 45-55 minutes per session). Each person pays $250, for a total of $1,000 ($50 per session).

Pricing by the session is a common way to sell personal training, but again, it is not the only way. One challenge with this approach is that you constantly need to sell clients new packages as they use up their purchased number of sessions. Additionally, in these situations people are able to use the sessions as they see fit. If they want to take a couple days off or a couple months off in the summer, they can do so, leaving trainers with a gap in their schedule and in their expected income.

There are personal training studios that have had success pricing their sessions by the month. In these situations, clients agree to a set amount each month and also commit to a specific number of sessions in a week. If clients miss a session, they have no way to get their money back. On the positive side, clients may be more committed to their programs knowing that they can't use the sessions at a later date. Clubs may also offer a greater discount to clients who agree to longer contracts with monthly payments. There are many ways to set up monthly payment plans; the one described here is just an example.

As you can see, there are many ways to structure the price of your sessions. In the end it will come down to you and your club deciding what is best based on your situation and the marketplace you are in.

Promotions

You can promote your business in many ways. The following are the most popular ways for Personal Training Specialists to promote themselves:

- Direct mail
- Print ads
- E-marketing
- Social media
- General networking
- Guerilla marketing
- Media relations

When determining which methods are the most appropriate for you, always consider who your target market is. When you start out as a Personal Training Specialist you may not know exactly who you want your target market to be. More than likely, in the beginning, you will work with a variety of clients simply out of availability and necessity. With experience over time, you will develop a better understanding of the type of training you enjoy doing and the particular characteristics you look for in a client. This will help you define your specific target market. Potential target markets for Personal Training Specialists include seniors, athletes, people who have exercised in the past, current exercisers, businesspeople, people who belong to certain organizations, people who subscribe to certain publications, and any other group you can identify. Understanding how your target audience feels about exercise is important as you consider your marketing message. For example, if you work at a downtown fitness club with a large business crowd, your message to this audience will be very different than the message that would be targeted to a residential area with a higher proportion of seniors and families.

Regardless of the method you choose, keep in mind that people may need to see your message numerous times before they will actually remember it and take action. If you are not able to send out numerous messages to your market, then you will need to make sure you have a unique message that will get people to take action right away. For example, you might give a special offer to the first 20 people who call you or give a special discount to anyone who mentions seeing your ad.

Your potential clients are bombarded with marketing messages from thousands of companies each day. What will make you stand out? What will cause your audience to take action by calling you or coming in to see you? You need to ask specific questions before deciding which type of marketing you will choose.

Direct Mail

Direct mail is a form of marketing that is sent directly to potential clients. In general, the more focused or specifically targeted the direct mail is, the better. In this text, we consider direct mail to be anything sent via regular mail, and the actual flyer, letter, or document you design is referred to as a *marketing piece*. This type of marketing is very effective because you are able to focus on specific characteristics. An example of a targeted piece of direct mail is one that is sent to all the postal codes within an 8- to 12-minute drive of your location. If you look at a map of your area and determine how far you can get in all directions in 8- to 12-minutes, you have just found what is referred to as your *isochrone*. Your isochrone is where you will get the majority of your clients. Experts agree that prospects will travel a maximum of around 8- to 12-minutes to join a fitness club. Specifically, your primary market is normally within an 8-minute drive and your secondary market is within a 12-minute drive. Keep in mind that isochrones are based on travel time. If you are in a downtown area where people will walk, then it is an 8- to 12-minute walk.

The isochrone allows you to send marketing pieces to the clients who are most likely to join your club. Experienced Personal Training Specialists might argue that they have clients who travel much farther than this. The reality is that the relationship a trainer has with clients is a unique one. Once you are established, you might find that people do come from much farther, but the isochrone is still the best place to start your marketing efforts.

Other potential targets of direct mail include the following:

- People at a certain income level
- People who belong to a particular group (e.g., downtown business association or employees of a hospital)
- People who attended a particular event (health and wellness show at a local convention centre)
- Past members of a fitness club
- Teachers, lawyers, and so on

The key to direct mail is to get the right offer to the right person. You will need to carefully consider the characteristics of your potential clients as you decide on the most appropriate offer for them.

Advantages

- You can target your message as much or as little as you want.
- You decide how many people you want to send your marketing piece to.
- Marketing pieces can be sent in many ways, including an insert with newspapers and a separate piece mailed through the postal service.

Disadvantages

- Postage and mailing costs can be high if you want to send mail to a large number of people. The more people you send mail to, the higher the cost.
- If you are not comfortable designing your marketing piece, you will need to get help from someone who is.
- If the piece is included as an insert with other material, it may not get enough attention because it is competing against other marketing pieces.

Print Ads

Print or space ads are a form of advertising normally found in newspapers, magazines, and newsletters. With this form of advertising, you have a dedicated space that is normally priced based on size. The bigger the ad, the more expensive it will be. In addition, colour ads are also more expensive than black-and-white ads. Discounts are normally given to those who commit to advertising over a period of time; that is, it is cheaper per ad if you commit to six ads as opposed to just one ad. When advertising in larger newspapers becomes cost prohibitive, you may want to consider smaller magazines and neighbourhood newspapers. These smaller publications might not get your message to as many people, but they might actually be more beneficial. Smaller publications are normally more focused in their content or geographic area, so depending on your goals, they might be more appropriate for you.

Advantages

- Space ads reach more people at a lower price than direct mail. The larger the audience, the more cost effective space ads become.
- Print ads may establish a certain level of credibility for your business if you advertise in publications that are well respected.
- Print ads may be very targeted if you choose a subject-specific magazine (e.g., fitness and health).

Disadvantages

- Costs can be significant for larger publications.
- Marketing research indicates that people need to see an ad numerous times before they actually respond to it.
- Ads may get lost when someone is looking at a page with many things on it.
- You need to have a message that will attract people's attention right away; otherwise, they will simply turn the page.

E-Marketing

In this text, the term *e-marketing* refers to anything that uses technology. Because technology is constantly changing and growing, we focus on the most popular methods.

E-mail is a great way to market your services if you are able to obtain reliable e-mail lists of potential customers. In this way, e-mail is similar to direct mail since you are choosing whom you want to send your message to and then catering that message specifically to them. The major difference between direct mail and e-mail is that e-mail is normally much quicker as well as much more cost effective since you are not paying for postage. On the other hand, e-mail has its limitations since potential prospects and customers likely have software programs known as *spam filters* that limit incoming e-mail from unknown sources. Some very good e-mail marketing companies and software programs are available that can be used at a reasonable price for those who are not technologically savvy. E-mail and traditional direct mail both have the same challenge of overcoming a barrage of competing messages in their given medium. Current and future legislation may also limit your ability to use e-mail because stiff fines may be applied to those who send unsolicited e-mails to prospective clients. It is imperative that you obtain permission to send these people e-mail to ensure you do not put yourself or your business at risk of breaking the law.

Developing your own website is also a great way to use technology in your business. Many great programs are available for those who are not comfortable designing their own web pages. Websites are a great way to provide an unlimited amount of information. Most of the formats we have talked about thus far have space limitations, but space is not an obstacle when it comes to the Internet. We are not saying that you should have so much information on your site that people feel overwhelmed, but you do have many more options with respect to the amount and type of information you can include.

Websites are a great way to post updated information about your business. Many people use their websites as an educational tool to keep their clients motivated and informed. Your options are unlimited when it comes to developing your own site. In the beginning, it is best to keep the site relatively simple. This will allow you to see what your clients are interested in and how they will use the site. One challenge with websites is ensuring the information is up to date and accurate. This is your responsibility. If you want people to use your site for specific reasons, then you will need to make sure those areas are constantly kept up to date. For example, if you are trying to educate people on good eating habits by posting articles every two weeks, then you will need to make sure you do this. Your clients will quickly move away from your site if certain areas are not updated as you intended. Your website is also one of the best place for you to obtain and collect elec-

tronic leads, which also ensure permission has been obtained for sending e-mail. As with e-mail, many companies and software programs are available that can help you with website design and ongoing maintenance.

Advantages
- It is cost effective.
- It allows for quick delivery.
- Responses are easy to track.

Disadvantages
- Spam filters may prevent your message from ever being read.
- Approximately 20% of e-mail users change their address each year.
- Design elements are limited because of spam filters.

Social Media

Social media can be used to supplement, or as an alternative to, creating and maintaining your own website. Generally, social media is free to use but many platforms provide additional paid-for options that allow you to boost your messages and advertising. Social media allows you to connect with your contacts in a more passive way. While not as customizable as email, social media allows you to send large amounts of information at little or no cost. Keep in mind that even though you may post information to social media, your clients may not see the information right away or at all. It is dependent on how often they use social media and how much other information is competing for their attention.

Advantages
- It is cost effective.
- It is targeted.
- Audience or followers can spread the word to a larger network.

Disadvantages
- It requires continual updating.
- It requires creativity.
- Negative comments are not always removable.

General Networking

Making yourself known in your community is another important element of promoting your business. Personal Training Specialists should not feel nervous about letting friends and acquaintances know what they do for a living. This is a great (and free!) way to promote yourself. Close friends and acquaintances are a part of what is known as your *circle of influence,* the group of people you have some sort of contact with or influence over. This influence may be very minor in most situations, but these are still people you know and will most likely want to help you if they can. In these situations it is critical that you have business cards. It is a good rule to always carry a supply of business cards because you never know when you might be able to acquire a new customer or simply get the word out about what you are doing. A common technique for identifying everyone in your circle of influence is to list all friends, family, people you do business with, and so on. A form in the web resource will help you get started. This list is simply a starting point for you to think about all the people you come into contact with. The majority of these people will be more than happy to tell others about what you are doing. If you don't come into personal contact with all of these people regularly, it would be a good idea to send out a note letting them know what you are now doing.

 See the web resource at www.HumanKinetics.com/FoundationsOfProfessionalPersonalTraining for a list to help you identify the people in your circle of influence.

While a list of the people you come into contact with regularly is a great starting point, do not hesitate to mention your services to anyone you meet, if the time and place are appropriate. Remember that you are working in a field that everyone needs to be able to access. The most successful Personal Training Specialists develop a 30-second "elevator pitch" that can be delivered at any time. A well-formulated pitch enables you to quickly convey to a potential client exactly who you are, what you do, and why you do it. This allows people you meet to learn a lot about you in a safe environment without feeling pressured or wasting their time. Many potential clients are held back or nervous because they have no idea where to start, or some might even have negative images of exercise and fitness clubs in their minds. If you can make them feel comfortable, both of you will have the opportunity

to be successful—you because you are getting a new client and them because of the results they will see.

Advantages

- Costs are minimal.
- People in your circle of influence will normally pass the word on to their own circle of influence.
- People are normally more comfortable purchasing from someone they trust, so this obstacle should already be taken care of if you are working within your own group of contacts.

Disadvantages

- Your circle of influence may not be receptive to your business.
- Some people may think you are crossing the line in your relationship with them by trying to sell them something.

Guerilla Marketing

Guerilla marketing is a type of nontraditional marketing that normally you do not have to pay for. The possibilities are limited only by your imagination and the message you want to send to prospective clients. The following are a few examples.

- **Guest passes** or complimentary sessions are a great way to get people to come into your establishment or try your services for the first time. They are normally given free of charge and allow the person to work out with you for free. It is generally suggested that you include a reasonable expiration date on these passes to create a sense of urgency in the potential clients' mind; otherwise, the pass is likely to be put aside and forgotten. Take care in the types of guest passes you use for general marketing and the type of passes you give to actual clients. If too many of the same guest passes are given out, they will eventually lose their value because people will feel they are getting something that anyone can get. One way to overcome this problem is to give one type of pass to prospects and save some special passes for friends of current clients. You should place a higher value on guest passes given to your current clients, partly as a thank-you to them but also because your clients will probably bring a potential client who is more likely to pay for your services after using the guest pass since your current client has most likely spoken highly of you.

- **Information tear-off sheets** are simple information sheets with phone numbers that can be torn off at the bottom. The sheets promote your business in some way and encourage people to call you if they want more information. They can be posted in all kinds of locations, like grocery stores, schools, or any other place that has a community events board. Owners may have restrictions on what they want posted, so it is always a good idea to check with them before posting anything.

- **Joint marketing,** which involves finding other businesses that can help to promote your business, is a great way to attract new clients. Some examples of complementary businesses are nutrition stores, weight-loss clinics, massage therapists, and chiropractors. Other businesses might include grocery stores or other retail outlets. They promote your business (by giving out flyers, posting signage, giving out free passes, and so on), and you in turn promote their business to your clients in some way. In the beginning when you do not have any clients, you may choose to give people some free personal training sessions in exchange for helping you. It's a good idea to implement some type of reward system for the businesses you are working with. For example, whenever someone comes to you based on seeing your information in another business, you could give that business owner a free personal training session. What you give them is not really that important, and you may choose not to give them something every time. The idea is that you are thanking them for helping you so that they are encouraged to keep promoting your business.

- **Lead boxes** are often used in joint marketing initiatives and are a great way to get a high volume of prospects. They are normally placed on countertops at other businesses. Prospects fill out a ballot for a chance to win something, such as 10 free training sessions. Everyone who fills out a ballot is offered something, such as 10% off or one free training session. The more closely the business is aligned with yours, the better. For example, a weight-loss clinic might give you better prospects than a dry cleaner. Either way, you will get a lot of ballots that are difficult to read or that have been filled out by people who are not interested in your service. Be prepared to make lots of phone calls and know that you will need to make many calls to get a few people who are interested in your services.

These are just a few examples of what you can do outside traditional forms of marketing avenues. Some forms of marketing may leave potential customers with a negative image of you and your business, so you will need to carefully consider this possibility when deciding what approach to take. Focus on attracting new clients through your marketing approach and your ability to connect and build relationships.

Advantages

- It has a low cost.
- Many potential clients are available.
- An unlimited number of potential marketing ideas are available.

Disadvantages

- Potential clients may have negative perceptions of some approaches (e.g., leaving guest passes in phone booths or on windshields).
- Some options will require constant follow-up to ensure your partner business is keeping up with their end of the agreement.

Media Outreach

Similar to guerilla marketing, media outreach is normally done for free or at a low cost. The key to successful media outreach is getting your name in the media or in front of a large audience. This can be done in many ways, but here are a few:

- Send out a press release to all media in the area about a particular event.
- Establish yourself as an expert by writing in local publications, speaking on the radio, or getting interviewed on TV.
- Hold open houses and invite the media and influential people from the area.
- Work with well-known people who are in the local news regularly. You might consider giving some of these people free sessions and promoting your program to the media.
- Testimonials from clients are a great way to generate publicity when done correctly.

Advantages

- It should normally come with little cost.
- There is a potential to reach a large audience.
- Information about your business may be presented by a respected person in the media.

Disadvantages

- It might be difficult to establish yourself with local media.
- If events are not planned properly, negative publicity may result.
- You might not see immediate results if publicity is not on a large scale.

Tracking Your Promotion Efforts

All good marketers track the results of their promotion efforts. How else will you know if the time and money you have invested have been well spent? When people call you or come in to see you, you should always ask how they heard about your business.

Each month you should have a running total of where your new clients are coming from. If all of your clients are coming from referrals, is it really necessary to spend a lot of money on direct mail or newspaper ads?

Place

The fitness industry is not unlike many other retail industries in that the location of your business will play a major role in your initial success or failure. You already know that people will not normally drive more than 12 minutes to join a fitness club. Other factors to keep in mind when choosing a location are traffic flow, parking, signage, perception of the neighbourhood, and future potential for expansion. Whether you are looking at opening your own personal training studio or working in a fitness club, your choice of location is an important one.

Successful trainers agree that once you have a dedicated client base, your location is not as important. If your clients have been with you for a long time, they will be willing to drive a little farther to stay with you. This might sound contradictory to the earlier statement about people not being willing to drive more than 12 minutes. This is true of new clients, but if you have a loyal group of clients, the regular rules do not always apply when it comes to location. However, this is not to say that people will be willing to drive an extra hour to an area of the city with no parking and a high crime rate.

Selling Your Services

When most new Personal Training Specialists hear that they have to sell their services, the initial reaction is normally a negative one, and images of pushy, insincere salespeople come to mind. The good news is that if you are to be successful as a Personal Training Specialist, the high-pressure sales approach is not something you need to worry about. This approach might work in the short term, but it will eventually turn people off and hurt your business.

Marketing will bring people to you, but you need to be comfortable selling your services if you want to make a living in this industry. The key to being comfortable with sales is getting people to trust you. If you know and believe in your product and can show prospective clients how it will benefit them, then you have the potential to be good at sales. Luckily, exercise is something that everyone needs, so you do not have to worry about trying to sell people something that they will not benefit from.

The following is a great way to approach people about personal training:

- If you are approaching someone you do not know, it is always a good idea to introduce yourself and tell the person that you are a Personal Training Specialist.
- Next, ask about the person's reasons and goals for working out.
- With this information, you should then be able to determine whether this is someone who might be interested in personal training.
- Once you have a sense of whether the person might be interested, ask if you can tell the person about what you do and how you might be able to help out. Be careful not to assume that people are not interested in your services. We are not suggesting that you be pushy, but you should be optimistic about the prospects of this person becoming a potential client.
- Once you have opened the discussion and you are confident that the person is interested in what you have to say, you can move to the next step, selling your personal training services.

Here is an example of the steps you can follow when selling your services:

1. Focus on the prospective clients and what they want.
2. Show them how you can help them achieve their goals.

3. Develop an action plan that outlines what you will do and the results they will see.

4. Ask for feedback on the plan.

5. Present your prices and ask for the sale.

6. Overcome any objections.

7. Follow up.

Focus on Potential Clients and What They Want

Your first priority should be the prospective clients and what they want to achieve. You need to find out as much as you can about them before trying to sell them anything. This includes not only their specific fitness goals but also their perceptions, fears, and expectations. Throughout this information-gathering stage, you should focus on building trust and getting the client to feel comfortable with you and the surroundings. Remember, people are much more likely to buy from someone they like and trust. Once you have collected all of this information and gotten to know the person, you are ready to talk about your services.

Show How You Can Help Them Achieve Goals

The key to this step is differentiating between features and benefits. Features are characteristics that are specific to you, your services, or your facility, such as a 20-minute workout, five treadmills, and qualified staff. These characteristics are the same regardless of the potential client. Benefits are those characteristics that are specific to the person. A benefit of a 20-minute workout for busy people is that they will be able to fit in a workout. A benefit of qualified staff is that clients do not have to worry about starting a program that will hurt them or that will not work. Benefits should be specific to the information you gathered in step 1 in focusing on potential clients. People will buy from you because of the benefits they perceive they will get. If you build trust with people and show them how they will benefit by working with you, you are well on your way to gaining new clients.

Develop an Action Plan

Once you have communicated the benefits of your program to prospective clients, you will need to tell them exactly what you will do and the results they can expect. When developing this action plan, it is best to use SMART goals. Remember from chapter 1 that SMART stands for the following:

S   specific

M   measurable

A   attainable

R   realistic

T   time sensitive

Use this acronym when setting goals for prospective clients. It is always best to break long-term goals into smaller short-term goals. For example, if your client has the long-term goal to lose 10 kilograms of body fat, a realistic and attainable short-term goal would be to lose 3 to 4 kilograms of body fat in 6 weeks by exercising 4 times a week with a Personal Training Specialist. As another example, here's a goal for a person whose energy level is currently at a 5 on a scale of 1 to 10 and who wants to have more energy: Get to an energy level of 8 in 6 weeks by exercising for at least 30 minutes 4 times a week.

Ask for Feedback

Once you have described the action plan, ask if the client has any questions about it. Several techniques can be used at this point. Many experts will tell you that you should never ask a question that you don't know how the client will answer. Some experts suggest asking only questions where yes is the answer, such as "Wouldn't you feel great if you lost those 4 kilograms in 6 weeks?" It is up to you to use whatever techniques you are comfortable with. You want to make sure you have answered any major concerns or questions before moving on to the next step.

Present Your Prices and Ask for the Sale

Once you have answered all of the questions related to the action plan and your program, it is time to present your prices. It is important that you do not review your prices before this step because people will not have any idea what they are getting for the price. People are much more likely to buy from you if they trust you and understand the benefits of what you can offer them. If you give your prices right away, you have not addressed the most important parts of the sale process. When presenting your prices, many techniques are available. Following are just a few.

Alternate Close

In this situation, you present two options and then ask which is best for the person. The idea is that you are letting potential clients choose the package, but you are also not allowing them to easily say no. By asking which is best for the client, you are taking "no" out of the possible answers.

Assumptive Close

In this technique, you are assuming the person will purchase from you. Examples of questions you could ask after presenting your prices are "When can we get you started?" and "How would you like to pay?" Both of these questions assume the person will buy from you.

Suggestive Close

In this method, you suggest what the person should purchase. The logic is that you are the expert and you should know what is best for the client since you are the one with the knowledge and experience.

Trial Close

This method is normally used before the actual sales presentation and before asking for the sale. The idea behind this method is that you are asking people what they think of things throughout the process. This allows you to gauge whether or not the person is likely to purchase from you. Following are some examples of trial closes:

- Could you see yourself working out in this fitness club?
- Could you fit in a 30-minute workout three times a week?
- Is your spouse or partner in favour of your purchasing personal training sessions?

If the person answers no to any of these questions, you want to be able to address these obstacles before presenting the prices.

Asking for the sale is difficult for many people. These are popular techniques that can make the process a little smoother for many new Personal Training Specialists; however, many other methods can work for you. As long as you give your prices in a confident but sincere manner that is consistent with how you have been communicating with the person, the prospective client will be receptive.

Overcome Objections

Once you have presented your prices, many people will not respond favourably at first. Some of the most common objections are as follows:

- I want to think about it.
- It's too much money.
- I need to talk it over with someone.

As a Personal Training Specialist getting started in the business, you need to accept that objections will happen. If you view objections as someone simply needing more information, then you will be comfortable dealing with them. Some experts suggest that potential clients may give up to five objections before they make a purchase from you. If you are not comfortable dealing with objections, you will miss out on potential clients. There are many ways to deal with objections, but we will consider a very simple method to start with.

The majority of objections can be dealt with ahead of time through the use of proper trial closes. Asking people how long they have been thinking about working out and whether they are ready to get started is a great way to deal with the objection of wanting to think about it. Asking people if their spouse or significant other is in favour of them doing this is another good way to address a potential objection ahead of time.

Assuming you have covered these questions before giving prices, the first thing to do when you hear an objection is to clarify it. You can do this by asking *why* or *what* types of questions. An objection normally comes from people who aren't ready to buy because they do not have all the information they need in order to be confident in their decision. If someone says, "I want to think about it," one potential response is "What is it you want to think about?" This clarification will normally get the person to tell you something else, such as "I'm not sure I can afford it" or "I'm not sure I can make the time." The idea is not to be pushy but to find out exactly what you have not answered or what you need to focus on. Whether the person buys from you is not the major concern. The point is that you want to make sure you have answered all of the person's questions and concerns and discussed all of the possibilities you have to offer. For example, if potential clients say that they can't afford your services and you don't tell them about a payment plan you offer that allows them to pay over the next three months, you may have lost clients simply because you didn't understand what their objection really was. It wasn't that they couldn't afford your training; it was that they couldn't afford to pay for it all at once.

How you deal with objections is up to you. The approaches you use need to be ones that you are comfortable with. The techniques given previously are just a few examples of how you can close the sale.

Follow Up

Whether someone purchases from you or not, it is important to follow up with that person. There are many ways this can be done, such as the following:

- Call to thank new clients for trusting you with their business.
- Call them to see if they have any questions and to find out what needs to happen to get them back in.
- Call them to see how they are feeling after their first workout.

Maintaining and Building Your Clientele

When it comes to maintaining your client base, the bottom line is that it is always less expensive to keep an existing client than it is to find a new one. You do not need to spend any money or time marketing to current clients, and you don't need to spend a lot of time trying to convince them that you are the right trainer for them. They are already your clients; you simply have to take care of them and give them what they want.

The key to long-term success in the fitness industry is the ability to generate referrals from your current clients. If you place as much focus on the relationship as you do on the actual program, you will develop loyal clients who will bring all of the future clientele you will ever need. This will not happen immediately since building any relationship takes time, but if you take the time to focus on all the people you are training and take care of them and their needs, you will reap the benefits both in client retention and referrals.

The most successful Personal Training Specialists do not actively seek new clients; instead, they have a waiting list of clients who are interested in being trained by them. This waiting list was not created by some great marketing piece that was sent out or that someone saw in a newspaper. It occurred because the trainer's clients were happy with the service. In general, referral sources can be organized into internal (current clients, past clients, other members) and external (friends, family, other health professionals, coaches) sources.

It is true that clients often send you referrals without your asking for their assistance, but more times than not you will need to ask your clients for some help in this area. The easiest way to do this is through guest passes. Anytime is a great time to ask a client for a referral, but the best times are when clients start and when they are happy with the results they have been getting, normally after 6 to 8 weeks. If you want to be proactive, you can even ask people to leave the names and phone numbers of their friends so you can call them to personally invite them, as long as it does not violate Do Not Call List legislation. You may not be comfortable with this at first, but when presented properly it can be very effective. Asking for this information allows you to follow up with people. When you simply give guest passes to clients, the passes might be forgotten or lost. If you have been working as a trainer for more than a year and you are not getting at least 75% of your new clients from referrals, you need to address this area of marketing.

Here are some things to keep in mind when asking for referrals outside your fitness centre or client base:

- Think of everyone as a potential client, but respect people's time and space.
- Build partnerships whenever you can. People will be more likely to refer others to you if they are getting something in return, such as a free session or a program designed for them.
- To come up with creative ways to work with people, use the marketing techniques mentioned previously in this chapter.

Whenever you ask for referrals, keep the following in mind:

- No one wants to be sold, so look at this as an opportunity to share some information or educate the person on what you are doing.

- Focus on the person's goals and then tailor your conversation around them.
- Let the person know that it would be helping you.

There are lots of creative ways to get referrals from your clients. As long as you ask in a professional manner and in a way that respects your clients, you will be successful.

Advantages

- It is low in cost.
- The buying decision is made easier for potential clients because of the referral.

Disadvantages

- You may need to get out of your comfort zone if this is not something you are comfortable doing.

Your Professional Image

One sure way to fail in the industry is to look and act the way most people perceive personal trainers—that is, muscle bound, unprofessional, intimidating, and unrelatable to the average person. It is important that you continue to enhance the reputation of the fitness industry by dressing appropriately and always presenting yourself in a professional manner.

When you are training a client, that person should be your entire focus. You should not have conversations with other people around you, and you should not be distracted by your phone. All of your energy should be focused on your client. This means giving feedback and encouragement based on how they are performing and being mentally and physically available to them.

Client–Trainer Relationship

Your relationship with your clients is another key to long-term success in the personal training field. As discussed, referrals can have a major impact on your business.

One of the keys to a good client–trainer relationship is that both parties know what to expect from each other. A great way to formalize these expectations is in an agreement. This document outlines the important business components of the client–trainer relationship. Common topics in this agreement include the following:

- **Term of the agreement**—Establishes time span of the agreement or what is included.
- **Fees and payment structure**—What methods of payment will you accept and over what amount of time will clients be able to pay you? It is up to you whether you want people to pay in full or in installments.
- **Cancellation policy**—It is strongly recommended that you include and enforce this policy. If you do not follow through on it, your clients will assume it is acceptable to cancel appointments without appropriate notice.
- **Late policy**—Similar to the cancellation policy, this is an area that needs to be enforced before it becomes a common occurrence.
- **Refund policy**—Many trainers provide a money-back guarantee for the unused portion of their sessions.
- **Informed consent**—This common stipulation ensures the client understands the risk of exercising.

 See the web resource at www.HumanKinetics.com/FoundationsOfProfessionalPersonalTraining for a sample personal training agreement that will keep your clients informed of their responsibilities.

Client–trainer agreements can be formatted in many ways. The example in the web resource covers the key elements, but you may need to modify it to suit your needs. The formal part of the client–trainer relationship is only one of the many areas that you need to consider. Some other areas that you need to pay attention to are as follows:

- **Professional image**—If you want to be treated and paid like a professional, you need to look and talk like a professional. Many people who purchase personal training sessions are professionals who are accustomed to being around certain types of people. If you want to attract this crowd, you need to keep these expectations in mind. Your professional image applies not only to professional clientele. All people who are paying you for your services deserve the same level of service and attention to detail.
- **Integrity**—Do what you say you will do and keep your promises. The formal agreement spells

out many areas, but there are still many things not mentioned in it. For example, if you tell clients you are going to bring in an article on cutting calories, do it. If you tell clients you are going to follow up with them if they miss a session, do it. And, if you tell clients you are going to help them get healthier in all aspects of their life, do it! At the time it may seem like a minor event if you forget to do something, but the reality is that your clients will notice and eventually lose faith in your ability to do the things you have promised.

• **Motivation and attitude**—Your clients are paying for you. They can most likely go anywhere to get a program. If you are not in a peak state each time you are with clients, then they are not getting what they paid for. If you are easily put off by people or certain types of situations and you can't overcome this when you are with clients, then personal training is not for you. When you are with your clients, you need to be 100% present. This means all of your energy needs to be focused on them. Anything else that is going on in your life or at work needs to be put on hold.

• **Personality types**—Most of us are comfortable around people who are like us. In our personal lives, we will normally choose our friends this way. Unfortunately, you will not always be able to choose your clients as a Personal Training Specialist, so you must be able to adjust your personality style to that of your clients. The same approach does not work for every client. You will need to be flexible in your approach, but there may be times when you choose not to take on new clients based on their personality because you will have to act in a way that you are not comfortable with. Regardless of the situation, it will normally be up to you to decide whether the client is compatible with your style.

• **General communication**—Clients need to feel comfortable with you so that they are willing to share any thoughts or concerns that will affect their session and their overall results. Listening is a key skill that all Personal Training Specialists need to master. This means listening without the intent of responding and trying to understand what people are saying and why they feel a certain way. When you do this, you not only listen to what they say, but you also watch body language and potentially find out even more information. There are times when clients simply need someone to talk to. They may

not need or want you to give them a solution. With experience you will become a good judge about when you should respond and when you should simply be a sounding board.

Terminating the Relationship

Unfortunately, some client–trainer relationships need to come to an end before clients reach all their goals. There are many reasons for this, but a major one is an incompatibility between the two people. As stated earlier, it is critical that the trainer seriously assess potential clients' personality and whether they are the right fit for one another. Even when this is done, however, things can go wrong.

When it comes time to end the relationship, take great care in ensuring that the client is treated with respect and with a genuine interest in what is best for both of you. It might be a good idea to suggest another trainer, assuming you know of another trainer who would be suited for the client. It is also important to explain the reasons for the termination. If the person wants to see results and you are not the best trainer to help with this, then it is in both of your best interests to get this out in the open. If the client is the one terminating the relationship, then it is important for you to find out exactly why so that you can incorporate this feedback with future clients. Whether or not you agree with the reasons, you should act professionally and thank the person for working with you. In either of these scenarios, the Personal Training Specialist and client must reach a mutual agreement on a refund for any prepaid sessions that have not been delivered.

Risk Management

Your clients place a great deal of trust in you as a Personal Training Specialist. It is your professional responsibility to be aware of the risks your client and you are exposed to. To protect your clients and yourself, adhere to the following guidelines:

• Always act within the canfitpro *Professional Member Code of Ethics* and *Standards of Practice for Personal Training Specialists*, which is in this book's preface. The canfitpro Personal Training Specialist certification has given you the ability to work with your client in certain ways, as outlined in this manual. Anytime you start to move outside of these abilities, you are getting outside of your *Standards of Practice* as a canfitpro Personal Training Specialist, and you could be held liable if a problem occurs unless you have received further education or certifications.

• *Negligence* is the failure to act as another reasonable, prudent professional would have acted in a similar situation. As a Personal Training Specialist, it is your responsibility to act in a reasonable and prudent manner.

• Ensure that all of your clients have filled out a comprehensive health history (PAR-Q+) questionnaire (see chapter 9).

• Ensure that all clients have signed a waiver. This waiver is limited in terms of its actual protection of the Personal Training Specialist, but it is still a good idea to use it.

• Ensure that you have followed up with your clients on any areas in the health history that are of concern, and make sure that clients get written authorization from a physician when you are not able to assess the severity of an injury or condition.

• Ensure that your clients are always safe and working within their own capabilities and that you are prescribing an exercise program that is specific to their unique background and goals.

• After the initial assessment and program design, it is your responsibility to continually reassess your clients to ensure that they are able to make changes to their program and to ensure that they can handle increased intensities or new exercises.

• Ensure that your cardiopulmonary resuscitation (CPR) certification is always up to date.

• If you are not an employee of a company, you are required to have your own liability insurance. Read the following section for further information on insurance needs.

Insurance

Personal Training Specialists often work as employees in a health club where coverage may already be provided by the insurance policy of the club. If trainers do any training outside the club or on their own time, they are not covered by the club, so they will need to purchase their own insurance. What determines whether Personal Training Specialists are employees of a club or are working on their own is who collects the money. Normally, if a Personal Training Specialist is being paid directly by the club for providing services, they are covered under the policy of the club as an employee or subcontractor. If this is your situation, check with the club owner to make sure that you are covered. If, on the other hand, you are being paid directly by the client, you are working as an independent contractor and the club insurance does not cover your personal training, even if you use the club facilities to do the workouts.

Litigious Situations

Following are some situations that could lead to litigation:

• Working outside of your set of abilities or not abiding by your *Standards of Practice*

• Prescribing exercise for clients who have injuries or conditions that you are not trained to work with

• Designing meal plans, analyzing nutrition plans, or giving specific nutrition counseling (unless you have the required qualifications)

• Exposing clients to unsafe or overly risky exercises based on their level of experience and capabilities

• Making false claims that cannot be supported by research

Policies and Procedures

Developing policies and procedures for your business enables you to identify potential problem areas ahead of time so that everyone is aware of what will be done in specific situations. Here is a list of policies that canfitpro recommends all trainers follow:

• Establish a fixed pricing policy and don't sway from this unless it is absolutely critical.

• Establish a fair and equitable cancelation policy, agree on it, and maintain it.

• Offer a money-back guarantee for all clients if they are not happy with the results or level of service they are getting. This guarantee would apply only to the unused remaining sessions.

Summary of Main Points

1. There are many options for new Personal Training Specialists, which include working in a fitness centre, in a privately owned studio, or as a freelance trainer.

2. The marketing process can be divided into four areas, known as the 4 Ps of marketing: product, price, promotions, and place.

3. To set yourself apart from your competition, consider the three factors when looking at your product: differentiation, development, and positioning.

4. Many factors determine your price and promotional efforts, including location, target demographic, number of competitors, and marketing cost.

5. A well-formulated elevator pitch will assist you in confidently sharing your product and services to anyone at any time.

6. Referrals are the best way to build your clientele and are the key to long-term success in the fitness industry.

7. Implement the necessary steps to manage risk, such as acquiring insurance, staying within your scope of practice, and developing policies and procedures.

Key Concepts for Study

4 Ps of marketing

Differentiation

Development

Positioning

Marketing piece

Isochrone

E-marketing

Circle of influence

Elevator pitch

Closing the sale

Referrals

Professional image

Negligence

Review Questions

1. List the 4 Ps of marketing.

2. What is not one of the three factors to consider when looking at your product?

   a. Differentiation

   b. Influence

   c. Positioning

   d. Development

3. Define isochrone and explain its significance to your marketing efforts.

4. True or false: Referrals are the best way to ensure your long-term success in the fitness industry.

5. Explain the steps you can take to maintain a quality professional image.

 Web Resource Contents

Form to identify circle of influence

Sample personal training agreement

Answers to review questions

PART IV Case Study Questions

1. Using the program card template provided (canfitpro INTERACTIVE), create a program for each of the three case study clients to use for the first two weeks of their personal training. (Keep in mind the unique requests, assessment results, and time constraints of each client.)

2. Catherine is concerned about moving too quickly and having to learn all new exercises as she progresses through her program. Select three resistance training exercises from the program card you've prepared for Catherine and describe how you could increase the level of challenge for her without her having to learn an entirely new exercise.

3. Lisa shows up to a training session complaining of pain in her elbow and forearm. She says it is no big deal and that she used to feel the same type of pain when she was on the volleyball team. She says that the pain is a 4 out of 10 and that it usually goes away after a few days. She wants to continue training as usual and says she can work through the pain. How do you proceed?

4. Thomas has requested an additional workout that he can complete at home between his personal training sessions with you. He has a limited variety of equipment at home—an upright stationary bike, a full set of dumbbells, a stability ball, and a flat bench. Create a 30-minute full-body workout that Thomas can complete at home using the equipment available and his own body weight for resistance.

Exercises

Mike Bates, MBA

UPPER BODY

CHEST

 Barbell Chest Press

Movement—horizontal adduction and elbow extension

Primary muscles worked—pectoralis major, anterior deltoid, triceps brachii

How to Perform

Starting Position

- Lie in a supine position with the eyes roughly in line with the barbell. Hold the bar with a common grip and with the hands slightly wider than shoulder-width apart so that the elbows are slightly bent.
- Maintain five points of contact with the floor and bench (i.e., left foot, right foot, lower back and buttocks, upper back and shoulder blades, and back of head) while keeping a natural arch in the back.

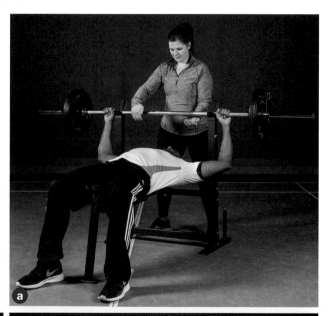

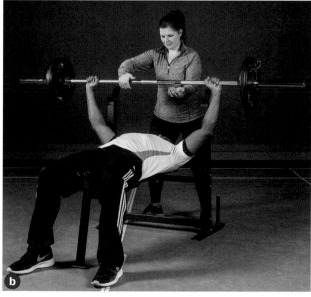

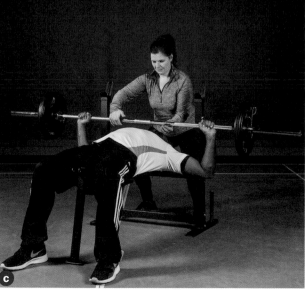

- Stabilize throughout the movement by maintaining scapulae in a neutral position (avoid excessive protraction or retraction).
- Extend the elbows to push the bar straight up.

Eccentric Phase

- Lower the bar so that the elbows bend to about 90° and the upper arm is approximately parallel to the ground. The bar should be just above the sternum without making contact with the sternum itself.
- Note: Clients may increase the range of motion beyond the 90° flexion point if the shoulders and scapulae are properly stabilized and clients experience no pain or discomfort during the full movement.

Concentric Phase

- Push the bar back up to the start position, straightening the arms but not locking the elbows or rotating the shoulders.

How to Spot

- Position yourself at the head of the client so that you can assist with the initial push off and monitor the movement throughout the exercise. Keep your hands close to bar at all times and use a mixed grip (overhand and underhand) to assist in returning the bar to the rack if required.
- Ensure that the client maintains five points of contact at all times and look for changes in alignment of the spine, arms, and neck.

Examples of Exercise Alternatives and Variations

- Machine chest press (seated)
- Body bar chest press
- Dumbbell chest press

- Incline dumbbell chest press
- Incline barbell chest press (wide grip)

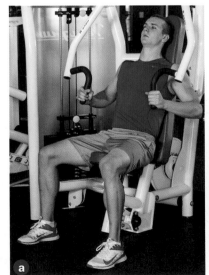 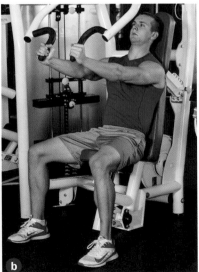

Machine chest press (seated)

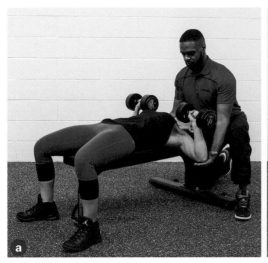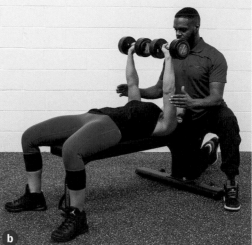

Dumbbell chest press

Dumbbell Chest Fly

Movement—horizontal adduction

Primary muscles worked—pectoralis major and anterior deltoid

How to Perform

Starting Position

- Lie in a supine position and retract the scapulae to set position.
- Hold the dumbbells above the body with a neutral grip and align the arms straight up from the shoulders.
- The arms should be slightly bent at the elbows, and the wrists should be in a stable position.

Eccentric Phase

- Lower the arms down to about parallel to the floor, keeping a slight bend in the elbow throughout the entire movement.

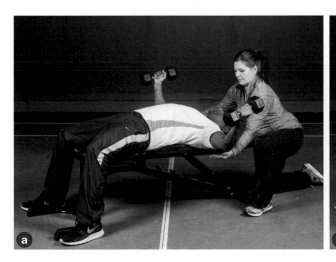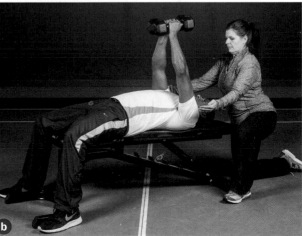

Concentric Phase

- Pull the arms up and together while contracting the muscles of the chest without extending the elbows or rotating the shoulders.

How to Spot

- Position yourself at the head of the bench in a kneeling lunge position. Spotting should be at the elbows. If the client becomes unstable, you may need to move your hands up to the client's wrists or as close to the weight as possible, without obstructing the movement.
- Monitor the five points of contact and proper alignment throughout the exercise.

Examples of Exercise Alternatives and Variations

- Machine chest fly
- Incline cable fly

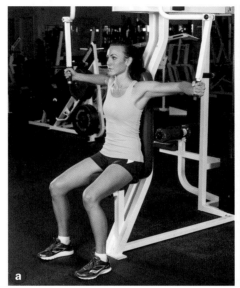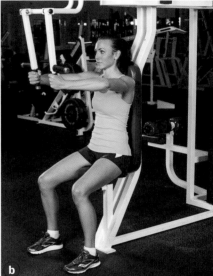

Machine chest fly

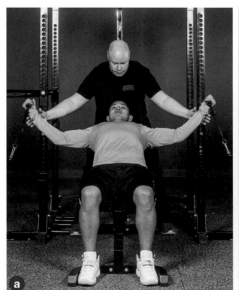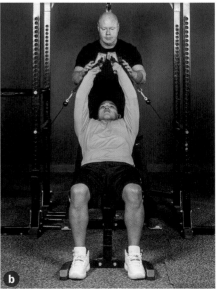

Incline cable fly

Push-Up (Hands and Toes)

Movement—horizontal adduction, elbow extension

Primary muscles worked—pectoralis major, anterior deltoid, triceps brachii, and core and trunk stabilizers

How to Perform

Starting Position

- In a prone position, place the hands wider than shoulder-width apart, feet about hip-width apart, and toes curled under.

Eccentric Phase

- Bend at the elbows to lower the body down toward the bottom position while maintaining proper alignment throughout the movement. The torso and legs should not touch the floor, and the nose should be slightly above the floor.

Concentric Phase

- Engage the muscles of the core and push up through the hands to lift the torso and legs off the floor while maintaining good posture throughout. Keep the shoulders, hips, knees, and ankles aligned.
- Push up until the elbows are fully extended.

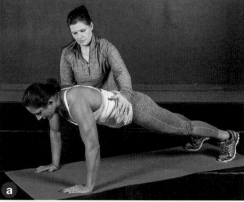

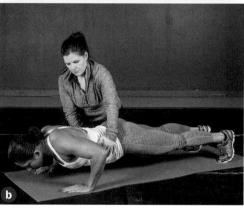

How to Spot

- Kneel in a lunge position next to the exerciser and watch for proper alignment throughout each phase of the movement.

Examples of Exercise Alternatives and Variations

- Push-up (on knees)
- Push-up (narrow hands, on knees)
- Push-up (standing, against wall)
- Push-up (wide hands, feet elevated)

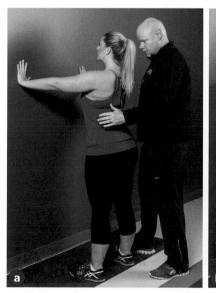

Push-up (standing, against wall)

BACK

 ## Cable Lat Pull-Down (Wide Grip)

Movement—combination of shoulder adduction and extension, scapular retraction, scapular depression and downward rotation, elbow flexion

Primary muscles worked—latissimus dorsi, teres major, posterior deltoid, rhomboids, mid- and lower trapezius, biceps brachii

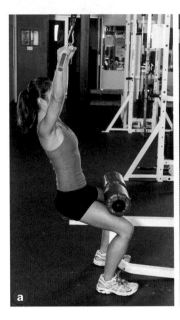
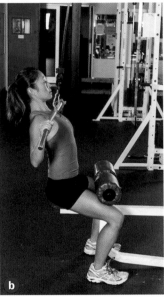

How to Perform

Starting Position

- Hold the bar with a wide, pronated grip so that when the upper arms are parallel to the ground they form an angle of approximately 90°.
- The knees should be secure under the pad, and you should lean back slightly (15° to 45°) while keeping the core muscles engaged.

Concentric Phase

- Pull the bar toward the chest until the arms are just below parallel to the ground.
- Pull the scapulae down and together, allowing a natural arch in the lower back.
- Keep the scapulae depressed and retracted

Eccentric Phase

- Control the arms as you let them slowly back up to the original starting position while keeping tension on the latissimus dorsi.
- No change should occur in the angle at the hips after the original degree of lean is established
- Pulling the bar behind the head can be stressful on the shoulder joint and is not advised.

How to Spot

- Position yourself behind the client with both hands on the bar.

Examples of Exercise Alternatives and Variations

- Cable lat pull-down (narrow supinated grip)
- Cable lat pull-down (medium grip)
- Double cable lat pull-down

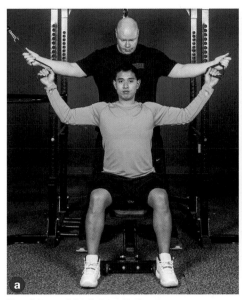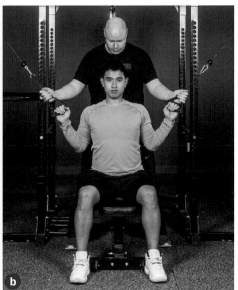

Double cable lat pull-down

Cable Lat Row (Seated With V-Bar)

Movement—scapular retraction, shoulder extension, elbow flexion

Primary muscles worked—rhomboids, midtrapezius, latissimus dorsi, teres major, posterior deltoid, biceps brachii

How to Perform

Starting Position

- Plant the feet firmly against the machine with the knees slightly bent.
- Lean back slightly and keep a natural arch in the lower back.
- While holding the handles, keep the wrists in a neutral position and the elbows slightly bent.

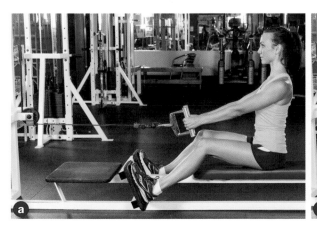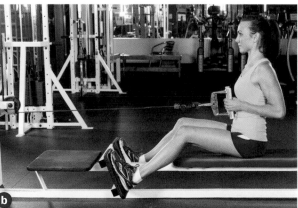

Concentric Phase

- Keeping the arms slightly bent, contract the rhomboids and pull the shoulder blades together and down (scapular retraction and depression).
- Pull the arms back, keeping them close to the side of the body until the elbows are aligned approximately below the shoulders.

Eccentric Phase

- Slowly return the arms and shoulders to the original position, keeping a neutral spine.

How to Spot

- Position yourself beside the client in a kneeling lunge position.
- Monitor spinal, scapular, and arm positioning. Ensure that the natural arch in the lower back is not compromised.

Examples of Exercise Alternatives and Variations

- Cable row (underhand, standing)
- Tubing lat row (standing)
- Tubing high row (standing)
- Cable lat row (wide pronated grip)
- Cable lat row (single arm)
- Cable lat row (standing, with rope)

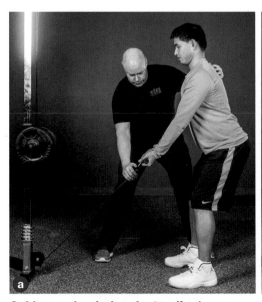 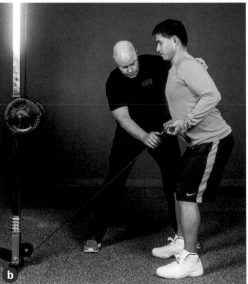

Cable row (underhand, standing)

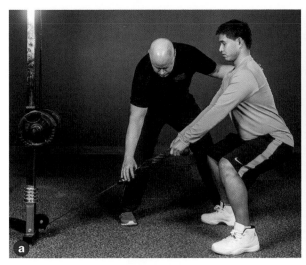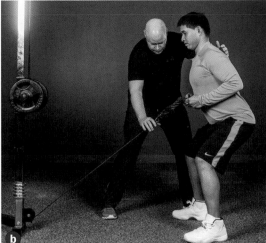

Cable lat row (standing, with rope)

Barbell Lat Row (Bent Over)

Movement—scapular retraction, shoulder extension, elbow flexion

Primary muscles worked—latissimus dorsi, teres major, rhomboids, midtrapezius, posterior deltoid, biceps brachii

How to Perform

Starting Position

- Hold the barbell with a pronated grip and the hands wider than shoulder-width apart.
- Lean forward about 45°, keeping the back and neck in a neutral position at all times.
- The knees should be slightly bent, and the feet should be shoulder-width apart.

Concentric Phase

- Pull the bar in toward the lower sternum until the elbows make a 90° angle.
- The scapulae should be in a retracted position.

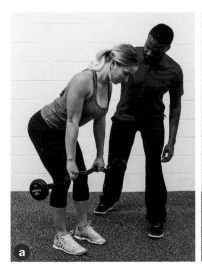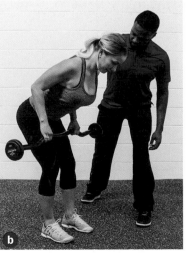

Eccentric Phase

- Lower the weight back to the starting position.

How to Spot

- Monitor body alignment from all angles while being prepared to assist with the barbell if needed.

Examples of Exercise Alternatives and Variations

- Dumbbell lat row (one arm on bench)
- Tubing lat row (bent over)
- Body bar lat row
- T-bar lat row (standing)

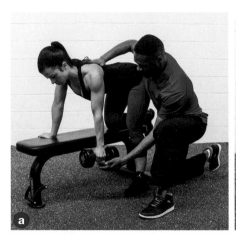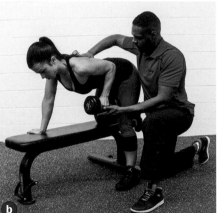

Dumbbell lat row (one arm on bench)

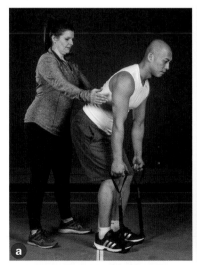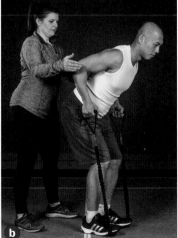

Tubing lat row (bent over)

Dumbbell Trap Shrug

Movement—scapular elevation

Primary muscles worked—levator scapulae, upper trapezius, midtrapezius, rhomboids

How to Perform

Starting Position

- Sit with the feet shoulder-width apart and hold one dumbbell on either side of the body with the palms facing the midline.
- The scapulae should be retracted to set position with the elbows extended but not locked.

Concentric Phase

- Pull the shoulders up toward the ears by contracting the upper trapezius and levator scapulae.

Eccentric Phase

- Lower the weights to the starting position, keeping the scapulae retracted.

How to Spot

- Monitor the lifter's alignment while spotting from behind.

Examples of Exercise Alternatives and Variations

- Dumbbell trap shrug (standing)
- Barbell trap shrug (standing)
- Cable trap shrug (seated)

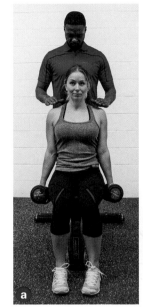
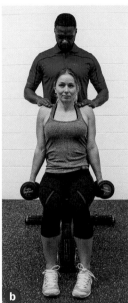

SHOULDERS

Shoulder Press (Seated)

Movement—shoulder flexion, elbow extension

Primary muscles worked—anterior deltoids, pectoralis major, triceps brachii, upper trapezius

How to Perform

Starting Position

- Sit with the feet firmly on the ground, the knees at about 90°, and a natural arch in the back.
- Bring the arms up and out to the side with the upper arms parallel to the floor and the elbows flexed.

Concentric Phase

- Press the arms up and over the head until the elbows are extended directly over the shoulders.
- Attempt to elevate the shoulder blades as they rotate upward while maintaining proper posture.

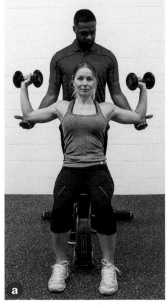
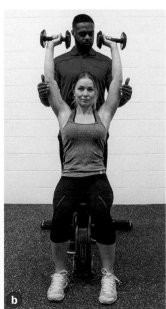

Eccentric Phase

- Lower the weight back to the starting position while maintaining posture.

How to Spot

- Position yourself directly behind the client spotting at the elbows but prepared to assist at the wrists if the lifter becomes unstable.

Examples of Exercise Alternatives and Variations

- Barbell shoulder press (standing, anterior)
- Body bar shoulder press (standing)
- Machine shoulder press (seated)
- Tubing shoulder press (standing, single arm)

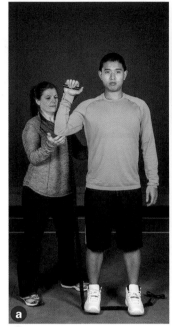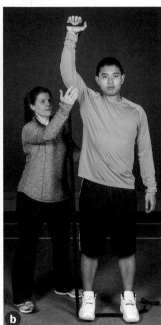

Tubing shoulder press (standing, single arm)

Dumbbell Shoulder Raise (Seated, Lateral)

Movement—shoulder abduction

Primary muscles worked—deltoid (medial head), trapezius

How to Perform

Starting Position

- Sit with the feet firmly on the ground, the knees bent at approximately 90°, and a natural arch in the back.
- Hold the dumbbells on either side of the body toward the outer part of the upper leg with the palms facing inward.
- Bend the elbows approximately 90°.

Concentric Phase

- Lift the dumbbells by abducting the shoulders while keeping the 90° angle at the elbows.

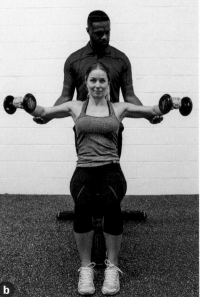

- Lift the weights until the dumbbells and elbows are parallel to the ground and in line with one another.

Eccentric Phase

- Lower the weights to the starting position, maintaining the 90° angle at the elbows.

How to Spot

- Position yourself behind the client with your arms close to the client's upper arms or elbows.

Examples of Exercise Alternatives and Variations

- Tubing shoulder raise (standing, anterior)
- Cable shoulder raise (standing, lateral, single arm)

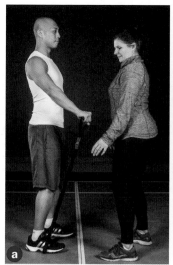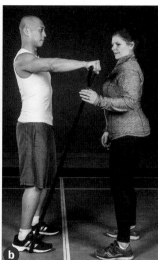

Tubing shoulder raise (standing, anterior)

Tubing Rotator Cuff External Rotation (Standing)

Movement—shoulder external rotation

Primary muscles worked—infraspinatus, teres minor, posterior deltoid

How to Perform

Starting Position

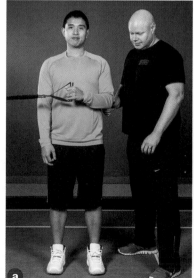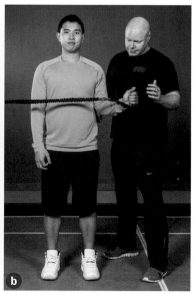

- Stand in good posture with the shoulders in set position and the feet shoulder-width apart.
- Grip the handle and flex the elbow 90°, holding the tubing at elbow height.

Concentric Phase

- Externally rotate the shoulder, pulling the arm out and across the body while keeping the elbow fixed at 90°.
- Continue rotating the arm while keeping the wrist neutral and the elbow in tight against the torso.

Eccentric Phase

- Return the tubing to the starting position while maintaining posture and elbow flexion at 90°.

How to Spot

- Spot on the forearm while monitoring the client for proper positioning.

Examples of Exercise Alternatives and Variations

- Dumbbell rotator cuff external rotation (semiprone)
- Cable rotator cuff external rotation (supine)
- Manual rotator cuff external rotation (standing)

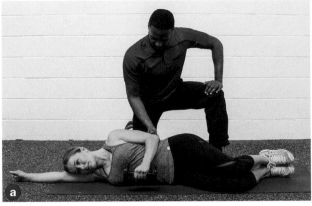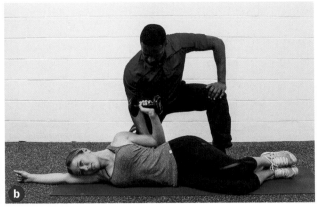

Dumbbell rotator cuff external rotation (semiprone)

Tubing Rotator Cuff Internal Rotation (Standing)

Movement—shoulder internal rotation

Primary muscles worked—subscapularis, anterior deltoid, pectoralis major, teres major

How to Perform

Starting Position

- Stand in good posture with the shoulders in set position and the feet shoulder-width apart.
- Grip the handle, flex the elbow at 90°, and hold the tubing at elbow height.

Concentric Phase

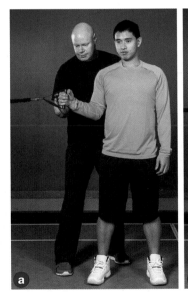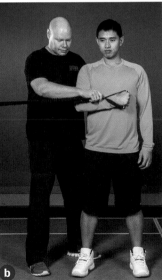

- Internally rotate the shoulder, pulling the arm in and across the body while keeping the elbow fixed at 90°.
- Continue pulling the arm in, keeping the wrist neutral and the elbow in tight against the torso.

Eccentric Phase

- Return the tubing to the starting position while maintaining posture and elbow flexion at 90°.

How to Spot

- Spot on the forearm while monitoring the client for proper positioning.

Examples of Exercise Alternatives and Variations

- Cable rotator cuff internal rotation (standing)
- Cable rotator cuff internal rotation (supine)
- Manual rotator cuff internal rotation (standing)

Barbell or EZ-Bar Biceps Curl (Standing, Supinated Grip)

Movement—elbow flexion

Primary muscles worked—biceps brachii, wrist flexors

How to Perform

Starting Position

- Grasp the barbell with a common supinated grip.
- Stand with the feet shoulder-width apart and maintain a neutral spine.
- The knees should be slightly flexed, and the scapulae should be retracted and depressed.

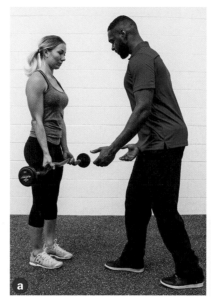
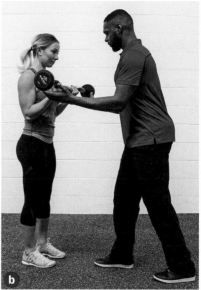

Concentric Phase

- Curl the bar up until the elbows are fully flexed and the barbell is in front of the chest. Keep the elbows close to the torso.

Eccentric Phase

- Lower the bar to the starting position until the elbows are extended with a slight bend.

How to Spot

- Stand directly in front of the client and spot the bar, inside the lifter's hands.
- Watch for proper alignment and posture throughout the movement

Examples of Exercise Alternatives and Variations

- Cable biceps curl (standing, straight bar)
- Tubing biceps curl (standing)
- Dumbbell biceps curl (standing)
- Machine preacher biceps curl
- Dumbbell biceps curl (seated with supination)

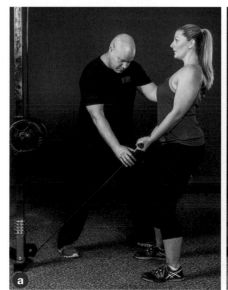
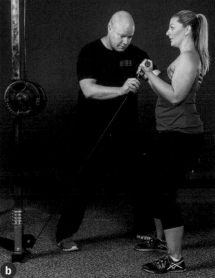

Cable biceps curl (standing, straight bar)

Dumbbell Biceps Concentration Curl (Seated)

Movement—elbow flexion

Primary muscles worked—biceps brachii

How to Perform

Starting Position

- Sit with the feet firmly on the ground.
- Hinge forward from the hip and rest the upper arm on the medial aspect of the thigh, grasping the dumbbell with a supinated grip.
- Engage the core muscles to stabilize the upper body.

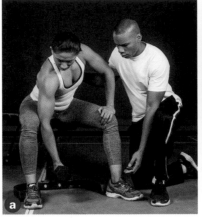
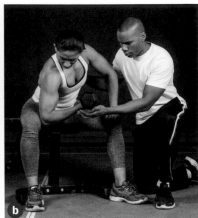

Concentric Phase

- Flex the elbow to raise the dumbbell toward the upper torso.
- Lift the dumbbell until the elbow is fully flexed and the weight is in front of the anterior deltoid.

Eccentric Phase

- Control the weight while lowering it back to the starting position.

How to Spot

- Spot in front of the client, as close to the weight as possible, without obstructing the lifter's movement.

Examples of Exercise Alternatives and Variations

- Cable biceps single-arm curl (standing)
- Tubing biceps curl

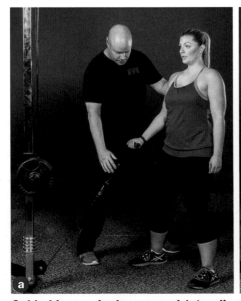
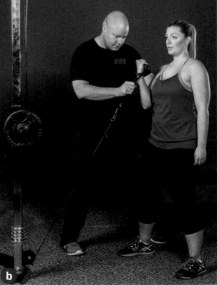

Cable biceps single-arm curl (standing)

Dumbbell Biceps Curl (Seated, Hammer Grip)

Movement—elbow flexion

Primary muscles worked—brachioradialis, biceps brachii

How to Perform

Starting Position

- Sit with the feet firmly on the ground.
- Hold dumbbells on either side of the body with the palms facing in.
- The elbows should be against the torso and slightly flexed.

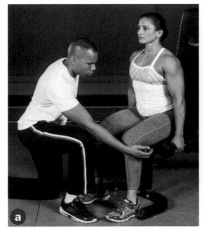
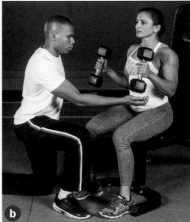

Concentric Phase

- Raise the dumbbells up until the elbows are fully flexed and the weights are in front of the anterior deltoid. Keep the palms facing in at all times.

Eccentric Phase

- Lower the dumbbells back to the starting position.

How to Spot

- Position yourself in front of the client, spotting as close to the weight as possible without obstructing the movement.

Examples of Exercise Alternatives and Variations

- Tubing hammer curl (standing)

Cable Triceps Extension (Standing, Rope)

Movement—elbow extension

Primary muscles worked—triceps brachii

How to Perform

Starting Position

- Stand with the feet shoulder-width apart and the knees slightly flexed.
- Grasp the rope with a pronated grip so that the elbows are against the torso.

Concentric Phase

- Push the rope handles down, fully extending the elbows but not locking them out.

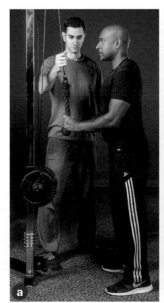
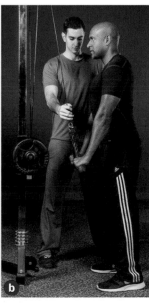

Eccentric Phase

- Return the rope to the starting position, using a full, pain-free range of motion.
- Maintain an upright posture with the scapulae in set position throughout the movement.

How to Spot

- Spot the client from both the side and behind.
- Be aware of proper alignment and posture throughout the exercise.

Examples of Exercise Alternatives and Variations

- Dumbbell triceps kickback (standing)
- Dumbbell triceps kickback (kneeling on bench)
- Barbell triceps extension (seated, pronated grip, straight bar)
- Cable triceps extension (standing, straight bar)
- Cable triceps extension (standing, V-bar)
- Tubing triceps extension (standing/overhead)

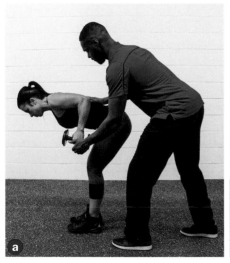
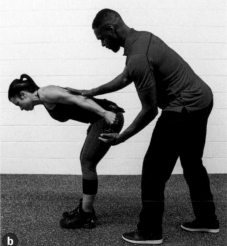

Dumbbell triceps kickback (standing)

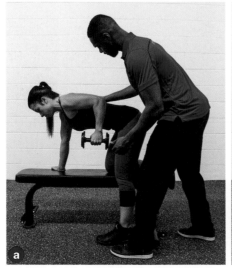
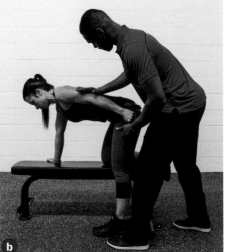

Dumbbell triceps kickback (kneeling on bench)

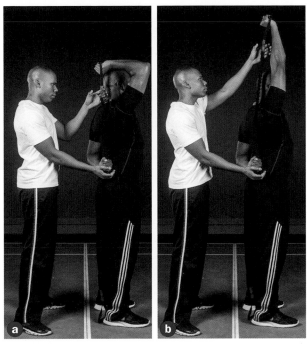

Tubing triceps extension (standing/overhead)

Bench Triceps Dips

Movement—elbow extension, scapular retraction

Primary muscles worked—triceps brachii, pectoralis major, anterior deltoid

How to Perform

Starting Position

- Place the body so that the hands are on the edge of a bench and the legs are extended out in front with the heels on the ground and minimal flexion at the knee.
- Lower the torso until the upper arms are about parallel to the ground.

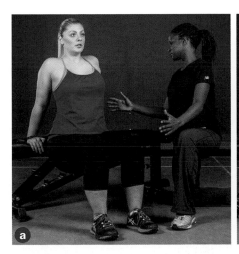
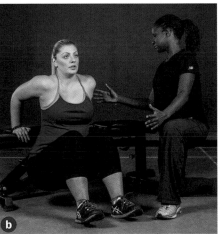

Concentric Phase

- Push down with the hands and fully extend the elbows to raise the torso.

Eccentric Phase

- Lower the torso back to starting position.

How to Spot

- Position yourself at the side of the exerciser in a kneeling lunge position.

Examples of Exercise Alternatives and Variations

- Barbell or body bar triceps press (supine, narrow grip)
- Machine-assisted triceps dips
- Parallel bar triceps dips

Barbell Triceps Extension (Seated, Overhead)

Movement—elbow extension

Primary muscles worked—triceps brachii

How to Perform

Starting Position

- Sit upright with the feet firmly on the ground.
- Grasp the bar above the head with an overhand grip, set the elbows at approximately 90°, and hold the hands and bar behind the head.
- The elbows should be facing forward or slightly outward.

Concentric Phase

- Press the bar overhead until the elbows are fully extended.

Eccentric Phase

- Return the bar to starting position.

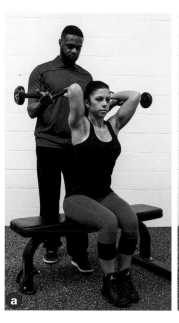 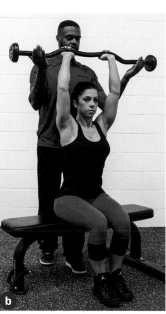

How to Spot

- Stand behind the client with your hands at the elbows but be prepared to assist at the bar if needed.

Examples of Exercise Alternatives and Variations

- Dumbbell triceps extension (seated, overhead)
- Tubing triceps extension (standing, overhead)
- Body bar triceps extension (supine)
- Cable triceps extension (kneeling, rope)

LOWER BODY

HIPS

Barbell Squat

Movement—hip extension, knee extension, plantar flexion

Primary muscles worked—hip extensors (gluteus maximus, hamstrings), hip adductors, gastrocnemius, quadriceps, spinal extensors

How to Perform

Starting Position

- Place the bar just above the scapulae with the hands placed comfortably on the bar and the elbows pointed down.
- The feet should be wider than shoulder-width apart and angled out slightly.
- The knees and hips should be slightly flexed, and the spine and neck should be held in neutral position.

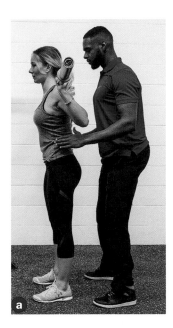
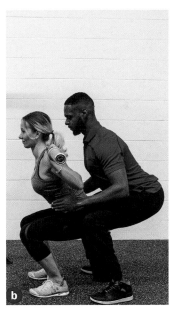

Eccentric Phase

- Push the hips back, allow the knees to bend naturally, and let the trunk lean forward slightly.
- Lower your body until the upper legs are parallel to the ground or as far down as you can comfortably go.
- Maintain proper posture throughout the movement.
- The eyes should be forward throughout the movement.
- Weight should be on the heels of the feet.
- Be careful that the knees do not go too far beyond the front of the toes.

Concentric Phase

- Return to the starting position by maintaining posture and pushing from the heels, keeping the eyes looking forward.

How to Spot

- Position yourself behind the exerciser with your arm at the lifter's torso.
- Look for proper alignment. Weight should be in the heels, and the knees should track over the top of the feet.
- Ensure that the squat rack safety is in place at the bottom range for the lifter so that he or she can safely exit the squat rack in the event of a muscle failure.

Examples of Exercise Alternatives and Variations

- Barbell deadlift
- Dumbbell stationary lunge (split squat)
- Body bar stationary lunge (split squat)
- Machine leg press
- Body bar squat

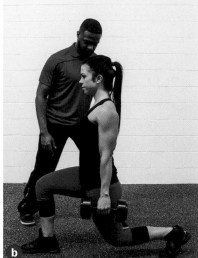
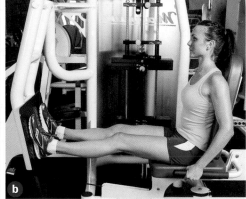

Dumbbell stationary lunge (split squat)

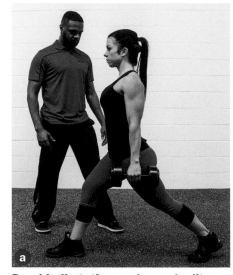
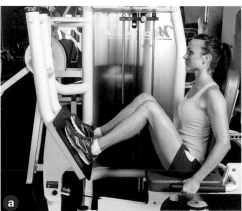

Machine leg press (seated, horizontal)

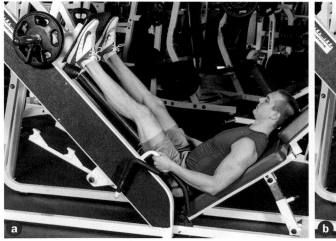
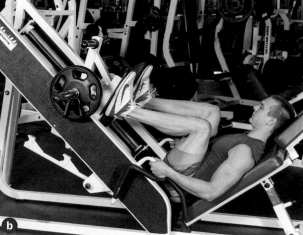

Machine leg press (incline)

Barbell Deadlift

Movement—hip extension, knee extension, plantar flexion

Primary muscles worked—hip extensors (gluteus maximus, hamstrings, hip adductors), psoas, spinal extensors, latissimus dorsi

How to Perform

Starting Position

- Stand behind the bar and assume a squat position with the hips and knees flexed.
- The feet should be wider than shoulder-width apart and angled out slightly.
- Hold the bar with the hands shoulder-width apart in an alternate (i.e., overhand and underhand) grip.
- Keep the torso upright and hold the spine and neck in a neutral position.

Concentric Phase

- Keeping the bar as close to the shins as possible, push the body up by driving weight through the heels and simultaneously extending the knees and hips.
- Engage the muscles of the back and core to maintain an upright posture and be sure not to round the back.
- Contract the gluteal muscles at the top of the movement.
- Maintain proper posture throughout the movement.

Eccentric Phase

- Return to the starting position by flexing the hips and knees while maintaining a stabilized posture.

How to Spot

- Position yourself beside the exerciser.
- Look for proper alignment. Weight should be on the balls of the feet, the knees should track over the top of the feet, and the torso should be upright in a stabilized posture.

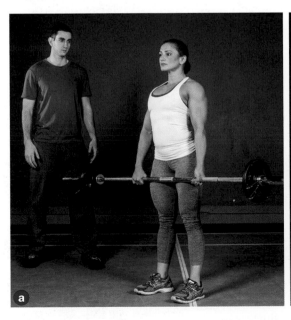
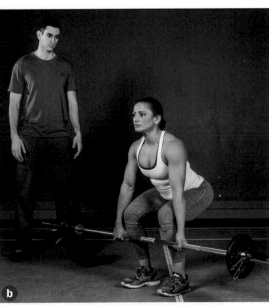

Examples of Exercise Alternatives and Variations

- Dumbbell deadlift
- Barbell squat
- Machine leg press
- Dumbbell stationary lunge (split squat)

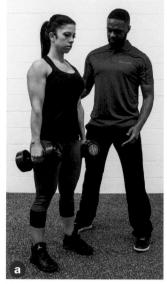
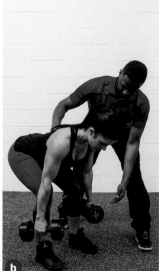

Dumbbell deadlift

UPPER LEG

Machine Leg Extension

Movement—knee extension

Primary muscles worked—quadriceps

How to Perform

Starting Position

- Sit so that the knee joints are aligned with the axis of the machine and the pad is pressing against the lower shins.
- The lower back should be firm against the seat.
- Sit upright with a natural arch in the lower back.

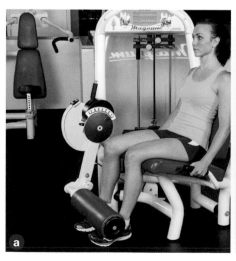
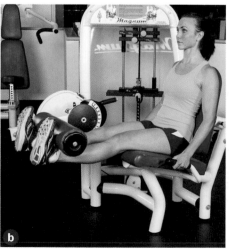

Concentric Phase

- Engage the quadriceps to raise the pad until the legs are almost fully extended.
- Maintain good posture throughout the movement.

Eccentric Phase

- Lower the legs to the starting position.

How to Spot

- Spot at the pad in a kneeling lunge position.
- Ensure that the client's knees do not lock out on extension.

Examples of Exercise Alternatives and Variations

- Tubing leg extension
- Cable hip flexion
- Machine hip flexion

Machine Leg Curl (Prone)

Movement—knee flexion

Primary muscles worked—hamstrings

How to Perform

Starting Position

- Lie prone on the bench so that knee joints are in line with the axis of the machine and the pad is below the gastrocnemius (but above the Achilles tendon).
- Position the trunk and neck in a neutral posture.

Concentric Phase

- Press the pelvis against the bench and flex the knees to raise the weight.
- Continue flexing at the knees until they form an angle of 90° or less.

Eccentric Phase

- Lower the weight to the starting position, taking care not to lock the knees.

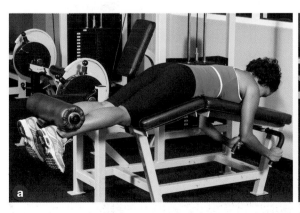
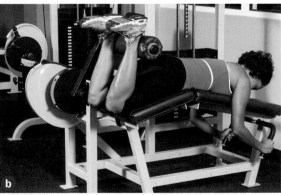

How to Spot

- Position yourself at the side to spot on the pad and watch for proper alignment.
- Be ready to assist with the weight if necessary.

Examples of Exercise Alternatives and Variations

- Machine leg curl (seated)
- Cable hip extension (standing)
- Stability ball hamstring curl

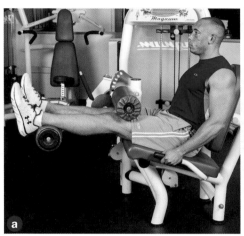 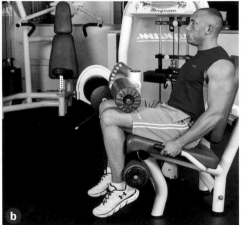

Machine leg curl (seated)

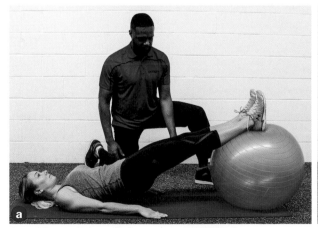 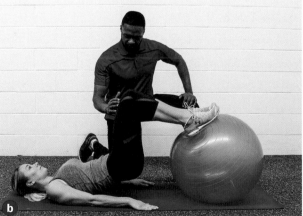

Stability ball hamstring curl (beginner)

Barbell Stiff-Legged Deadlift

Movement—hip extension

Primary muscles worked—hamstrings, spinal extensors

How to Perform

Starting Position

- Stand with the feet shoulder-width apart and the torso straight.
- Hold the bar with the hands shoulder-width apart in an overhand or alternated grip.
- Keep the spine and neck in a neutral position.

Eccentric Phase

- Keeping the knees extended (but allowing a slight bend), hinge forward at the hip to lower the bar below the level of the knees.
- Engage the muscles of the back and core to maintain a stable posture.

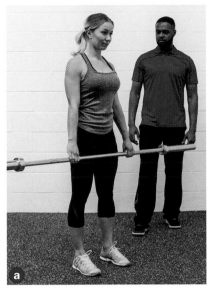
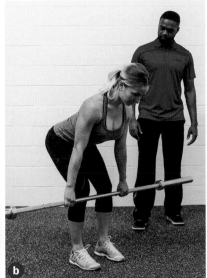

Concentric Phase

- Maintaining straight legs, extend at the hips to return to the starting position.

How to Spot

- Position yourself beside the exerciser.
- Look for proper alignment and a stabilized posture.

Examples of Exercise Alternatives and Variations

- Dumbbell stiff-legged deadlift

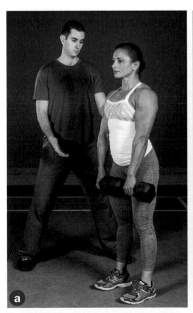
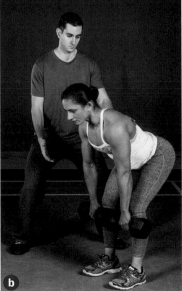

Dumbbell stiff-legged deadlift

Standing Hip Adduction (Tubing)

Movement—hip adduction

Primary muscles worked—hip adductors

How to Perform

Starting Position

- Strap one end of the tubing to the inside ankle and stand with the opposite foot straight ahead, aligned directly under the hip and with the knee slightly bent.
- Begin with the moving leg about 45° out from the body.
- Maintain good posture and keep the pelvis level throughout the movement.

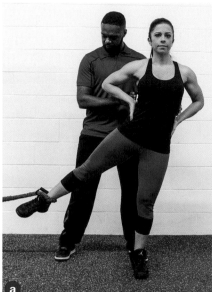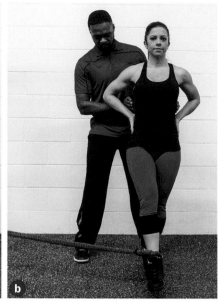

Concentric Phase

- Pull the leg across the body.

Eccentric Phase

- Return the leg to the starting position.

How to Spot

- Position yourself directly behind the exerciser in a standing position with your hands monitoring the client's pelvis.

Examples of Exercise Alternatives and Variations

- Machine hip adduction (seated)
- Cable hip adduction (standing)
- Hip adduction (semiprone)

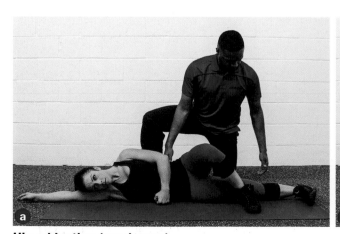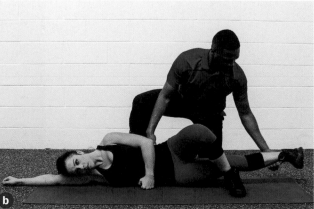

Hip adduction (semiprone)

Cable Hip Abduction (Tubing)

Movement—hip abduction

Primary muscles worked—hip abductors (gluteus medius)

How to Perform

Starting Position

- Strap one end of the tubing to the outside ankle and stand with the opposite foot straight ahead and the knee slightly bent.
- Position the outside leg slightly across the body and in front of the stationary leg.

Concentric Phase

- Pull the leg across and out from the body as far as possible while maintaining good posture and pelvic position.

Eccentric Phase

- Return the leg to the starting position.

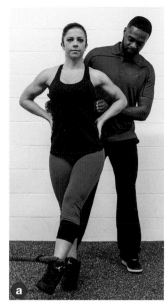
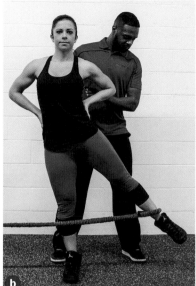

How to Spot

- Position yourself behind the exerciser with your hands at the client's hips, monitoring the level of the pelvis and overall alignment.

Examples of Exercise Alternatives and Variations

- Machine hip abduction (seated)
- Cable hip abduction (standing)
- Hip abduction (semiprone)

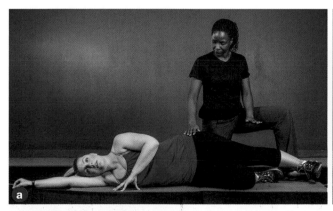
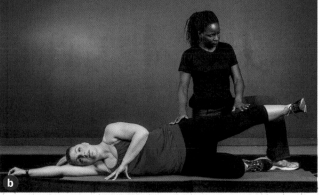

Hip abduction (semiprone)

Dumbbell Heel Raise (Standing)

Movement—plantar flexion

Primary muscles worked—gastrocnemius and soleus

How to Perform

Starting Position

- Stand with the toes on the edge of the platform and hold dumbbells on either side (or on one side only, using the other hand for support).
- Begin with a slight knee bend and the heels close to the floor.

Concentric Phase

- Raise the heels by plantar flexing the ankles, keeping the weight over the balls of the feet.
- Raise the heels as far as possible while maintaining good posture.

Eccentric Phase

- Lower the body down to the starting position.

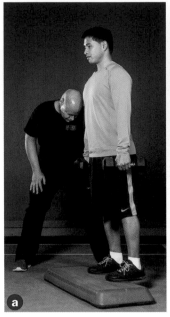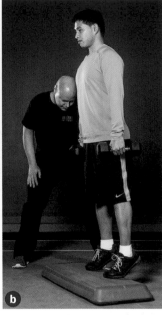

How to Spot

- Position yourself beside the exerciser to monitor movement.

Examples of Exercise Alternatives and Variations

- Machine heel raise (standing)
- Machine heel raise (seated)
- Smith machine heel raise (standing)

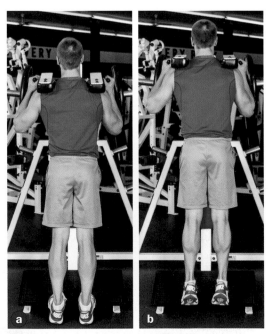

Machine heel raise (standing)

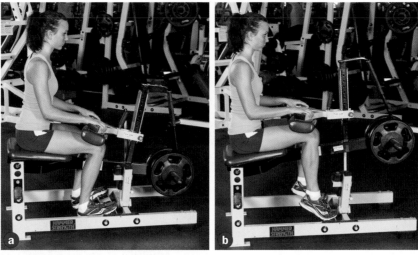

Machine heel raise (seated)

CORE EXERCISES

 ## Back Extension (Prone, Upper Body)

Movement—trunk extension

Primary muscles worked—erector spinae

How to Perform

Starting Position

- Lie in a prone position with the hands next to the ears on the mat, the elbows at the torso, and the head slightly lifted.

Concentric Phase

- Move up slowly by lifting the upper torso off the floor and retracting the scapulae.
- Maintain neutral alignment of the head throughout the movement and take care not to hyperextend the lower back.

Eccentric Phase

- Gently lower the body to the start position.

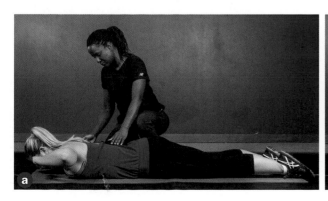
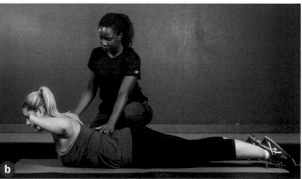

How to Spot

- Position yourself beside the client in a kneeling lunge with your hand on the client's lower back to monitor the movement.

Examples of Exercise Alternatives and Variations

- Modified back extension
- Roman chair back extension (prone, upper body)
- Machine back extension (seated)
- Stability ball back extension

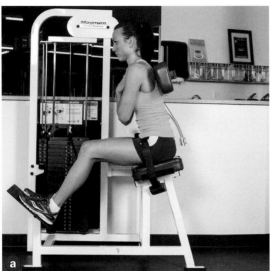 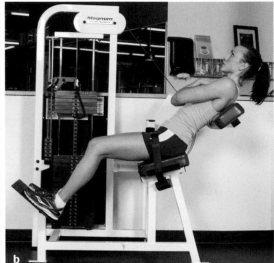

Machine back extension (seated)

RECTUS ABDOMINIS

Partial Abdominal Curl-Up

Movement—spinal flexion

Primary muscles worked—rectus abdominis

How to Perform

Starting Position

- In a supine position with the arms fully extended along the torso, bend the knees so that the feet are flat on the floor.

Concentric Phase

- Curl up the torso by bringing the ribs toward the pelvis and moving the fingertips straight down toward the feet.

Eccentric Phase

- Return to the starting position.

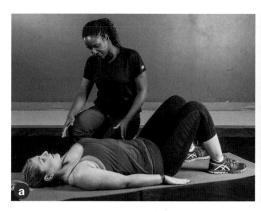
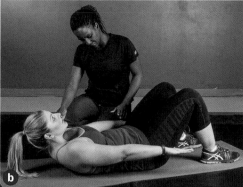

How to Spot

- Position yourself in a kneeling lunge next to the exerciser and monitor the alignment throughout the movement.

Examples of Exercise Alternatives and Variations

- Reverse abdominal curl
- Stability ball abdominal curl

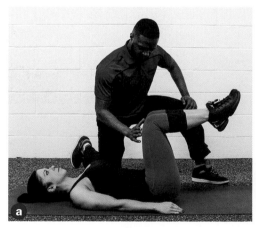
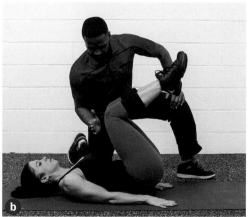

Reverse abdominal curl

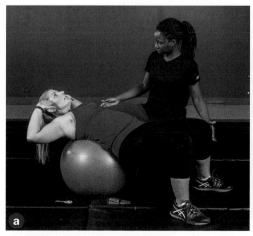
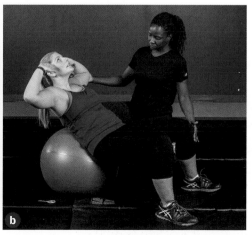

Stability ball abdominal curl

Shoulder to Knee Curl-Up

Movement—Spinal flexion and rotation

Primary muscles worked—Rectus abdominis and obliques

How to Perform

Starting Position

- In a supine position, place both hands behind the head and have one leg straight and the other knee at a 90° angle.

Concentric Phase

- Bring the elbow to the opposing knee by flexing the torso and pulling the ribs toward the pelvis.
- Keep the neck in a neutral and relaxed position throughout the movement.

Eccentric Phase

- Return to the starting position.
- Continue movement by alternating sides.

How to Spot

- Position yourself in a kneeling lunge next to the exerciser and monitor the alignment throughout the movement.

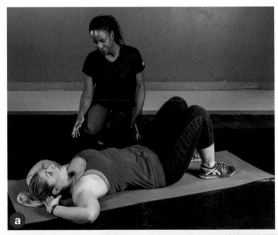

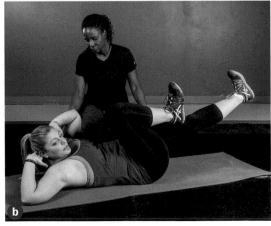

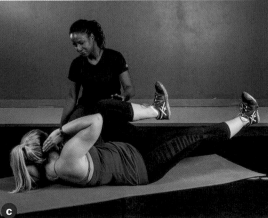

Examples of Exercise Alternatives and Variations

- Oblique lateral flexion (semiprone)
- Dumbbell oblique lateral flexion (standing)
- Stability ball oblique lateral flexion (semiprone)
- Side plank

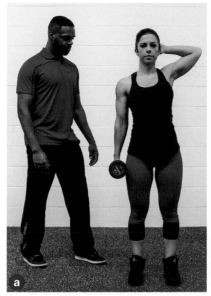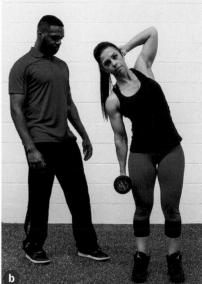

Dumbbell oblique lateral flexion (standing)

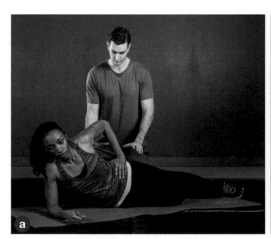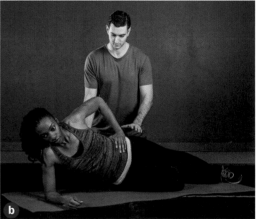

Side plank (knees)

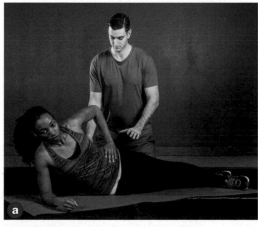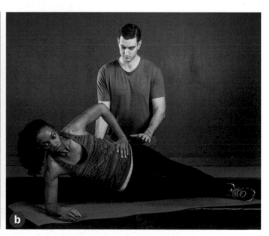

Side plank (toes)

Plank (From Elbows, on Toes)

Movement—shoulder flexion, hip extension

Primary muscles worked—core, hip extensors (gluteus maximus, hamstrings), erector spinae

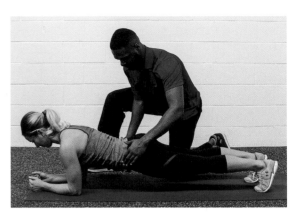

How to Perform

Starting Position

- In a prone position with the neck and back in proper alignment, place the elbows at a 90° angle along the torso.
- Point the toes down.

Concentric Phase

- Lift up the upper and lower body by engaging the core muscles and pushing up from the elbows.
- Maintain posture and alignment while holding your body weight with the elbows and toes.

Eccentric Phase

- Lower the body back to the starting position.

How to Spot

- Position yourself in a kneeling lunge position next to the exerciser and watch for proper alignment throughout the movement.

Examples of Exercise Alternatives and Variations

- Plank (semiprone, from elbows, on knees or toes)
- Plank (from elbows, on knees)
- Plank (from elbows, contralateral)
- V-sit

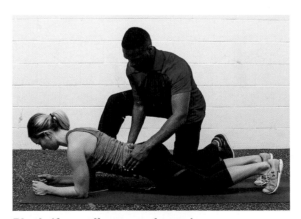

Plank (from elbows, on knees)

Plank (From Elbows, Contralateral)

Movement—shoulder flexion, hip extension, spinal flexion

Primary muscles worked—core, hip extensors, shoulder flexors, erector spinae

How to Perform

Starting Position

- In a prone position with the neck and back in proper alignment, place the elbows at a 90° angle along the torso.
- Point the toes down.

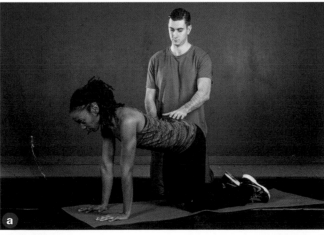

Concentric Phase

- Lift up the upper and lower body by engaging the core muscles and pushing up from the elbows.
- Raise one arm off the floor, extending at the elbow and pointing the fingers above the head.
- At the same time, lift the opposite foot off the floor, keeping the leg straight.
- Maintain posture and alignment throughout the movement.

Eccentric Phase

- Lower the body back to the starting position.
- Continue movement by alternating sides.

How to Spot

- Position yourself in a kneeling lunge position next to the exerciser and watch for proper alignment throughout the movement.

Examples of Exercise Alternatives and Variations

- Bird dog

- Dead bug

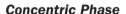

Bird dog

(continued)

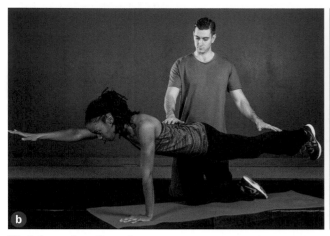
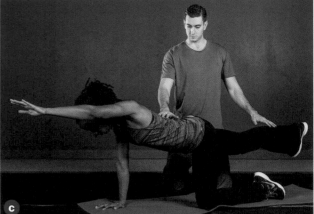

Bird dog *(continued)*

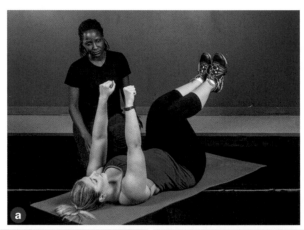

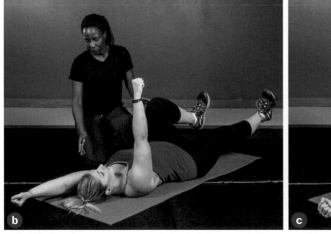
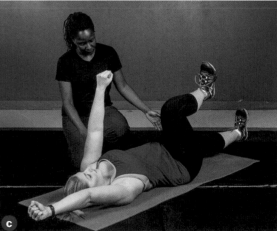

Dead bug

Stretches

CHEST

PECTORALS

Chest Expansion

Raise your arms and bend the elbows, holding your fingertips near the ears. Gently pull the elbows posteriorly and retract the scapulae until you feel slight tension in the muscle.

Tips

- If standing, keep your feet shoulder-width apart.
- Keep your spine neutral.
- Breathe out as you go into the stretch and continue to breathe comfortably as you hold.

Variation

This stretch can also be performed from a seated or kneeling position.

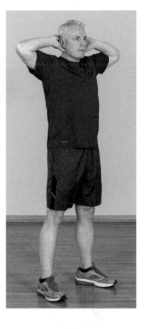

Doorway Stretch

Standing in front of a doorway, raise both arms out to the sides and begin to walk through the doorway until both arms feel gentle resistance from the doorway. Push forward until you feel slight tension in the pectoral muscles.

Tips

- Keep your feet shoulder-width apart and your spine neutral.
- Breathe out as you go into the stretch and continue to breathe comfortably as you hold.

Variation

Lower or raise the angle of the arm to stretch different parts of the pectorals.

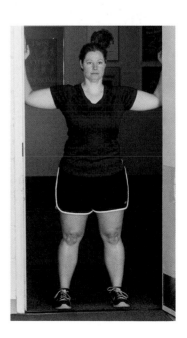

Chest Reach Back and Turn

Stand alongside a stationary object such as a door frame or wall. Raise one arm parallel to the ground and reach behind you. As you reach back with the arm, hold on to the stable surface and turn your head and body in the opposite direction until you feel slight tension in the pectoral muscle. Repeat on the other side.

Tips

- Keep your feet shoulder-width apart and your spine neutral.
- Breathe out as you go into the stretch and continue to breathe comfortably as you hold.

Variation

Lower or raise the angle of the arm to stretch different parts of the pectorals.

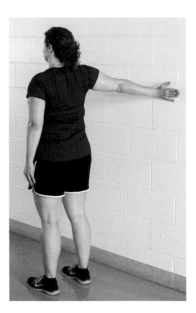

Arms Behind the Back

From a standing position, clasp your hands together behind your back. Ensure that your scapulae are in set position by moving the shoulders up, back, and then down. Gently lift the arms upward until you feel slight tension in the muscle.

Tips

- Keep your feet shoulder-width apart and your spine neutral (don't round the spine).
- Breathe out as you go into the stretch and continue to breathe comfortably.

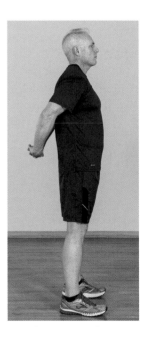

UPPER BACK

MID-TRAPEZIUS AND RHOMBOIDS

Upper Back Scoop

Raise both arms in front of you and interlace your fingers. While keeping the shoulders down and elbows slightly bent, reach your clasped hands forward and protract the scapulae to create a rounded shape in your back. Drop your head and push your arms forward until you feel gentle tension between your shoulder blades.

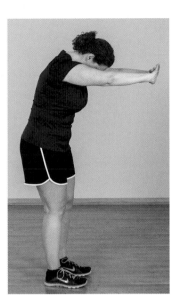

Tips

- If standing, keep your feet shoulder-width apart.
- Keep your hips neutral.
- Breathe out as you go into the stretch and continue to breathe comfortably as you hold.

Variation

If performing this stretch from a seated position, extend the legs, keep the knees slightly bent, and reach your hands around the back of the thighs to round out the upper back.

Bear Hug

In a standing position, wrap your arms around your body and with each hand grasp the opposite scapula. Drop your head and protract the scapulae to round out the back and create a gentle pulling sensation between your shoulder blades.

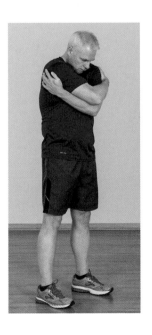

Tips

- If standing, keep your feet shoulder-width apart.
- Keep your hips neutral.
- Breathe out as you go into the stretch and continue to breathe comfortably as you hold.

Variation

This stretch can also be performed from a seated or kneeling position.

LATISSIMUS DORSI

Side Reach

Raise one arm and extend it over the side of your head and lean to the side. Allow your torso to flex gently to the side until you feel slight tension down the arm, side, and mid and upper back. Repeat on the other side.

Tips

- If standing, keep your feet hip-width apart.
- Keep your neck neutral and only allow lateral flexion of the spine.
- Breathe out as you go into the stretch and continue to breathe comfortably as you hold.

Variation

This stretch can also be performed from a seated or kneeling position.

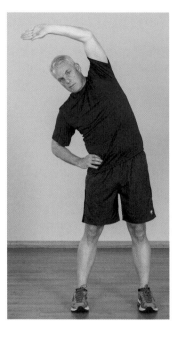

Pole Reach

Standing in front of a pole (or any stable object), grab it with both hands. When you are secure, drop your glutes back to create a straight line between your hands and your hips. Your back should remain neutral, and your arms should stay extended. Continue until you feel slight tension in the muscle.

Tips

- Keep your feet shoulder-width apart and maintain soft knees.
- Align your shoulders with your arms in the extended position and maintain a neutral spine. Breathe out as you go into the stretch and continue to breathe comfortably as you hold.

Variation

Perform the stretch with one arm at a time and lean your body toward the same side to increase the stretch.

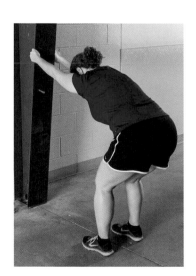

NECK

UPPER TRAPEZIUS

Shoulder Depression

While standing, tilt your head toward the left shoulder while depressing your right shoulder until you feel slight tension through the upper trapezius muscle on the right side. Repeat on the other side.

Tips

- Keep your feet shoulder-width apart and your spine neutral.
- Breathe out as you go into the stretch and continue to breathe comfortably as you hold.
- It may help to secure a light weight on the shoulder that is being depressed or to hold the wrist of that side with the other hand.

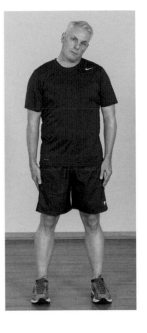

SHOULDER

ANTERIOR DELTOIDS

Reach Back and Turn

Stand alongside a stationary object such as a door frame or wall. Raise one arm parallel to the ground and reach behind you. As you reach back with the arm, hold on to a stable surface and turn your head and body in the opposite direction until you feel slight tension in the muscle. Repeat on the other side.

Tips

- Keep your feet shoulder-width apart and your spine neutral.
- Breathe out as you go into the stretch and continue to breathe comfortably as you hold.

Variation

Lower or raise the angle of the arm to stretch different parts of the deltoids.

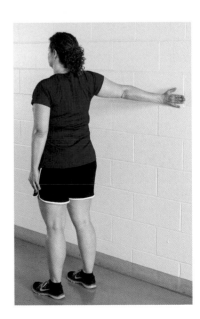

Arm Across Chest

Take one arm straight across your chest while holding it in place with the other forearm. Support the straight arm between the elbow and wrist, keep the shoulder down and away from the ears, and pull gently to create length in the mid and upper back. Continue until you feel slight tension in the muscles around your shoulder blade. Repeat on the other side.

Tips

- If standing, keep your feet shoulder-width apart.
- Keep the hips neutral.
- Breathe out as you go into the stretch and continue to breathe comfortably as you hold.

Variation

This stretch can also be performed from a seated or kneeling position.

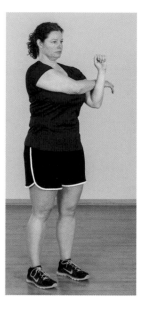

ARM

BICEPS BRACHII

Pronated Hand Reach Back and Turn

Stand alongside a stationary object such as a door frame or wall. Raise one arm parallel to the ground and then reach behind you with the hand pronated. Turn your head and body in the opposite direction until you feel slight tension in the biceps muscle. Repeat on the other side.

Tips

- Keep your feet shoulder-width apart, your arm parallel to the ground, and your spine neutral.
- Breathe out as you go into the stretch and continue to breathe comfortably.

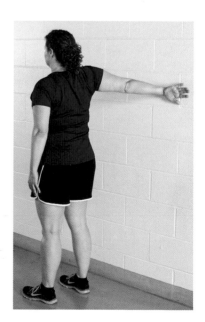

Elbow Bend and Push

While standing, take your right hand and place it between your shoulder blades. Slightly flex your neck. Use your left hand to pull the right elbow behind your head and across toward the opposite shoulder until you feel slight tension in the muscle. Repeat on the other side.

Tips

- Keep your feet shoulder-width apart and your spine neutral.
- Breathe out as you go into the stretch and continue to breathe comfortably.

Variation

This stretch can also be performed from a seated or kneeling position.

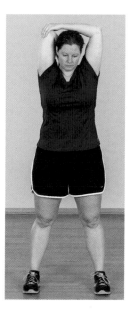

TORSO

RECTUS ABDOMINIS

Cobra Stretch

Lying in a prone position, place your hands directly under your shoulders. Pressing your hands into the floor, begin to lift your chest and ribs while keeping your hips on the ground. Rise until you feel a slight stretch in the abdominal muscle.

Tips

- Keep your legs shoulder-width apart.
- Be sure to keep your neck neutral and your chin and eyes forward.
- Do not hyperextend the spine or rise beyond the point that is comfortable for your lower back.
- Breathe out as you go into the stretch and continue to breathe comfortably as you hold.

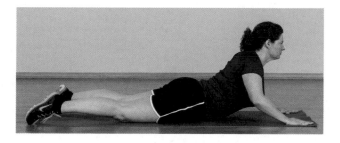

Lying Arch

While lying supine with your arms extending over your head and parallel to the ground, gently lengthen through your torso by pulling your body from your hands and feet until you feel a slight arch in your back and slight tension in the abdominal muscles.

Tips

- Be sure not to hyperextend the spine.
- Breathe out as you go into the stretch and continue to breathe comfortably.

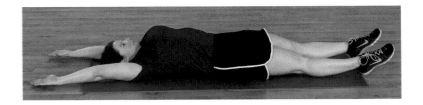

Standing Spinal Extension

While standing, extend your arms above your head and let your torso extend backward until you feel slight tension in the muscle.

Tips

- Keep your feet shoulder-width apart.
- Be careful not to hyperextend the spine.
- Breathe out as you go into the stretch and continue to breathe comfortably.

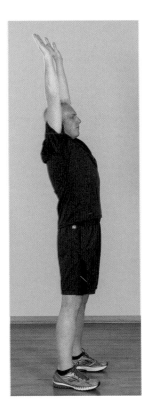

LOWER BACK

Back Spinal Flexion (Cat Stretch)

Kneel on the floor with your hands placed under your shoulders and your knees under your hips. Gently engage the abdominals and tuck your chin as you arch your back up toward the ceiling. Continue arching until you feel slight tension in the muscles of your back.

Tips

- Breathe out as you go into the stretch and continue to breathe comfortably as you hold.

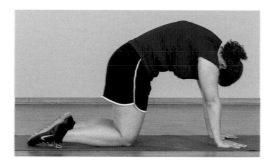

Seated Twist

Sit on the floor with both legs extended in front of you. Bend the right knee and place your foot on the floor, on the outside of the left knee. With your right hand on the floor behind your body and your left arm against the thigh of the bent leg, gently twist your torso and turn your head to look over the right shoulder. Repeat in the opposite direction.

Tips

- Maintain an upright posture before beginning to twist.
- Breathe out as you go into the stretch and continue to breathe comfortably as you hold.

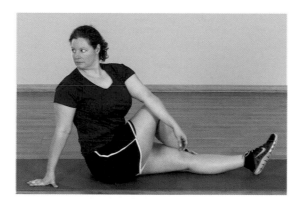

QUADRICEPS

RECTUS FEMORIS AND VASTUS GROUP

Kneeling Lunge (Rectus Femoris)

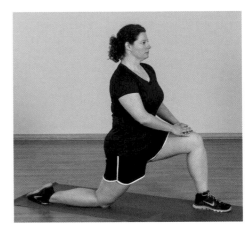

Kneel in a lunge position and gently lean forward while keeping your torso upright. Ensure that your front knee remains behind or directly above the ankle as you continue to lean forward until the point of slight tension in the quadriceps muscle of the back leg. Repeat on the other side.

Tips

- Keep your spine neutral.
- Breathe out as you go into the stretch and continue to breathe comfortably as you hold.

Knee Bend (Vastus Group)

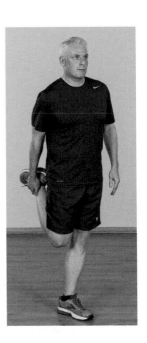

While in a standing position, flex the right knee and hold the front of the right ankle with your right hand. Continue to flex the knee by dropping it down and placing it parallel to the other knee. Gently pull on the ankle until you feel slight tension in the muscle. Be sure to keep your hips in a neutral position. Hold on to a stable object or wall for balance, if necessary. Repeat on the other side.

Tips

- Keep your feet shoulder-width apart and your spine neutral.
- Keep your knees aligned.
- Breathe out as you go into the stretch and continue to breathe comfortably as you hold.

Variation

Perform the same stretch in a side-lying position, making sure to maintain neutral spine and hips.

HAMSTRINGS

BICEPS FEMORIS, SEMITENDINOSUS, SEMIMEMBRANOSUS

Seated Hip Hinge

Sit on the floor with both legs extended in front of you. Bend forward at the hips until you feel slight tension in the muscle.

Tips

- Keep your spine neutral.
- Breathe out as you go into the stretch and continue to breathe comfortably as you hold.

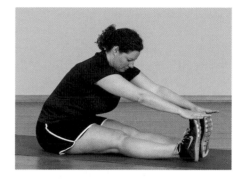

Leg Up

While in a standing position, lift the right leg and place the heel on the bench. Keeping a soft knee and a neutral spine, bend forward at the hips until you feel slight tension in the muscle. Repeat on the other side. (The height of bench will vary depending on the height and flexibility of the participant.)

Tips

- Keep your feet shoulder-width apart and your spine neutral.
- Breathe out as you go into the stretch and continue to breathe comfortably as you hold.

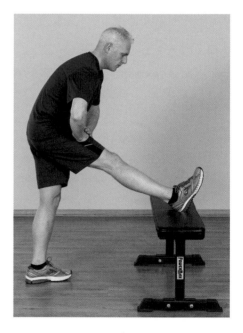

Modified Hurdlers Stretch

Sit on the floor with both legs extended in front of you. Flex one knee and externally rotate at the hip to rest that knee to the side while bringing the foot in contact with the adductors of the opposite leg. Lean forward at the hips, toward the straight leg, until you feel slight tension in the muscle. Repeat on the other side.

Tips

- Keep your spine neutral.
- Breathe out as you go into the stretch and continue to breathe comfortably as you hold.

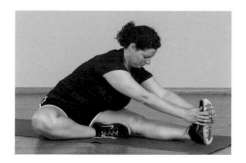

GLUTEAL MUSCLES AND ABDUCTORS

GLUTEUS MAXIMUS

Lying Knee Hug

While lying supine, flex your hip and bring one knee up and into your chest while holding the thigh with your hands. Gently pull the knee in toward your torso until you feel slight tension in the muscle. Repeat on the other side.

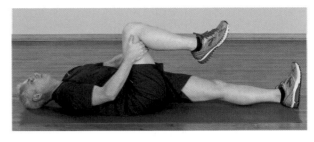

Tips

- Keep your spine and hips neutral.
- Breathe out as you go into the stretch and continue to breathe comfortably as you hold.

ABDUCTORS (GLUTEUS MEDIUS, PIRIFORMIS)

Seated Figure (Gluteus Medius)

While in a seated position, take your right leg across the left in a figure-four position. The lateral side of the ankle should rest on the thigh, slightly above the left knee. While maintaining a neutral spine, begin to lean your torso forward, flexing at the hips, until you feel slight tension in the muscle. Repeat on the other side.

Tips

- Keep your spine neutral.
- Place your hands behind you on the floor to provide support, if necessary.
- Breathe out as you go into the stretch and continue to breathe comfortably.

Variation

Perform the stretch while lying supine and use your hands to support the supporting leg.

Lying Leg Crossover (Gluteus Medius, Piriformis)

Lie on your back with your arms out to the sides and your legs extended. Flex one knee and bring it across your body toward the opposite side. Use your opposite hand to pull the knee gently toward the floor, keeping your shoulders, elbow, and head on the floor. Repeat on the other side.

Tips

- Keep your spine neutral.
- Breathe out as you go into the stretch and continue to breathe comfortably.

Variation

Perform the stretch by bringing a straight leg across your body to the opposite side.

ADDUCTORS

Seated Butterfly

Sit on the floor with the soles of your feet together and knees out to the side. Place your forearms on your inner thighs and hinge forward from the hips, bringing your torso closer to your legs. Gently press down on your legs with your forearms as you ease into the stretch position. Lean forward and push only to the point where you feel slight tension in the muscle.

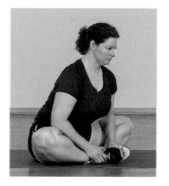

Tips

- Keep your spine neutral (avoid rounding out your back).
- Breathe out as you go into the stretch and continue to breathe comfortably as you hold.

Side Lunge

While in a standing position, step one foot out into a lateral lunge and lean into that side until you feel slight tension in the opposite adductors. Repeat on the other side.

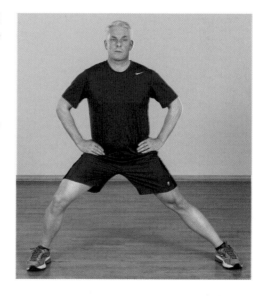

Tips

- Keep your spine neutral.
- Breathe out as you go into the stretch and continue to breathe comfortably.

Splits

While in a standing or seated position, simply move your legs apart until you feel slight tension in the adductors.

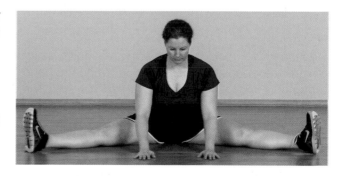

Tips

- Keep your spine neutral.
- Breathe out as you go into the stretch and continue to breathe comfortably.

CALVES

GASTROCNEMIUS

Heel Drop

Stand on a step or other slightly elevated object and position both feet overhanging it. The balls of your feet should be on the step, and the rest of your foot should be hanging over. Gently lower your ankles below the step to create slight tension in the muscle. Perform this on a stable surface that allows you to maintain a safe and sturdy position.

Tips

- Place your feet shoulder-width apart and keep your spine neutral.
- Breathe out as you go into the stretch and continue to breathe comfortably as you hold.

Variation

Perform one leg at a time.

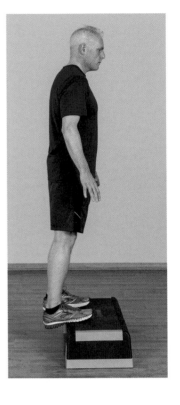

Toe Raise

In a standing position, place the ball of your foot against a stable surface and point the toes toward the ceiling. Lean in gently until you feel slight tension in the muscle. Maintain a straight knee. Repeat on the other side.

Tips

- Keep your feet shoulder-width apart and your spine neutral.
- Breathe out as you go into the stretch and continue to breathe comfortably as you hold.

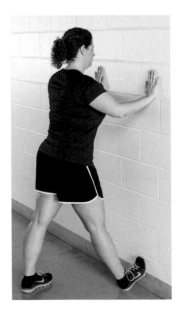

Bent-Knee Heel Drop

Stand on a step or other slightly elevated surface with both feet overhanging it and maintain a 30-degree bend in your knee. The ball of the foot should be on the step, and the rest of foot should be hanging over. Now simply drop your ankles below the step to create slight tension in the muscle being stretched. Be sure to perform this on a stable surface that allows you to maintain a safe and sturdy position. Perform one leg at a time or both at the same time.

Tips

- Keep your feet shoulder-width apart and your spine neutral.
- Breathe out as you go into the stretch and continue to breathe comfortably as you hold.

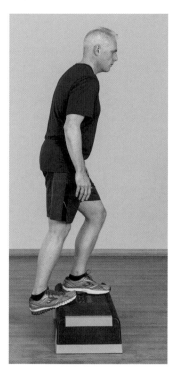

Bent-Knee Toe Raise

In a standing position, place the ball of your foot against a stable surface and point the toes toward the ceiling. Lean in gently until you feel slight tension in the muscle. Be sure to maintain a 30-degree bend in your knee. Repeat on the other side.

Tips

- Keep your feet shoulder-width apart and your spine neutral.
- Breathe out as you go into the stretch and continue to breathe comfortably as you hold.

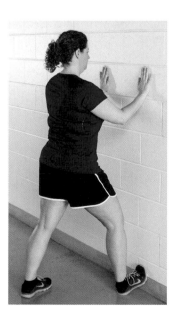

Wall Stretch

Position yourself in front of a wall with one foot in front of the other. Place both hands on the wall and step back so that the front leg is about 30 cm from the wall and the back leg is about a metre from the wall. Push into the floor with both feet and gently flex the back knee toward the floor until you feel slight tension in the muscle. Be sure to maintain at least a 30-degree bend in your knee. Repeat on the other side.

Tips

- Keep your spine neutral.
- Breathe out as you go into the stretch and continue to breathe comfortably as you hold.

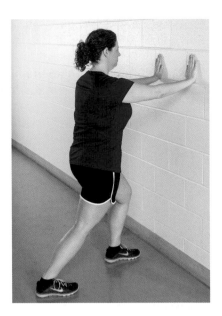

SHIN (TIBIALIS ANTERIOR)

Toe Drop

Point the toes of one foot and rest the top of the foot against the floor. Keep the other foot in front and lean forward gently through the back foot until you feel slight tension in the muscle. Stabilize yourself against a secure object, if necessary. Repeat on the other side.

Tips

- Keep your spine neutral.
- Breathe out as you go into the stretch and continue to breathe comfortably as you hold.

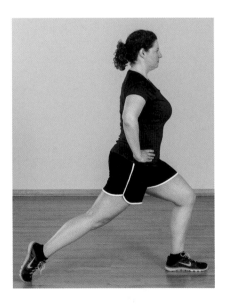

Fitness Norms for Health and Performance

CARDIOVASCULAR PROFILES

TABLE C.1 Resting and Maximal Heart Rates in Men and Women

	MEN					WOMEN				
%	20–29 yr	30–39 yr	40–49 yr	50–59 yr	>60 yr	20–29 yr	30–39 yr	40–49 yr	50–59 yr	>60 yr
RESTING HEART RATES (BPM)										
90	50	50	50	50	52	55	55	55	55	52
80	54	55	54	55	55	59	58	60	60	57
70	58	58	58	58	58	60	62	62	61	60
60	60	60	60	60	60	63	65	64	64	62
50	63	63	62	63	62	65	68	66	67	64
40	66	65	65	65	65	70	70	70	69	66
30	70	68	69	68	68	72	74	72	72	72
20	72	72	72	72	72	75	76	76	75	74
10	80	77	78	77	77	84	82	80	83	79
n	358	1,538	1,826	1,046	267	115	280	260	162	43
$\bar{X}$	64	63	64	63	63	67	68	68	68	65
SD	12.5	11.0	11.5	11.0	10.4	11.2	11.5	10.7	11.7	9.6
MAXIMAL HEART RATES (BPM)										
90	205	200	196	188	184	203	196	192	185	176
80	200	198	191	183	175	198	192	186	180	165
70	199	194	188	180	170	194	189	183	176	160
60	197	191	185	176	165	190	185	180	173	155
50	194	189	182	173	162	188	184	177	170	153
40	192	186	180	170	159	186	182	173	167	150
30	188	183	176	166	152	182	180	170	162	145
20	183	180	171	160	145	180	176	166	160	140
10	179	174	164	150	131	172	170	158	152	126
n	371	1,632	1,898	1,087	249	119	309	286	169	46
X	192	188	181	171	159	188	183	175	169	151
SD	12.2	11.7	13.3	15.9	19.5	11.8	14.8	14.8	14.5	17.5

n = number; X = sample mean; SD = standard deviation.

Reprinted, by permission, from J. Hoffman, 2006, *Norms for fitness, performance, and health* (Champaign, IL: Human Kinetics), 121. Data from the U.S. Department of Health and Human Services.

ANTHROPOMETRY AND BODY COMPOSITION

TABLE C.2 Waist-to-Hip Ratio and Heart Disease Risk for Men and Women

Age (yr)	LOW		MODERATE		HIGH		VERY HIGH	
	Men	Women	Men	Women	Men	Women	Men	Women
20–29	<0.83	<0.71	0.83–0.88	0.71–0.77	0.89–0.94	0.78–0.82	>0.94	>0.82
30–39	<0.84	<0.72	0.84–0.91	0.72–0.78	0.92–0.96	0.79–0.84	>0 .96	>0.84
40–49	<0 .88	<0.73	0.88–0.95	0.73–0.79	0.96–1.00	0.80–0.87	>1.00	>0.87
50–59	<0.90	<0.74	0.90–0.96	0.74–0.81	0.97–1.02	0.82–0.88	>1.02	>0.88
60–69	<0.91	<0.76	0.91–0.98	0.76–0.83	0.99–1.03	0.84–0.90	>1.03	>0.90

Reprinted, by permission, from J. Hoffman, 2006, *Norms for fitness, performance, and health* (Champaign, IL: Human Kinetics), 87. Adapted from G.A. Bray and D.S. Gray, 1988, "Obesity part I—pathogenesis," *Western Journal of Medicine* 149:432.

TABLE C.3 BMI Values by Height and Weight

BMI	19	20	21	22	23	24	25	26	27	28	29	30	31	32	33	34	35
HEIGHT (CM)	WEIGHT (KG)																
147 cm	41	44	45	48	50	52	54	56	59	61	63	65	67	69	72	73	76
152 cm	44	46	49	51	54	56	58	60	63	65	67	69	72	74	76	79	81
157cm	47	49	52	54	57	59	62	64	67	69	72	74	77	79	82	84	87
163 cm	50	53	55	58	61	64	66	68	71	74	77	79	82	84	87	89	93
168 cm	54	56	59	62	64	67	70	73	76	78	81	84	87	90	93	95	98
172 cm	57	59	63	65	68	72	74	78	80	83	86	89	92	95	98	101	104
178 cm	60	63	66	69	73	76	79	82	85	88	92	95	98	101	104	107	110
183 cm	64	67	70	73	77	80	83	87	90	93	97	100	103	107	110	113	117
188 cm	67	70	74	78	81	84	88	92	95	99	102	106	109	113	116	120	123
193 cm	71	74	78	82	86	89	93	97	100	104	108	112	115	119	123	127	130

Reprinted from NIH/National Heart, Lung, and Blood Institute (NHLBI), 1998, Evidence report of clinical guidelines on the identification, evaluation, and treatment of overweight and obesity in adults.

CARDIORESPIRATORY FITNESS

TABLE C.4 Cardiorespiratory Fitness Classifications: $\dot{V}O_2$max (ml/kg/min)

Age (yr)	Poor	Fair	Good	Excellent	Superior
WOMEN					
20–29	<35	36–38	40–43	44–48	>49
30–39	<33	34–36	37–41	42–46	>47
40–49	<32	33–35	36–38	39–44	>45
50–59	<28	29–31	32–35	36–40	>41
60–69	<26	27–28	29–32	33–36	>37
70–79	<25	26–27	28–29	30–36	>37
MEN					
20–29	<41	42–45	46–49	51–55	>56
30–39	<40	41–43	44–47	48–53	>54
40–49	<37	38–41	42–45	46–52	>53
50–59	<34	35–38	39–42	43–48	>49
60–69	<31	32–34	35–38	39–44	>45
70–79	<28	29–31	32–35	36–42	>43

Reprinted, by permission, from K. Heyward, 2014, *Advanced fitness assessment and exercise prescription,* 7th ed. (Champaign, IL: Human Kinetics), 81. Data from Cooper Institute for Aerobics Research 2005.

TABLE C.5 Age-Gender Norms for Combined Isometric Grip Strength

	GRIP STRENGTH (KG)*											
	15–19 YR		20–29 YR		30–39 YR		40–49 YR		50–59 YR		60–69 YR	
Rating	M	F	M	F	M	F	M	F	M	F	M	F
Excellent	>108	>68	>115	>70	>115	>71	>108	>69	>101	>61	>100	>54
Very good	98–107	60–67	104–114	63–69	104–114	63–70	97–107	61–68	92–100	54–60	91–99	48–53
Good	90–97	53–59	95–103	60–62	95–103	58–62	88–96	54–60	84–91	49–53	84–90	45–47
Fair	79–89	48–52	84–94	52–59	84–94	51–57	80–87	49–53	76–83	45–48	73–83	41–44
Needs improvement	<78	<47	<83	<51	<83	<50	<79	<48	<75	<44	<72	<40

*Combined right- and left-hand grip strength scores.

M = males; F = females.

Reprinted, by permission, from K. Heyward, 2014, *Advanced fitness assessment and exercise prescription*, 7th ed. (Champaign, IL: Human Kinetics), 157. Source: *Canadian Physical Activity Guidelines*, © 2011, 2012. Used with permission from the Canadian Society for Exercise Physiology, www.csep.ca/guidelines.

MUSCULAR STRENGTH

TABLE C.6   Age-Gender Norms for Push-Up Test

	AGE (YR)					
	15–19	20–29	30–39	40–49	50–59	60–69
MEN						
Excellent	>39	>36	>30	>25	>21	>18
Very good	29–38	29–35	22–29	17–24	13–20	11–17
Good	23–28	22–28	17–21	13–16	10–12	8–10
Fair	18–22	17–21	12–16	10–12	7–9	5–7
Needs improvement	<17	<16	<11	<9	<6	<4
WOMEN						
Excellent	>33	>30	>27	>24	>21	>17
Very good	25–32	21–29	20–26	15–23	11–20	12–16
Good	18–24	15–20	13–19	11–14	7–10	5–11
Fair	12–17	10–14	8–12	5–10	2–6	2–4
Needs improvement	<11	<9	<7	<4	<1	<1

Reprinted, by permission, from K. Heyward, 2014, *Advanced fitness assessment and exercise prescription*, 7th ed. (Champaign, IL: Human Kinetics), 168.
Source: *Canadian Physical Activity Guidelines*, © 2011, 2012. Used with permission from the Canadian Society for Exercise Physiology, www.csep.ca/guidelines.

TABLE C.7   Age-Gender Norms for Partial Curl-Up Test

	AGE (YR)					
	15–19	20–29	30–39	40–49	50–59	60–69
MEN						
Excellent	25	25	25	25	25	25
Very good	23–24	21–24	18–24	18–24	17–24	16–24
Good	21–22	16–20	15–17	13–17	11–16	11–15
Fair	16–20	11–15	11–14	6–12	8–10	6–10
Needs improvement	<15	<10	<10	<5	<7	<5
WOMEN						
Excellent	25	25	25	25	25	25
Very good	22–24	18–24	19–24	19–24	19–24	17–24
Good	17–21	14–17	10–18	11–18	10–18	8–16
Fair	12–16	5–13	6–9	4–10	6–9	3–7
Needs improvement	<11	<4	<5	<3	<5	<2

Reprinted, by permission, from K. Heyward, 2014, *Advanced fitness assessment and exercise prescription*, 7th ed. (Champaign, IL: Human Kinetics), 469.
Source: *Canadian Physical Activity Guidelines*, © 2011, 2012. Used with permission from the Canadian Society for Exercise Physiology, www.csep.ca/guidelines.

FLEXIBILITY

TABLE C.8 Percentile Ranks for the Sit-and-Reach Test (cm)

% rank	20–29 M	20–29 F	30–39 M	30–39 F	40–49 M	40–49 F	50–59 M	50–59 F	60–69 M	60–69 F
90	39	40	37	39	34	37	35	37	32	34
80	35	37	34	36	31	33	29	34	27	31
70	33	35	31	34	27	32	26	32	23	28
60	30	33	29	32	25	30	24	29	21	27
50	28	31	26	30	22	28	22	27	19	25
40	26	29	24	28	20	26	19	26	15	23
30	23	26	21	25	17	23	15	23	13	21
20	20	23	18	22	13	21	12	20	11	20
10	15	19	14	18	9	16	9	16	8	15

Reprinted, by permission, from K. Heyward, 2014, *Advanced fitness assessment and exercise prescription*, 7th ed. (Champaign, IL: Human Kinetics), 236. Source: *Canadian Standardized Test of Fitness (CSTF) Operations Manual*, 3rd ed., Public Health Agency of Canada, 1986. Adapted and reproduced with permission of the Minister of Public Works and Government Services, Canada, 2006.

TABLE C.9 Percentile Ranks for the Modified Sit-and-Reach Test

FEMALES

% rank	<18 YR in.	<18 YR cm	19–35 YR in.	19–35 YR cm	36–49 YR in.	36–49 YR cm	>50 YR in.	>50 YR cm
99	22.6	57.4	21.0	53.3	19.8	50.3	17.2	43.7
95	19.5	49.5	19.3	49.0	19.2	48.8	15.7	39.9
90	18.7	47.5	17.9	45.5	17.4	44.2	15.0	38.1
80	17.8	45.2	16.7	42.4	16.2	41.1	14.2	36.1
70	16.5	41.9	16.2	41.1	15.2	38.6	13.6	34.5
60	16.0	40.6	15.8	40.1	14.5	36.8	12.3	31.2
50	15.2	38.6	14.8	37.6	13.5	34.3	11.1	28.2
40	14.5	36.8	14.5	36.8	12.8	32.5	10.1	25.7
30	13.7	34.8	13.7	34.8	12.2	31.0	9.2	23.4
20	12.6	32.0	12.6	32.0	11.0	27.9	8.3	21.1
10	11.4	29.0	10.1	25.7	9.7	24.6	7.5	19.1

MALES

% rank	<18 YR in.	<18 YR cm	19–35 YR in.	19–35 YR cm	36–49 YR in.	36–49 YR cm	>50 YR in.	>50 YR cm
99	20.1	51.1	24.7	62.7	18.9	48.0	16.2	41.1
95	19.6	49.8	18.9	48.0	18.2	46.2	15.8	40.1
90	18.2	46.2	17.2	43.7	16.1	40.9	15.0	38.1
80	17.8	45.2	17.0	43.2	14.6	37.1	13.3	33.8
70	16.0	40.6	15.8	40.1	13.9	35.3	12.3	31.2
60	15.2	38.6	15.0	38.1	13.4	34.0	11.5	29.2
50	14.5	36.8	14.4	36.6	12.6	32.0	10.2	25.9
40	14.0	35.6	13.5	34.3	11.6	29.5	9.7	24.6
30	13.4	34.0	13.0	33.0	10.8	27.4	9.3	23.6
20	11.8	30.0	11.6	29.5	9.9	25.1	8.8	22.4
10	9.5	24.1	9.2	23.4	8.3	21.1	7.8	19.8

Fitness and wellness by Hoeger, Werner W.K., Hoeger, Sharon A. Reproduced with permission of Thomson/Wadsworth in the format Republish in a book via Copyright Clearance Center.

TABLE C.10 Shoulder Flexibility Test Norms

Rating	Score (cm, average of left and right sides)
Poor	<−2.5
Below average	−2.5 to −0.5
Average	−0.5 to 4.4
Above average	4.5 to 12.0
Excellent	>12.0

acute injury—An injury that occurs because of a single application of force, has a sudden onset, and generates immediate pain.

action stage—The stage of behaviour change in which a person takes appropriate steps toward achieving the desired change.

adaptation—The physiological response of the human body initiated by a programmed activity.

adenosine triphosphate (ATP)—The energy currency of the body. A chemical compound made up of adenosine and three phosphate molecules.

aerobic metabolism system—One of the body's energy production systems in which chemical reactions take place with oxygen. Energy is created by the metabolism of oxygen and glucose, or oxygen and fatty acids, depending on the intensity of the activity.

agility—A secondary component of fitness; it involves the ability to change direction effectively and efficiently.

all-around development—The training principle that suggests that people who are well developed through all components of fitness are less prone to injury, and more likely to have performance increases in sport and in life.

anaerobic metabolism system—One of the body's energy systems in which chemical reactions take place in the absence of oxygen. Energy is created by the metabolism of stored creatine phosphate, or glucose depending on the intensity of the activity.

antagonist—Muscle that performs the opposite movement to the primary mover. Antagonist muscles act to stop or slow the moving muscle, assisting in a controlled movement.

appendicular skeleton—The portion of the skeleton consisting of the upper and lower limbs, the pelvic girdle, and the shoulder girdles.

arterioles—Microscopic blood vessels that branch from the arteries and lead to the capillaries.

arthrology—The study of the joints in the human body.

articulation—The area within a joint where two bones are attached for the purpose of movement.

atria—The two upper chambers of the human heart (singular: atrium). The left atrium and the right atrium receive blood returning to the heart through the veins.

atrophy—The wasting away or diminution in size of a cell, tissue, organ, or body part.

axial skeleton—The portion of the skeleton consisting of the skull, spine, ribs, and sternum.

balance—A secondary component of fitness; it involves the ability to maintain a specific body position in a stationary or dynamic situation.

bioelectric impedance—A body composition analysis that is often used to measure a person's percentage of body fat. This assessment measures the strength and speed of an electric signal sent through the human body. The values given by a bioelectrical impedance analysis are based on the speed of the signal, which is affected by water, air, adipose tissue, and bone tissue within the body.

bioenergetics—The scientific study of how energy is created and used in the human body.

biomotor ability—A movement skillset that a person is born with, and can maintain or advance with little instruction.

blood pressure (BP)—The measure of the force of blood exerted on the walls of the veins and arteries by the heart.

body composition—The proportion of fat-free mass (i.e., muscle, bone, blood, organs, and fluids) to fat mass (adipose tissue deposited under the skin and around organs) in the human body.

bursa—A fluid-filled sac found in an area of high friction, typically under a tendon.

bursitis—The inflammation of a bursa pad because of the overuse of an associated muscle or tendon.

calisthenic exercise—Exercises performed with the weight of the body without using any equipment or apparatus, typically incorporating rhythm and coordination. These exercises can involve jumping, swinging, rotating, and bending.

cam—A component of exercise equipment that varies the resistance of movements performed with pulleys, levers, or belts so that the exerciser maintains a challenging level of tension through the entire phase of an exercise.

capillaries—The smallest and most numerous blood vessels within the body. Capillaries branch off from arterioles and participate in the transport of blood on the cellular level. The location of gas exchange with cells.

cardiac output (Q)—The amount of blood that the heart ejects in one minute; the product of heart rate and stroke volume, represented mathematically as Q= SV \x\ HR.

cardiorespiratory capacity—The ability of the body to take in oxygen (respiration), deliver it to the cells (circulation), and use it at the cellular level to create energy (bioenergetics) for physical work (activity).

carpal tunnel syndrome—An overuse injury that occurs when the median nerve is entrapped through the carpal tunnel; a common injury that affects multiple muscles within the hand.

cartilaginous joints—Joints that act to separate bones and are composed of cartilage. These joints are static and do not provide large movements.

central nervous system—Composed of the brain and spinal cord.

central training effects—The primary physiological responses to exercise training a specific component of fitness.

circulatory system—The system in the human body that allows the movement and dissipation of oxygen around the body. Also known as the oxygen transport system.

closed kinetic chain exercises (CKCE)—An exercise performed with the distal end of the moving limb fixed in place. The remainder of the body moves about the fixed appendage through a specific movement pattern.

coaching—Providing reinforcement and encouragement to help clients push themselves toward success and achievement of their goals.

concentric contraction—A muscular contraction that involves the shortening of a muscle against a load.

contemplation stage—The stage of behaviour change in which a person develops increased belief and confidence in the possibility of change.

coordination—A secondary component of fitness; it involves the ability to use multiple body parts to create smooth and fluid movement patterns.

creatine phosphate (CP)—A high-energy chemical compound stored in the muscle cell. With the aid of an enzyme called creatine kinase, CP splits to create ATP and provide energy.

cue—A coaching prompt that focuses the learner's attention to a given aspect of movement. Delivered verbally, visually, or through kinesthetic (physical) prompts.

diagnosed disease—A preexisting medical condition diagnosed by a medical professional and disclosed to a Personal Training Specialist by the client.

diastolic blood pressure—The pressure exerted on the walls of the veins and arteries as the heart relaxes and fills again. In a blood pressure reading, the diastolic pressure is represented as x in y/x.

duty of care—The legal and ethical obligation of every Personal Training Specialist and facility to ensure that clients are reasonably safe.

dynamic postural stability—The ability to maintain control and remain stable while the body moves through space.

dynamic stretching—A type of stretching that is performed through various common movements at a specific joint.

eccentric contraction—A muscular contraction that occurs as a muscle lengthens with a force or load.

elasticity—A characteristic of muscles that allows them both to stretch and to return to original form without tearing.

endurance—The ability to withstand periods of exertion.

energy—The ability to do physical work.

energy continuum—A bioenergetics concept that suggests that the energy systems in the human body do not function on their own and are constantly working in conjunction with one another.

excess postexercise oxygen consumption (EPOC)—The process by which the body continues to take in extra oxygen postexercise, to recover the cell and repay the oxygen deficit that occurred while active.

equilibrium reflexes—The body's ability to maintain a constant state of equilibrium (from a biomechanical point of view) while on a surface that is constantly changing.

exercise adherence—The act, or actions, of consistently participating in the assigned physical training activities.

extrinsic risk factors—The risk factors external to the client's physical and psychological status. These external risk factors include environmental factors such as temperature and humidity, exercise equipment, fitness apparel, and footwear.

fascia—A layer of fibrous tissue that wraps around and between all muscles, tendons, ligaments, organs, and systems of the body.

fast-twitch muscle fibers—The muscle fibers that perform quick and intense contractions. These muscle fibers contract quickly, fatigue quickly, and work anaerobically.

FITT—The training principle that suggests that when designing a personal training program, the frequency, intensity, time, and type of exercise must be considered.

flexibility—Refers to absolute range of motion, or relative range of motion, of a joint as a result of muscles that cross the joint.

foundational movement sequences—The basic movements required by the human body to survive. The ability to perform movements such as pushing, pulling, squatting, lunging, twisting, and lifting, as well as running, climbing, and throwing.

frontal plane—The plane of movement that cuts the body into an anterior portion and posterior portion. Movements occurring along this plane include abduction, adduction, and lateral flexion.

functional movements—The movement patterns in program design that are intended primarily to improve function in daily activities. Exercise movements that replicate real-life movements.

functional training—An approach to training in which the primary goal is a client's improvement in daily function.

golgi tendon organs (GTO)—The sensory receptors in tendons that monitor changes in muscle tension.

heart rate (HR)—The speed of the heart beat measure in beats per minute.

homeostasis—A state of balance and stability within the human body. The body's ability to maintain an overall balance of metabolic processes to adapt to the changing environment.

hypermobility—A state of excessive range of motion capacity at a particular joint. Can be a potentially injurious state because of increased instability at the joint site.

hypertrophy—A type of resistance training with the intention of increasing overall muscle size by enlargement of the muscle cells.

hypotrophy—A loss of muscle tissue size because of the deterioration of the muscle cells.

individualization—The training principle that suggests that program designs must be made to accommodate every client's individual needs.

integration—The systematic blending of the primary components of fitness—cardiorespiratory, muscular, and flexibility components.

intervertebral disc—A fibrous cartilaginous disc between the vertebrae that keeps them separate and allows the creation of the vertebral joint.

intrinsic risk factor (IRF)—The risk factors of physical activity that are internal to the person and occur because of the unique physiology of the exercise participant.

kinesiology and biomechanics—The study of human movement and the knowledge base that pertains to human movement.

kinesthetic—The body's detection of its position and weight or movement of the muscles, tendons, and joints.

kyphosis—A spinal posture characterized by an exaggerated rounding of the spine, usually at the upper thoracic and lumbar regions.

lactate threshold—The point at which the lactic acid begins to accumulate in the blood.

lactic acidosis—The point at which the lactic acid within a muscle reaches a level high enough to cause temporary muscle failure.

ligaments—The short bands of fibrous tissue that connect bone to bone.

lordosis—A spinal posture characterized by excessive curvature of the spine in the lumbar region. The spine appears hyperextended, and the thoracic cavity is extended upward.

lower crossed syndrome—A typical postural stress resulting primarily from imbalances in the muscles connecting the lumbar spine, pelvis, and femur.

maintenance stage—The stage of behaviour change in which, after change has occurred, the person continues with the behaviours required for success.

macrocycle—The largest component of the periodized program, usually consisting of several months to several years.

mastery—Learning methodology conceived by Benjamin Bloom in the late 1960s. Anyone could learn and subsequently master a task or subject if given the opportunity to do so at an appropriate pace.

mechanical pain—Pain that is created by a mechanical action or motion (e.g., falling) and is the result of damage to the musculoskeletal system.

mental capability—A person's ability to concentrate during exercise to improve training effects.

mesocycle—The intermediate component of the periodized program, usually consisting of one to several months.

metabolism—The sum of all chemical reactions in the body that either use or create energy.

microcycle—The smallest component of the periodized program, usually consisting of one to several weeks.

mobility—The body and its ability to move.

motor unit—Composed of a muscle fiber and a motor neuron, the motor unit is the group of muscle fibers that contracts when the associated motor neuron is stimulated.

muscle fiber—The term used to describe the thousands of elongated, rod-shaped muscles cells that make up skeletal muscle.

muscle spindle—The sensory receptor cells within a muscle that detect changes in muscle length.

muscular capacity—The full spectrum of muscular capability, including endurance, strength, and power.

muscular endurance—The ability of a muscle to exert or withstand force repeatedly over a period of time.

muscular power—The product of the strength and speed of movement that a muscle can produce. Muscular power is described in terms of explosive muscular contraction.

muscular strength—The maximum amount of force that a muscle or muscle group can generate against a force or load.

myofascial sling—The chain of interconnected fascial tissue that crosses multiple muscles and allows continuous movement between multiple muscles.

myology—The study of the structure, function, and diseases of muscle tissue.

nonnormative tests—Tests that do not possess any data for comparison and therefore have no established ratings. In these tests, the data obtained for the individual client are compared with the client's own past performance to quantify improvement.

normative tests—Tests that have normative data available for comparison, allowing a rating of the client's level of performance relative to his or her age population.

open kinetic chain exercises (OKCE)—An exercise performed with the distal end of the moving limb moving freely. The moving appendage moves the body about through a specific movement pattern.

optimal health perspective—Includes the pursuit of enhanced quality of life, personal growth, and individual potential through positive lifestyle behaviours and attitudes.

osteoarthritis—A chronic disease involving joints in which destruction of articular or hyaline cartilage is accompanied with by overgrowth, creating pain or immobility within the joints.

osteology—The study of and knowledge base pertaining to the bones and skeleton.

osteoporosis—A chronic disease caused by low bone mass and deterioration of bone tissues that increase the risk of fractures and overall injury risk.

overuse injury—An injury with long-term onset caused by repetitive strain on a tissue, resulting in continuous breakdown of tissue with little to no recovery time.

oxygen deficit—The cellular situation in which the body does not have the required amount of oxygen to maintain homeostasis and meet the needs of the increased level of activity.

performance training—Movement patterns in program designs for exercisers with a particular athletic expression as a goal of the training. This training is sport specific and not related to daily living.

periodization—The systematic organization of training periods (measured in time) to facilitate the most efficient path from goal setting to goal attainment.

peripheral nervous system—Part of the nervous system that lies outside the brain and spinal cord and is made up of nerves that connect the extremities to the brain.

planes of movement—The system by which the body can be divided into three planes of function to describe the directions in which the body moves. The three planes, or dimensions, are the frontal, sagittal, and transverse planes.

plasticity—The ability of a muscle tissue to change shape in response to a continued stimulus.

pneumatic machines—The resistance training machines in which resistance comes from compressed air and remains constant throughout the entire range of motion.

postural stability—The ability of the body to control its position within a specific base of support.

power—The product of speed and strength expressed by the muscular or cardiorespiratory systems.

pre-contemplation stage—The stage of behaviour change in which a person might develop increased awareness of an opportunity but is not yet thinking seriously about making the change.

preparation stage—The stage of behaviour change in which a person becomes informed about the requirements for success and makes plans to implement change.

prime mover—The muscle that provides the initial and primary source of a movement.

program card—A personal training tool used to design and chart a client's program that typically contains the client's name, date, exercises, sets and set performance, reps and tempo of reps, rest between sets, and other relevant information.

progression—The practice of making an activity more challenging or beneficial by adjusting a program component.

progressive overload—Suggests that to improve, clients must continually challenge their fitness. This occurs through gradually increasing the volume or intensity of the program to realize ongoing adaptations.

proprioception—The unconscious perception of the relative position and spatial orientation of body parts, coming from stimuli within the body.

proprioceptors—Specialized sensory receptors found in joints, muscles, and tendons that respond to stimuli produced within the body, allowing maintenance or adjustment of the relative position of the body.

protocols—A set of standardized procedures intended to ensure consistent performance of an activity or procedure.

pulmonary circulation—The movement of deoxygenated blood from the body into the right atrium and right ventricle of the heart.

range of motion (ROM)—The degree of motion possible in a particular joint.

rating of perceived exertion (RPE)—A scale for rating the perception of physical effort on a 15-point (6–20) or 10-point (0–10) scale.

reaction time—The time required for a person to respond to a specific stimulus.

recovery—The training principle that suggests that a postworkout recovery period must allow the client to return to the next workout at least as fit as the previous one, if not more.

regression—The practice of making an activity easier by adjusting a program component.

reversibility—The training principle that suggests that after training ceases, the body gradually returns to its pre-training state.

RICE—An approach to managing acute injuries with rest, ice, compression, and elevation.

righting reflexes—Reactions that are expressed when the body attempts to move or maintain a position on a stable or fixed surface.

sagittal plane—The plane that divides the body into left and right sides. The movements that occur in this plane are primarily flexion and extension movements.

sarcomere—The basic unit of muscular contraction, which is composed of two types of protein: actin and myosin.

scar tissue—A type of body tissue that replaces the original tissue after injury.

scope of practice—The predefined actions, procedures, and processes defined for a specific profession.

segmentation—A program design method that keeps the primary components of fitness (cardiorespiratory, muscular, and flexibility) and their performance separate from one another.

sign—Objective evidence of an abnormal situation in the body, which is verifiable by an external monitor.

slow-twitch muscle fibers—The muscle fibers that perform slow and controlled muscle contractions. These fibers contract slowly, are resistant to fatigue, and work aerobically.

SMART goals—Goals expressed in a specific, measurable, attainable, realistic, and time-sensitive manner.

specificity—The training principle that suggests that if clients want to improve an aspect of their performance, they have to train that aspect deliberately.

spinal stabilization system—A system containing the nerves, joints, and muscles of the spine, which allows proper spinal function and lower back health.

speed—The rate of change in position of a person.

spinal column—The overall structure of the vertebrae, also known as the spine, consisting of the cervical, thoracic, lumbar, and sacral spinal sections.

spotting—The act of closely following the movement of the client with hands on either the client or the equipment to intervene if the client begin to fail in the movement or is at risk of injury.

sprain—The deformation of ligamentous tissue under loading resulting in pain or dysfunction.

standardization—The process of determining established normative behaviours, standards, and procedures to act as a standard reference point for future results.

static postural stability—The ability to show control and remain stable for a certain length of time while muscle length remains constant or the body moves minimally or not at all.

static stretching—The practice of stretching in which the muscle is held at a constant elongated length with the purpose of increasing flexibility.

strain—The deformation of tendon or muscle tissues under loading resulting in pain or dysfunction.

strength—The ability to produce or break movement against a force or load.

stretch reflex—The automatic muscular contraction caused by a muscle resisting passive stretch or sudden loading to maintain a certain length.

stroke volume (SV)—The volume of blood being ejected to the body by the left ventricle of the heart in one beat.

structural tolerance—The principle of physical fitness that suggests that the strengthening of tissues in and around joints will result in the ability to sustain subsequently greater stresses in training with greater resistance to injury.

submaximal test—A testing procedure used to determine fitness level in exercise participants that measures proficiency at submaximal exertion.

sum of training effect—The total effect of physical training on the body.

supercompensation—A phase of physical training characterized by an improvement in performance from the previous attempt at the physical activity.

symptom—Subjective evidence of an abnormal situation in the body that is described or felt by the injured party.

synovial joint—A common joint in the human body that connects two bones and allows the movement of the bones associated with it.

systemic circulation—The movement of oxygenated blood from the left atrium and left ventricle to the body tissues.

systemic pain—Pain that is a result of a disease, infection, or medical condition.

systolic pressure—The pressure exerted on the walls of the arteries as the heart contracts. Represented as y in y/x.

target heart rate—A desired heart rate range selected by a Personal Training Specialist to encourage clients to exercise hard enough for cardiorespiratory gains yet not so hard that the aerobic energy system is unable to provide enough energy.

tendinitis—The inflammation of a tendon because of prolonged, repetitive use.

tennis elbow—An overuse injury associated with lateral forearm (wrist extensors) muscles. Continuous use of these muscles results in pain on the lateral side of the elbow joint.

training zone—A range of heart rate targets in a program design to meet cardiorespiratory training goals.

transverse plane—The plane that divides the body into upper and lower halves. Movements occurring along this plane typically involve twisting and rotation

upper crossed syndrome—A typical postural stress resulting primarily from imbalances in the muscles that bridge and connect the head, neck, shoulder girdle, and thorax.

ventilation—The exchange of air between the lungs and the atmosphere through the contraction and relaxation of the diaphragm and intercostal muscles.

ventricle—The two lower chambers of the human heart, composed of the left ventricle and the right ventricle. The ventricles expel blood to the lungs and the body.

visceral fat—The adipose tissue in the torso that is concentrated around the organs.

$\dot{V}O_2max$—The maximal capacity of the body to transport and use oxygen during exercise. Reflects a person's physical fitness.

work-to-rest ratio—The systematic organization of the time spent between exercise performance and rest during physical activity.

References

Chapter 1

Howley, E.T., and B.D. Franks. 2003. *Health fitness instructor's handbook*. 4th ed. Champaign, IL: Human Kinetics.

O'Connor, J. 2001. *NLP workbook: A practical guide to achieving the results you want*. Hammersmith, London: HarperCollins.

Whitworth, L., K. Kimsey-House, H. Kimsey-House, and P. Sandahl. 2007. *Co-active coaching*. 2nd ed. Mountain View, CA: Davies-Black.

Chapter 2

Greenberg, J.S., G.B. Dintiman, and B. Myers Oakes. 2004. *Physical Fitness and Wellness: Changing the Way You Look, Feel, and Perform*. 3rd ed. Champaign, IL: Human Kinetics.

Zaryski, S. and D.J. Smith. 2005. Training principles and issues for ultra-endurance athletes. Current Sports Medicine Reports 4(3): 165-170.

Bibliography for Chapter 2 Nutrition Recommendations

Bellisle, F., R. McDevitt, and A.M. Prentice. 1997. Meal frequency and energy balance. *British Journal of Nutrition* 77:S57–S70.

Berkey, C., et al. 2005. Milk, dairy fat, dietary calcium, and weight gain: A longitudinal study of adolescents. *Archives of Pediatrics & Adolescent Medicine* 159 (6):543–50.

Bowen, J., M. Noakes, C. Trenerry, and P.M. Clifton. 2006. Energy intake, ghrelin, and cholecystokinin after different carbohydrate and protein preloads in overweight men. *The Journal of Clinical Endocrinology & Metabolism* 91:1477–83.

Brooks, D. 2004. *The complete book of personal training*. Champaign, IL: Human Kinetics.

Campbell, T. 2005. *The China study*. Dallas, TX: BenBella Books.

Chen, C.Y., P.E. Milbury, K. Lapsley, and J.B. Blumberg. 2005. Flavonoids from almond skins are bioavailable and act synergistically with vitamins C and E to enhance hamster and human LDL resistance to oxidation. *The Journal of Nutrition* 135:1366–73.

Clifton, P. 2012. Effects of a high protein diet on body weight and comorbidities associated with obesity. *British Journal of Nutrition* 108 Supplement 2:S122–S129.

Covington, C. 2012, March 14. Sugarwise: How Fruit Stacks Up. *Greatist* (blog). http://greatist.com/health/sugar-wise-how-fruits-stack.

Cummings, J.H., and A.M. Stephen. 2007. Carbohydrate terminology and classification. *European Journal of Clinical Nutrition* 61:S5–S18.

Dahlen, G.H., L. Weinehall, H. Stenlund, J.H. Jansson, G. Hallmans, F. Huhtasaari, and S. Wall. 1998. Lipoprotein (a) and cholesterol levels act synergistically and apolipoprotein AI is protective for the incidence of primary acute myocardial infarction in middleaged males. An incident case-control study from Sweden. *Journal of Internal Medicine-Oxford* 244:425–30.

DHA/EPA Omega-3 Institute. n.d. Conversion efficiency of ALA to DHA in humans. www.dhaomega3.org/Overview/Conversion-Efficiency-of-ALA-to-DHA-in-Humans.

Dhiman, T.R., G.R. Anand, L.D. Satter, and M.W. Pariza. 1999. Conjugated linoleic acid content of milk from cows fed different diets. *Journal of Dairy Science* 82:2146–56.

Enig, M., and S. Fallon. 1999. *The skinny on fats*. The Weston A. Price Foundation.

Farr, G. 2006, December 31. What are fats? www.become-healthynow.com/article/fats/39.

Ferrucci, L.M., R. Sinha, M.H. Ward, B.I. Graubard, A.R. Hollenbeck, B.A. Kilfoy, and A.J. Cross. 2010. Meat and components of meat and the risk of bladder cancer in the NIH-AARP Diet and Health Study. *Cancer* 116:4345–53.

Fuhrman. J. n.d. Nutrient density. www.drfuhrman.com/library/article17.aspx.

Harper, A. 2003. Contributions of women scientists in the U.S. to the development of Recommended Dietary Allowances. *The Journal of Nutrition* 133:3698–702.

Hu, F.B., M.J. Stampfer, J.E. Manson, E.B. Rimm, G.A. Colditz, B.A. Rosner, and W.C. Willett. 1998. Frequent nut consumption and risk of coronary heart disease in women: Prospective cohort study. *BMJ* 317:1341–5.

Hyson, D.A., B.O. Schneeman, and P.A. Davis. 2002. Almonds and almond oil have similar effects on plasma lipids and LDL oxidation in healthy men and women. *The Journal of Nutrition* 132:703–7.

Ippagunta, S., et al. 2011. Dietary conjugated linoleic acid induces lipolysis in adipose tissue of coconut oil-fed mice but not soy oil-fed mice. *Lipids* 46 (9):821–30.

Jakobsen, M.U., E.J. O'Reilly, B.L. Heitmann, M.A. Pereira, K. Bälter, G.E. Fraser, and A. Ascherio. 2009. Major types of dietary fat and risk of coronary heart disease: A pooled analysis of 11 cohort studies. *The American Journal of Clinical Nutrition* 89:1425–32.

Karl, J., and E. Saltzman. 2012. The role of whole grains in body weight regulation. *Advanced Nutrition* 1;3 (5):697–707.

Long, C. 2009, March 5. Free range vs. pastured: Chicken and eggs. www.motherearthnews.com/homesteading-and-livestock/free-range-versus-pastured-chicken-and-eggs.aspx#axzz2Z9DvCTn4.

Li, C., and M. Uppal. 2010. Clinical update on dietary fibre in diabetes: Food sources to physiological effects. *Canadian Journal of Diabetes* 34:355–61.

Lu, X., X. Zhao, J. Feng, A.P. Liou, S. Anthony, S. Pechhold, and S. Wank. 2012. Postprandial inhibition of gastric ghrelin secretion by long-chain fatty acid through GPR120 in isolated gastric ghrelin cells and mice. *American Journal of Physiology-Gastrointestinal and Liver Physiology* 303:G367–G376.

Mercola, J. 2010, February 25. Saturated fat is not the cause of heart disease. http://articles.mercola.com/sites/articles/archive/2010/02/25/saturated-fat-is-not-the-cause-of-heart-disease.aspx.

Mercola, J. 2012, June 28. Red meat can be part of a healthful diet. http://articles.mercola.com/sites/articles/archive/2012/06/28/grass-fed-beef-a-healthy-diet.aspx.

Morrow, W.J., Y. Ohashi, J. Hall, J. Pribnow, S. Hirose, T. Shirai, and J.A. Levy. 1985. Dietary fat and immune function. I. Antibody responses, lymphocyte and accessory cell function in (NZB x NZW) F1 mice. *The Journal of Immunology* 135:3857–63.

Munro, I., and M. Garg. 2013. Prior supplementation with long chain omega-3 polyunsaturated fatty acids promotes weight loss in obese adults: A double-blinded randomised controlled trial. *Food and Function* 25;4 (4):650–8.

Nishi, T., H. Hara, T. Hira, and F. Tomita. 2001. Dietary protein peptic hydrolysates stimulate cholecystokinin release via direct sensing by rat intestinal mucosal cells. *Experimental Biology and Medicine* 226:1031–6.

Simopoulos, A. 2002. The importance of the ratio of omega-6/omega-3 essential fatty acids. *Biomedicine and Pharmacotherapy* 56 (8):365–79.

Standing Committee on the Scientific Evaluation of Dietary Reference Intake. 2005. *Dietary reference intakes for water, potassium, sodium, chloride, and sulfate.* Washington, DC: Institute of Medicine of the National Academies.

Thomas, D.E., E.J. Elliott, and L. Baur. 2007. Low glycaemic index or low glycaemic load diets for overweight and obesity. *Cochrane Database Syst Rev* 3.

Tohill, B. 2005. *Dietary intake of fruit and vegetables and management of bodyweight.* Atlanta, GA: Centers for Disease Control and Prevention.

Watkins, B.A., J.J. Turek, M.F. Seifert, and H. Xu. 1996. Importance of vitamin E in bone formation and in chrondrocyte function. In *AOCS Proceedings,* 101. Lafayette, IN: Purdue University.

Willett, W.C. 2012. Dietary fats and coronary heart disease. *Journal of Internal Medicine* 272:13-24.

World Health Organization. 2013. Obesity and overweight (fact sheet). www.who.int/mediacentre/factsheets/fs311/en.

Chapter 4

Garber, C.E., B. Blissmer, M.R. Deschenes, B.A. Franklin, M.J. Lamonte, I.M. Lee, D.C. Nieman, D.P Swain. 2011. American College of Sports Medicine position stand. Quantity and quality of exercise for developing and maintaining cardiorespiratory, musculoskeletal, and neuromotor fitness in apparently healthy adults: guidance for prescribing exercise. *Medicine and Science in Sport and Exercise* 43 (7):1334–59.

Warburton, D.E., C.W. Nicol, and S.S. Bredin. 2006. Prescribing exercise as preventative therapy. *Canadian Medical Association Journal* 174 (7):961–74.

Chapter 7

Alter, M.J. 2004. *Science of flexibility.* 3rd ed. Champaign, IL: Human Kinetics.

Frederick, A., and C. Frederick. 2006. *Stretch to win.* Champaign, IL: Human Kinetics.

Page, P. 2012. Current concepts in muscle stretching for exercise and rehabilitation. *International Journal of Sports Physical Therapy* 7 (1):109–19.

Schleip, R., ed., et al. 2012. Fascia: *The tensional network of the human body.* Edinburgh, Scotland: Elsevier.

Chapter 8

Bompa, Tudor. 2009. *Periodization. The theory and methodology of training.* 5th ed. Champaign, IL: Human Kinetics.

Chek, P. 2001. *Movement that matters.* Vista, CA: C.H.E.K. Institute.

Chapter 9

Myers, T.W. 2009. *Anatomy Trains: Myofascial Meridians for Manual and Movement Therapists.* 2nd ed. London: Elsevier Health Science.

Page, P., C. Frank, and R. Lardner. 2010. *Assessment and treatment of muscle imbalance: The Janda approach.* Windsor, ON: Human Kinetics.

Chapter 11

Bompa, T.O. 2009. *Periodization.* 5th ed. Champaign, IL: Human Kinetics, 16.

Selye, H. 1950. Stress and the general adaptation syndrome. *British Medical Journal* 1 (4667):1383–92.

Chapter 14

Houglum, P. 2010. *Therapeutic exercise for musculoskeletal injuries.* 3rd ed. Champaign, IL: Human Kinetics.

Appendix A

Aaberg, E. 2007. *Resistance training instruction.* 2nd ed. Champaign, IL: Human Kinetics.

Delavier, F. 2006. *Strength training anatomy.* 2nd ed. Champaign, IL: Human Kinetics.

Golding, L.A., and S.M. Golding. 2003. *Fitness professionals' guide to musculoskeletal anatomy and human movement.* Monterey, CA: Healthy Learning.

Index

NOTE: Page numbers followed by an italicized *f* or *t* indicate a figure or table will be found on those pages, respectively. Page numbers followed by italicized *ff* or *tt* indicate multiple figures or tables will be found on those pages, respectively.

About canfitpro

The organization canfitpro is a division of Canadian Fitness Professionals, Inc., which was established in 1993 to provide Canadian fitness professionals with continuing education and professional support. In 1998, canfitpro launched its national certification program that provides one standardized comprehensive certification body in Canada for specialists in fitness instruction, personal training, healthy eating and weight loss, and ongoing fitness education. Known for quality and positive results, a canfitpro certification establishes a benchmark for excellence and education in the fitness industry. *Foundations of Professional Personal Training* is used by canfitpro for their Personal Training Specialist certification program for candidates who work with clients on an individual basis and design exercise programs for improved health and fitness.

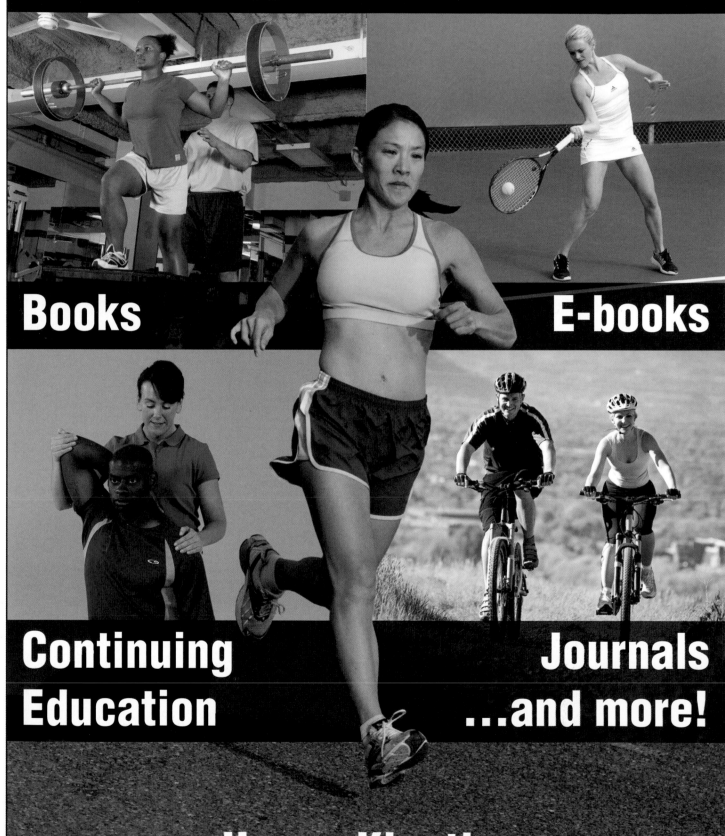

HUMAN KINETICS

Books

E-books

Continuing Education

Journals ...and more!

www.HumanKinetics.com